T0366867

EMERGENCY

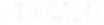

EMERGENCY

COVID-19 AND THE UNEVEN
VALUATION OF LIFE

CLAIRE LAURIER DECOTEAU

The University of Chicago Press
Chicago and London

The University of Chicago Press, Chicago 60637
The University of Chicago Press, Ltd., London
© 2024 by The University of Chicago
Published 2024
Printed and bound by CPI Group (UK) Ltd, Croydon, CR0 4YY

33 32 10 30 29 28 27 26 25 24   1 2 3 4 5

ISBN-13: 978-0-226-83686-7 (cloth)
ISBN-13: 978-0-226-83688-1 (paper)
ISBN-13: 978-0-226-83687-4 (e-book)
DOI: https://doi.org/10.7208/chicago/9780226836874.001.0001

Library of Congress Cataloging-in-Publication Data

Names: Decoteau, Claire Laurier, author.
Title: Emergency : Covid-19 and the uneven valuation of life /
Claire Laurier Decoteau.
Description: Chicago : The University of Chicago Press, 2024. |
Includes bibliographical references and index.
Identifiers: LCCN 2024011415 | ISBN 9780226836867 (cloth) |
ISBN 9780226836881 (paperback) | ISBN 9780226836874 (ebook)
Subjects: LCSH: COVID-19 Pandemic, 2020—Illinois—Chicago. |
Discrimination in medical care—Illinois—Chicago.
Classification: LCC RA644.C67 D4536 2024 |
DDC 362.1962/41440977311—dc23/eng/20240405
LC record available at https://lccn.loc.gov/2024011415

FOR PAM AND JACK

CONTENTS

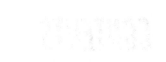

ABBREVIATIONS

ACA	Affordable Care Act
ACS	American Community Survey
ARPA	American Rescue Plan Act (2021)
CARES ACT	Coronavirus Aid, Relief, and Economic Security Act (2020)
CBO	community-based organization
CCVI	COVID Community Vulnerability Index
CDC	Centers for Disease Control and Prevention
CDPH	Chicago Department of Public Health
CHA	Chicago Housing Authority
COVID-19	Coronavirus Disease 2019
ERA	emergency rental assistance
FFCRA	Families First Coronavirus Response Act (2020)
FHA	Federal Housing Authority
FQHC	Federally Qualified Health Center
HIV	human immunodeficiency virus
ICE	Immigration and Customs Enforcement
IDES	Illinois Department of Employment Services
IHDA	Illinois Housing Development Authority
PPE	personal protective equipment
PRWORA	Personal Responsibility and Work Opportunity Reconciliation Act (1996)
RERRT	Racial Equity Rapid Response Team
SNAP	Supplemental Nutrition Assistance Program
SSI	supplemental security income
TANF	Temporary Assistance for Needy Families
UI	unemployment insurance

FIGURES AND TABLES

FIGURES

TABLES

PREFACE

Like many people around the world, I found the experience of being mandated to shelter at home at the outset of the COVID-19 pandemic both terrifying and unmooring. With a new and unknown pathogen in circulation, none of us had a compass to direct our thoughts and actions. My son was only three, and my parents were almost eighty. Not knowing how to protect the vulnerable people you love breeds a particularly desperate kind of fear. We couldn't find masks and we never left the house. For weeks on end. It was as boring as it was disorienting.

Then we slowly started to emerge from our domestic cocoons. And we had to relearn how to engage in a different kind of world, one whose edges were always dangerous. One in which we were always on guard. When George Floyd was brutally murdered by the police in Minneapolis in late May 2020, the nerves, fear, and anger people were harboring exploded into protests that rocked my hometown of Chicago. The mayor and police department responded with ruthless racial repression and manipulated the segregated landscape of Chicago to protect wealthy white residents and elite businesses, while letting neighborhoods on the West and South Sides of Chicago burn.

I started this project that summer of 2020—amid the panic, rage, and uncertainty. In August, I began interviewing people from the Chicago neighborhoods of Austin, Little Village, and Albany Park. These neighborhoods were extremely impacted by COVID-19 in part because most of the residents were rendered vulnerable by their race, nationality, and socioeconomic status. I continued interviewing Chicago residents until May 2022. Those interviews were important to me in ways I cannot fully express. They allowed me entry into the intimate lives of people who live in my city but experience it in a dramatically different way than I do because of the privilege my race, class, and nationality afford me.

Although I have always known and felt the power of ethnography to grant access to people's ontological landscapes, the phone was the conduit of connection in this case. Those phone calls allowed the people I interviewed to reflect, to remember, and to voice their deepest thoughts: their grief, their anger, their sadness, and their fear. Because of the risks of exposure and people's busy work schedules, the interviews had to be over the phone. But the phone also offered an intimacy and honesty that in-person interviews might have obscured. I could never have imagined how close I felt to the people I interviewed without ever seeing or meeting them, as I hunkered down in my living room after my son's bedtime, listening to their stories. And they offered me a glimpse of the vulnerability so many people were facing just blocks away from where I sat, safe in my home, protected by my wealth and racial privilege. It was through their voices on the phone that I understood the slow, deep emergencies that COVID-19 exposed and exacerbated.

These phone calls kept me grounded in a messy and confusing world. Yes, everything was newly scary, but each time I conducted an interview, I was reminded of my tremendous privilege and the protection it afforded me. And not just safety from this particular deadly pathogen but from devaluation and neglect, state violence, distrust of institutions meant to serve and offer respite, deadly work environments, and tremendous loss. The mitigation efforts and expert advice offered me a succor that was withheld from those on the other side of the phone. Hearing from them allowed me to glimpse the slow and immediate emergencies happening around me. And helped me understand why those emergencies were so unevenly distributed throughout the city.

People very generously shared their knowledge, fear, and pain with me. Some were initially wary of me, questioning why a white college professor wanted to hear about their difficulties and challenges. Others only did the interview because they needed the fifty dollars I offered as compensation. For the most part, however, people found the interviews cathartic. Many were surprised at how the interview let them process deep emotions they had locked away. Or allowed them to voice critiques about the city's mitigation policies that no one was listening to. They told me, in manifold ways, what precisely was wrong with the city's and the federal government's approach to the pandemic. The interviews presented an opportunity to reflect on how the pandemic was reshaping their lives.

This book is about the city of Chicago and how its mitigation policies failed its most vulnerable residents. But it is also about the *people* of Chicago and how they survived the slow and urgent emergencies of COVID-19. Obviously, my own theoretical and analytic lens refracts their experiences, but I am also indebted to their insight for helping me build my account. Any inconsistencies or failures in my analysis are my fault alone.

This book is about Chicago, but it is also about the slow and urgent emergencies of our current era: outbreaks, wars, hurricanes, famine. Each of these urgent crises is governed with temporary, technocratic fixes that obscure the ongoing slow emergencies that racial biocapitalism has unleashed over a longer historic arc. By responding with temporally bounded scarcity governance, the structural inequities that necessarily lead to disproportionate loss among the most vulnerable communities are reified and exacerbated. This book recounts how protracted devaluation and urgent crisis converge in the midst of emergency.

INTRODUCTION: CONVERGING COVID-19 EMERGENCIES

On April 7, 2020, after reviewing data published by Chicago's radio station WBEZ, which revealed that 72 percent of deaths and 52 percent of COVID-19 cases were concentrated in Chicago's Black communities, Mayor Lori Lightfoot declared, "Those numbers take your breath away. . . . We're all in this crisis together, but we are not experiencing this crisis in the same way. . . . Equity and inclusion . . . are an imperative that we must embrace as a city. And we see this even more urgently when we look at these numbers."[1] Almost exactly one year later, Mayor Lightfoot declared racism a public health crisis, noting that throughout "our city's history, racism has taken a devastating toll on the health and wellbeing of our residents of color—especially those who are Black. . . . Without formally acknowledging this . . . we will never be able to . . . fully provide our communities with the resources they need to live . . . healthy lives."[2] According to Mayor Lightfoot, racism is a long-standing crisis in Chicago that was revealed in breathtaking relief during the COVID-19 pandemic. In response, Lightfoot embarked on what she called a "racial equity" approach to the pandemic, which entailed prioritizing six racially marginalized neighborhoods with extensive testing and educational outreach and fifteen neighborhoods for vaccine distribution.

Under the administrations of both US presidents Donald Trump and Joe Biden, the federal government expanded the welfare safety net in unprecedented ways to protect citizens from the urgent impact of mass unemployment and economic shock. Five federal laws enacted between March 18, 2020, and August 2021 offered various extensions of federal aid to citizens, resulting in $3.4 trillion in spending.[3] These included stimulus payments, child tax credits, and increases and extensions for participation in unemployment insurance, food stamps, housing assistance, and Medicaid, among others.[4] As a result, poverty rates across all ages, races, and ethnicities declined from 2019 to 2020, child poverty was reduced by one-third, and the health care uninsurance rate declined to a record low of 8 percent.[5]

Despite the mayor's commitment to racial equity and the federal government's unprecedented expansion of social assistance, the Black and Latinx Chicagoans I interviewed for this book not only suffered higher rates of infection, hospitalization, and death from COVID-19 but also experienced housing, food, financial, educational, and welfare precarity during the pandemic.[6] For example, Shantal, a woman I interviewed from the predominantly Black neighborhood of Austin, explained that marginalized populations experienced COVID-19 as a series of converging "demics" leading to accumulated vulnerability: "Within this pandemic, we've had so many other demics. The violence-demic, the losin'-my-job-demic. It's just been so many demics to add on, which causes more mental health issues."[7] This book seeks to explain why a local commitment to racial equity and unprecedented expansion of federal welfare failed to protect Chicago's most vulnerable from a series of converging "demics."

At the federal and local levels, state actors implemented emergency policies that failed to reimagine welfare and simply bolstered already existing, patchwork, and means-tested systems; sacrificed frontline workers for the protection of the economy; and not only ignored but exacerbated ongoing endemic crises that lower-income and racially marginalized populations were already facing. I argue that this was done by delinking the *virus response*, as an urgent and spectacularized emergency, from the *causes* of its uneven racial and class impact.

In this book I focus on the case of Chicago, and I explain how a temporally urgent, spectacularized, data-driven approach described as "racially equitable" can obscure and reify ongoing structural abandonment and the devaluation of Black and Brown lives.[8] As evidence for my analysis, I draw on interviews conducted from August 2020 through May 2022.[9] I interviewed 65 state actors, policymakers, housing specialists and lawyers, epidemiologists, hospital administrators, clinic staff, alderpeople, and community organizers and 110 Black, Latinx, Asian, and white Chicagoans who were employed as frontline "essential workers" *or* who had lost work hours or employment during the pandemic from three racially marginalized neighborhoods in Chicago.[10] On the one hand, Chicago officials claimed a racial equity approach that prioritized the most vulnerable neighborhoods, incorporated community organizations into its response, and built a complex epistemic infrastructure to track population disparity trends. On the other hand, city officials failed to initiate policies that could have immediately helped those most vulnerable, such as citywide work protections and paid sick leave, immediate and extensive cash and rental assistance programs, or policies whereby private hospitals took on uninsured and Medicaid-reliant patients when *safety net hospitals* (care facilities that serve the uninsured, the underinsured, and people on Medicaid and Medicare) faced surges. Instead, city officials presumed that basic resources were scarce and failed to attend to entrenched structural inequality. City officials named racism a crisis and then disregarded its root causes. One community organizer explained, "'Vulnerable' kind of doesn't cover it. Some folks were on the edge before COVID. And then COVID kicked them off the side. Our systems, our governments, our policies, they are not meeting the needs."[11]

I analyze the causes of the uneven racial impact of COVID-19 and the governmental response to it as a convergence of multiple emergencies. First, I argue that the federal and local governments *governed through emergency*, enacting temporally bounded governmental strategies that presumed scarcity, triaged care, and naturalized structural inequality by delinking the effects of racism from its causes. While federal social assistance was expanded, and eligibility requirements extended, the US social safety net, delivered through multiple distinct programs, has always been fragmented, means-tested (requiring ongoing bureaucratic proof of eligibility) and largely work conditioned. The patchwork care infrastructure through which welfare, health care, housing, and food relief are provisioned was never reimagined, and many people fell through the cracks.[12] In Chicago specifically, the city prioritized the extension of certain technocratic resources such as testing and vaccines in selected neighborhoods, thereby triaging medical aid. The implementation of technocratic solutions to manage structural crisis was made possible by the expansion of disease surveillance infrastructure. Cash and rental assistance were slow to be implemented by city officials and, when they were rolled out, entailed tremendous bureaucratic proof to access. Existing infrastructural lacks and vulnerabilities were left intact, while exceptional forms of aid were triaged for only those deemed most worthy.

Second, while the declaration of the state of emergency (at the federal and local levels) enabled the expansion of welfare, it also actively *sacrificed frontline workers*, throwing them into immediate emergency. Laborers (many of whom were unable to access safety nets because they were undocumented or from mixed-status households) were forced to expose themselves to a deadly virus to protect the nation's norm.[13] The category of so-called essential work was bifurcated. Higher-income medical professionals were heralded for their selflessness and given greater protections for the risks they were taking. Lower-income workers who continued to labor in poorly remunerated and dangerous jobs in agriculture, meatpacking, delivery, food preparation, restaurants, janitorial services, transportation, and medical facilities were largely ignored and taken for granted. People working in these lower-paid, front-facing jobs were sacrificed to protect middle-class people from exposure and to keep the economy prospering.

Lastly, the spectacular governance of the emergency by state actors ignored and exacerbated ongoing *slow emergencies* that many lower-income and racially marginalized people were already facing. In his work on environmental disasters and chemical radiation, Rob Nixon discusses "slow violence" as an attritional lethality that often goes unnoticed because it is categorically unspectacular, which makes attributing blame difficult.[14] Because slow emergencies are unspectacular and mundane, they often fade into the background, making it easier for corporations and political actors to ignore and naturalize them.

As such, the COVID-19 pandemic was governed through emergency, which relied on the urgent sacrifice of workers and ignored and exacerbated ongoing slow emergencies. These are the converging emergencies that constituted the coronavirus crisis. Labor sacrifice and slow emergencies predate the COVID-19 pandemic, serving as deep causes for the pandemic's uneven racial and class impact. And yet, governing through emergency also accelerated and invisibilized these other forms of emergency already at work. In my analysis, I pay heed to the distinct depths, temporalities, and politics of visibility at play in examining the entanglement of emergencies that transpired during COVID-19.

As William Sewell notes, historical events that inspire radical structural ruptures are "interlaced with remarkable continuities" and combine "social processes with multiple different temporalities."[15] This is at least in part because events bring together conjunctures of structures that already operate at distinct depths, durations, and strengths. It is precisely the depth and duration of slow emergencies, caused by protracted historical processes, that allows them to fade into the structural background, so political actors can naturalize and invisibilize them. Similarly, the US economy's reliance on the sacrifice of low-wage workers and their exposure to premature death has long served to buoy and shape the economy, in often disavowed ways.[16] In analyzing COVID-19 as a historical event that brought together multiple emergencies—exposing some and obscuring others—the depth, visibility, and temporality of these existing emergencies must be analyzed.

So, too, must the *strategic* response mounted by state actors at multiple scales. Michel Foucault suggests that a strategic governmental "dispositive" or apparatus often emerges in response to urgent need. An *apparatus* is a heterogeneous ensemble of discourses, institutions, regulatory decisions, administrative measures, and scientific knowledges.[17] Although it may begin as a hodgepodge of various policies, discourses, and truths, it tends to congeal over time, gaining what Foucault called "functional overdetermination" as certain pathways are fortified and others are blocked. Yet, as Robin Wagner-Pacifici has convincingly shown, events are "restless" by nature; therefore, it takes tremendous political authority to forcibly bound them in time and space.[18] The governmental apparatus that was quickly mounted to respond to COVID-19 congealed over time into an emergency strategy that delinked the virus response from a broader reckoning with entrenched racial and class inequality. State mitigation strategies, while in some ways novel, kept existing government infrastructures (e.g., welfare and health policies) in place and simply expanded funding. And although structural inequality was discursively recognized by and through state policies and data projects, it was also left intact and naturalized. The pandemic response necessitated the sacrifice of workers, who have long been exploited to safeguard the norm. Therefore, the pandemic response relied on and reified existing systems of inequality, leaving those most vulnerable, once again, devalued and neglected.

While this book takes Chicago as its case, my analysis could equally describe mitigation efforts taken in multiple US cities during the pandemic. This book focuses on the COVID-19 pandemic, but all contemporary emergencies (wars, environmental disasters, climate change, financial crises) are increasingly governed with temporally bounded, data-driven, technocratic solutions that both obscure and exacerbate the ongoing slow emergencies experienced by lower-income and racially marginalized groups. The temporal arc of a viral threat, just like a hurricane or a bank crisis, is conceptualized by state actors and experts as short-term. Because a virus also poses an economic and political threat, it must be governed quickly (unlike chronic illness). Like other crises, viral emergencies also bring scientific experts into the policymaking arena. Even though crises are increasingly governed as temporary and urgent, their impact is shaped by slow and enduring emergencies created by racist, market fundamentalist policies enacted over the *longue durée*.[19]

In the rest of this introduction, I begin by providing essential background on theorizing emergencies, and then I explain my framework of governing through emergency by reviewing both the federal expansion of the social safety net and Chicago's "racial equity" mitigation strategy. Finally, I provide historical background on how slow emergencies and labor exploitation became endemic problems for the neighborhoods I studied (and for vulnerable Chicagoans more generally). In so doing, I describe the three neighborhoods from which I recruited participants for this project. The introduction wraps up with a brief outline of the book's six chapters and coda.

RACIAL BIOPOWER AND EMERGENCY GOVERNANCE

My analysis of entangled emergencies is inspired by the work of Foucault and Giorgio Agamben. This is perhaps ironic given Agamben's recent COVID-19 denialism, in which he labeled public health officials "Nazis" and celebrated conservative libertarians' evasion of mask and vaccine man-dates.[20] Beyond this recent controversy, however, Foucault's and Agamben's analyses of racial biopower are limited in their application to the US racial state.[21] Foucault forcibly illustrated how state racism, inscribed in the workings of all states, simultaneously optimizes the lives of the normative population, while condemning to slow or quick death those who live on the margins of the body politic.[22] The condemning to death of racialized oth-ers, who are seen as a threat to the dominant race, constitutes a caesura in the administration of life. Yet, as Agamben explains, the governance and valuation of life are marked not by outright elimination but by paradoxical forms of exclusionary inclusion.[23] Building on their work, my analysis fore-grounds the paradox of a white supremacist liberal order that names itself democratic and depends on the labor of racialized others for capitalist ac-cumulation, while treating racialized others as exceptions with regard to state recognition, rights, and resources. Both materially and symbolically, racial others constitute exceptions to the norm—they are necessary for its establishment yet threaten its stability.

Foucault argued that biopolitical technologies that foster population growth were inextricably linked to capitalist accumulation.[24] But they also establish and reproduce racial hierarchies. Drawing on the scholarship on racial capitalism, but adding attention to biopolitical governance, I suggest that racial biocapitalism operates through apparatuses of security, which link policing, surveillance, and disciplinary regimes *with* the provision of welfare and an incitement to labor.[25] According to Foucault, while sover-eign power *makes* die, biopower manages the healthiness of the norm by *letting* racial others die from lack of resources and rights.[26] Welfare states regularly make biopolitical investments in securing the health of the na-tional body politic, while introducing policy caesuras that exclude racial others from welfare protection, thereby "letting" them die.[27] Exclusionary inclusion denotes the various ways in which racialized others are governed and their lives devalued within a system of racial biocapitalism. Racial oth-ers have always been essential to the symbolism of the democratic liberal order *and* the material pursuit of capitalist accumulation, but their inclusion within the norm is conditional and paradoxical. They are often extended provisional recognition while being forced to subsist in conditions of racialized structural neglect.

The mechanisms by which exclusionary inclusion operates for diverse racial groups in the US shifts across history and location, especially in re-sponse to challenges from the racially marginalized. When racial others push back against their paradoxical treatment and demand recognition or resources, the boundaries of the norm shift and new mechanisms of exclu-sionary inclusion are operationalized. When exceptional state recognition or resources are extended to racially marginalized groups, those marginalized are often required to perform their identity or history in a way that forces them to violently translate their realities to achieve recognition, to undergo behavioral or capital regulation to sustain "rights" that have been made contractual, or to agree to terms that are almost impossible to achieve because they necessarily ignore the structural conditions in which people live.[28] Such are the costs of inclusion in a racial biocapitalist system.

One of the primary means by which exclusionary inclusion is operationalized is through invocations of emergency. My theorization of emergency as a technology of exclusionary inclusion builds on the work of political geographer Ben Anderson, who theorizes emergencies as a foundational biopolitical category that secures certain lives at the expense of others.[29] Anderson describes emergencies in two ways. First, he suggests that emergencies operate as modes of eventfulness that make particular diagnoses of the present possible, in order to foreclose alternative futures for the marginalized.[30] Second, Anderson and colleagues suggest that emergency can operate as a technique of liberal rule.[31] At the most basic level, the ability of the white middle-class majority to experience normality (that is only intermittently and sparingly disrupted by crisis) relies on the constancy with which racial others experience converging emergencies and accumulated vulnerability. Or, as Anderson explains, "the distinction between the everyday and emergency has only ever been available to some and is produced at the cost of making life into a perpetual emergency for others."[32] In the words of Shantal, whom I quoted earlier, people living in conditions of structural violence experience a series of converging "demics"—of unemployment, of imprisonment, of sickness, of death. To call these conditions emergencies highlights the political nature of their origins. Although state actors often discuss structural inequality as an unfortunate, ontological truth, slow emergency conditions were caused by converging racist policies that *can* be countered through political will. Slow emergencies are long in the making and have been caused by a series of historical racial projects, including neoliberal economic restructuring, policies that authorized racial segregation, the failure to build robust care and labor infrastructure for the working poor, police hypersurveillance, and punitive containment, to name a few.[33]

One of the primary emergency tactics deployed under neoliberalism is what Vinh-Kim Nguyen labels "government-by-exception."[34] According to Nguyen, global "emergencies" are increasingly managed by nongovernmental actors who intervene in spaces where there is gross infrastructural lack by providing certain populations (deemed to be exceptional) with technoscientific resources.[35] Specifically, Nguyen analyzes the provision of antiretroviral medication to people living with HIV in sub-Saharan Africa. The effort is not to meet basic resource needs but to provide one solution to one subgroup deemed to be in "emergency," without providing broader support. Proof of success comes from intensive accounting and data-collection efforts, and nongovernmental agencies often gain scientific merit and advancement as a reward. "Under the guise of emergency, triage is an automatic function that separates those who must live from those who might die, while only the former get counted," Nguyen argues.[36]

But in fact, I argue that governing through emergency has become a generalized response that state actors employ when disasters (e.g., the COVID-19 pandemic) arise. Governing through emergency may target an exceptional population category (e.g., those living with HIV), but it is always a *temporally* bounded governance strategy that seeks to bracket an instance of emergency, with the anticipation that the crisis will end and a return to "normalcy" will ensue. While Agamben suggested that the state of emergency develops permanency when the exception becomes the rule, I argue that it is important to document different temporalities of control.[37] State actors impose protracted, endemic emergencies that last for long periods and become ordinary and mundane *and* forge temporally bounded governing strategies to stem crisis conditions until the norm can be safeguarded and the emergency ended. These temporally bounded *instances* of emergency necessarily fail to attend to the history of inequality that inevitably causes racially and socioeconomically marginalized people to suffer the worst impact of any disaster.

In addition to temporally bounded strategies used to govern instances of emergency, federal, state, and city policies also create, over longer historical arcs, endemic emergencies to manage the paradoxes of racial biocapitalism. There are multiple types of endemic emergencies that enact distinct forms of exclusion, and I discuss three in this book. First, surveilling, policing, and imprisoning racially marginalized people (and especially the Black population) while simultaneously subjecting them to instances of spectacular state brutality (for example, police murders) combines immediate death making and slow violence. In a purportedly democratic state, entire populations are generally not exterminated but can be targeted with paradoxical yet consistent instances of spectacular death making, especially when they are combined with other forms of exclusionary inclusion. Second, the fragmented and corporatized approach to the provision of welfare and health care and the creation of patchwork care infrastructure creates slow emergencies, whereby those marginalized by race and class are slowly let die. And third, extinguishing racially marginalized workers in the pursuit of accumulated wealth constitutes exploitative sacrificial emergencies, whereby certain populations are deemed both essential and replenishable. Workers' social reproduction is withheld or threatened to the point of exhaustion, until others take their place in a system of renewable exploitation.

Racially and socioeconomically marginalized populations are subject to making die, letting die, and sacrificial logics through the endemic emergencies of racial biocapitalism. The same populations are often targeted by all three forms of exclusionary inclusion simultaneously, resulting in the convergence of emergency conditions and an accumulation of social vulnerability. The creation and sustenance of endemic emergencies is an ongoing strategy of the US racial state and constitutes the everyday operations of liberal white supremacy. Sometimes one of these endemic emergencies intensifies into a temporally bounded, spectacular emergency to which the state must mount a specific legislative or governmental response—for example, after the murder of George Floyd. During these instances, an endemic emergency is given spectacular governmental attention for a limited amount of time. Often state actors acknowledge the enduring quality of the crisis but respond with a temporary, exceptional solution.

The state response to the pandemic sanctioned the immediate sacrifice of frontline workers *and* invisibilized and naturalized ongoing slow emergencies. Because events are "restless," temporally bounding them requires tremendous political capital.[38] Determining the beginning and end of the "emergency" of COVID-19—being able to temporally bound the crisis, end the aid extended to mitigate its impact, and determine when normalcy has been restored—is a powerful governmental act. But it also detaches this particular emergency, and the exceptional response to it, from the ongoing emergencies that determined who was most affected. As Yarimar Bonilla explains about Hurricane Maria, "it is the 'slow violence' of colonial and racial governance which sets the stage for the accelerated dispossession made evident in a state of emergency."[39] Next I will explain how the federal government expanded the social safety net to govern the COVID-19 pandemic emergency.

GOVERNING THE COVID-19 EMERGENCY

The widespread expansion of the US social safety net by the federal government, the implementation of direct cash transfers (in the form of stimulus payments), and the expansion of state and city coffers to deepen social assistance with fewer federal limitations *did* attempt to counteract, to some degree, the disproportionate impact of the pandemic caused by entrenched racial and class inequality. While the unemployment shock negatively impacted Latinx and Black Americans more substantially and for longer periods than other racial groups, the rates of poverty did drop in 2020, for the one year in which social assistance benefits were deepened and expanded.[40] Why did this unprecedented expansion of the social safety net fail to make more of a dent in the accumulated vulnerability of the most marginalized Americans?

First, the public sector was already incredibly decimated from years of budgetary cutbacks.[41] Despite the windfall of new federal funding, the emphasis was placed on orchestrating a response to immediate crisis and not attending to converging endemic emergencies. In chapter 2, I provide details on how existing fault lines and fragmentation in health care, public health, and mental health infrastructure in the US left the most vulnerable Americans without basic health resources during an infectious pandemic. The Chicago public health department, for example, had to outsource a lot of its response to other programs, as well as to community organizations, as one community organizer explained in late 2021:

> We have to understand that . . . under the previous administration, and this current administration, investment in public health had decreased and [remained] dismally low . . . so all of a sudden, you have a global pandemic playing out in your city, and the department of public health is very limited in its own capacity. So what does it do? Right? The very conscious decision was made, instead of building up the public health system, you're outsourcing to the nonprofit sector.[42]

Second, the existing social safety net was largely kept in place. Certain programs received extensions so slightly more people qualified for them, people were not required to show ongoing proof of eligibility, or the highest amount paid out was extended to everyone who qualified. For example, unemployment insurance (UI) was increased for one year by $600 monthly, paid for by the federal government and not state budgets, and people who had previously been ineligible (the self-employed, people working part-time or in the gig economy) were included.[43] Medicaid coverage was expanded to more families during the COVID-19 pandemic. People registered for Medicaid when they lost work and income, states expanded their eligibility requirements, and the continuous enrollment stipulation meant that families did not need to requalify for Medicaid until the public health emergency was terminated.[44] With Supplemental Nutrition Assistance Program (SNAP) benefits, all families who qualified were given the maximum payout, as opposed to linking benefit payouts to household income.[45] Because SNAP is an entitlement program whose benefits are fully federally funded (as opposed to state administered) and any household that becomes eligible based on loss of income gets paid within thirty days, it is the social assistance program best structured to respond to immediate crisis.[46]

And yet, as a whole, the US safety net allows the most vulnerable Americans to fall through its cracks. There are basically two kinds of aid: social insurance (which is tied to work history or old age) *or* means-tested transfers for those with low income or assets (also often tied to work requirements or the dependency of children). Robert Moffitt and James Ziliak report that before the pandemic, "among very-low-income, non-disabled, non-elderly families in the country, fewer than half receive[d] benefits from any major program . . . and among the childless families, only 20–25% d[id]."[47] And even when the federal government extended aid during the pandemic, these benefits often did not alleviate social suffering. Marianne Bitler, Hilary Hoynes, and Diane Whitmore Schanzenbach, for example, found that the extension of SNAP benefits better assisted white families, who experienced a "larger percentage increase in their benefits" than Black and Latinx families, because the latter were already receiving the maximum allotment before the pandemic.[48] In chapter 3, I review the various ways in which the Chicago residents I interviewed suffered from gaps and fragmentations in the patchwork pandemic aid extended to them.

Part of the problem is that the social safety net is porous and does not meet the needs of those facing multiple converging social crises associated with housing, health care, welfare, employment, and childcare precarity. Endemic, slow emergencies run deep and cannot be countered by spectacularized emergency governance. Candice, a Black woman from the Austin neighborhood of Chicago, was awed by the support she saw—food banks, additional unemployment checks, stimulus payments—but then questioned why this could not be the norm instead of the exception.

> What my problem was, it took a pandemic for them to do it. Whatever they was giving, eventually it was going to stop. So all that stimulus money they gave us . . . they was only gonna give it to us them couple of times; it was going to stop. What about before the pandemic and after the pandemic? That's what I'm talking about. These same people need help, not just 'cause it's COVID. [*Pause.*] Where was all this assistance, all this free food and all this free money, and extra food stamps? You got people out here that need this stuff *way* before the pandemic and still need it after the pandemic! So . . . that was my thing with the government. Not that they ain't give enough . . . [but] they *should* have been doing this all the time.[49]

Candice indicates the precise problem with approaching vulnerability in a piecemeal, emergency fashion. In the next section, I turn toward explaining broadly how the City of Chicago's approach also failed to attend to the real emergencies many Chicago residents were experiencing.

CHICAGO'S "RACIAL EQUITY" RESPONSE

Why are rates of death "three or four times more so for the Black community as opposed to other people?" President Donald Trump asked in a press conference on April 7, 2020. Dr. Anthony Fauci, director of the National Institute of Allergy and Infectious Diseases, added, "*There is nothing we can do about it right now* except to try and give" African Americans "the best possible care to avoid complications."[50] Responding to the disproportionate toll of Black death in Chicago in May 2020, Mayor Lori Lightfoot said, "Now, *we're not going to be able to erase decades of health disparities in a few days or weeks*, but we have to impress upon people in these communities that there are things they can do ... to help themselves."[51] Similarly, Illinois Governor JB Pritzker commented in May 2020, "Decades of institutional inequities and obstacles for members of our Latinx communities are now amplified in this pandemic. And while *we can't fix generations of history in the span of a few months*, we must advance equity in our public health response today."[52]

In each of these instances, federal, state, and local leaders decry the uneven impact of COVID-19 on Latinx and Black communities, recognizing that it stems from deep, underlying structural inequality, *while simultaneously* disavowing any political power to address it. Rather, in these speeches, each speaker provides evidence of the medical policies implemented to stem the virus's spread. Up to a point. Workers, however, were asked to put themselves directly in the pathway of the virus, without protection. When asked about outbreaks in Tyson Foods processing plants on April 7, 2020, Vice President Mike Pence simply acknowledged that workers "are giving a great service to the people of the United States of America, and we need you to continue, as part of what we call critical infrastructure, to show up and do your job."[53]

In these quotations, political leaders *recognize* the causes of the massive differential in infection and death among the racially marginalized in the US: long histories of racist social, economic, and health policies and the need to rely on "essential" workers. Then, they suggest that deep-rooted problems *cannot* be addressed through urgent, emergency policies—excusing themselves from responsibility and naturalizing race and class inequity. Instead, they offer technocratic *medical* resources which fail to attend to the deep, intertwined emergencies that low-income and racially marginalized groups were facing. When pushed in an interview, one epidemiologist working alongside Chicago city officials on their racial equity response admitted, "Yeah. I think we're so focused on the urgent. We struggled with some of the underlying factors."[54]

Slow emergencies are caused by protracted processes that are difficult to pinpoint. This often invisibilizes structural determinants, which are then more easily explained away via scientific and political discourses that point to biological determinants (e.g., preexisting health conditions) and behavioral norms (e.g., not masking) and that highlight medical, technocratic solutions (e.g., testing and vaccines). Lightfoot's directive that marginalized communities should "help themselves" urges people to enact self-responsibility, placing blame on individuals, even as she recognizes historical disadvantage. Because slow violence is spatially and temporally distanced from its causes, it is easy to point to it in political rhetoric but to completely avoid addressing it in policy initiatives. As such, "decades of health disparities" simply become intransigent, historic truths, impossible for any administration to actually remedy.

In a city like Chicago, which is a Democratic stronghold and majority-minority city where Latinx, Black, and white residents each make up approximately one-third of the population, addressing racial disparities is paramount for political legibility and capital. Therefore, calculating racial disparities through epidemiology and enacting a "racially equitable" response was a crucial effort to gain political and symbolic capital, especially for a Black mayor. Other scholars have argued that liberal political actors often invoke "woke credentials" by championing social movements such as Black Lives Matter while simultaneously voting against policies that might address the legacies of structural racism.[55] This use of antiracist rhetoric to garner political capital constitutes a move away from "colorblind neoliberal" policies to more race-conscious strategies that nonetheless reentrench neoliberal hegemony and reify structural, racial inequalities.[56] In this way, race-conscious policies obscure deeply embedded, institutionalized racism that was exacerbated by colorblind rollbacks.[57] In this section, I illustrate *how* race-conscious discourse and a reliance on "data-driven" policy become a new kind of racial project that *names* racism a crisis but continues to nonetheless support white supremacist power structures.[58]

In May 2020, Mayor Lightfoot created the Racial Equity Rapid Response Team (RERRT), which incorporated representatives from three predominantly Black neighborhoods with high rates of death from COVID-19 and three predominantly Latinx neighborhoods with the highest infection rates, to sit on a task force. Members included city officials and epidemiologists, hospital administrators and clinic staff, members of the Chicago Department of Public Health (CDPH), and one large nongovernmental organization from the region. Members of this task force designed and operationalized testing, educational programs, and vaccine distribution in these neighborhoods. But because only six neighborhoods out of seventy-seven were selected, and vulnerability moved as resources were allocated, keeping up on epidemiological metrics of COVID-19 vulnerability was key to triaging what the city considered "scarce resources." As one CDPH official explained, "Unfortunately, when you have a very scarce resource, and you want to give it to folks who are most likely to get the least of it, there ends up being a fighting-for-the-scraps phenomenon."[59]

In chapter 3, I provide extensive evidence of the city of Chicago's approach, but here I highlight three racial projects associated with the pandemic through which city agents claimed "equity" but nonetheless exacerbated or ignored structural inequalities, thereby ontologizing racial difference. First, the city *invested heavily in technocratic, medical responses to infectious disease* spread *instead* of broader expansions in its social safety net, which also required investing in the building up of a robust epistemic infrastructure. Epidemiological modeling was used to determine which neighborhoods were *most* vulnerable at any given time to allocate testing or vaccine resources. Once an area's positivity or death rate fell, those resources were retracted and repurposed elsewhere. So, communities were pitted against one another for limited public health resources. The shifting spatial patterns of outbreaks thus became cause for activating an epidemiological surveillance infrastructure to manage geographic disparities in the epidemic while it precluded sustained, broad public health supports.

Second, by investing in and circulating racial disparity statistics, to drive its triaged approach to the pandemic, officials *delinked the epistemic effects of racism* (population metrics of racial disparities) *from its causes*. Quantifying racism reduces its historical complexity into something that can be legible and usable within an administrative apparatus. Investment in lowering the numbers (of case and death rates in Black and Latinx neighborhoods) became a technical exercise that was detached from people's grounded experiences of racial harm and neglect. One epidemiologist who worked on the city task force explained why racial statistics were so important to the city's response:

> I'm a fan of saying what gets measured is what gets done. . . . Probably our first-year bachelor students would've predicted which communities got impacted. So, why do you have to measure it? I don't know. I guess partly because I'm an epidemiologist. I do think people wanna see the data. They wanna see the evidence.[60]

A CDPH director explained that racism should be considered a *public health* crisis *because* epidemiologists can prove racism with quantifiable metrics:

> Can we quantify structural racism? . . . Public health would say we have been [doing so for] a long time. When you look at the inequities and the disparities in . . . life expectancy . . . or maternal . . . morbidity and mortality . . . I think public health offers measurement in a way that, you know, can be resonant.[61]

Such a focus on numbers allows officials to show they are addressing racism without attempting to redress the historic causes of racism. It is governing through emergency—choosing certain technocratic interventions to provide to those deemed *most* vulnerable at a given moment, while ignoring infrastructural disinvestment and lack.

By eschewing investment in direct services and abstracting individual experiences into statistical variables, certain lives are prioritized over others based on how they are represented with data. Residents felt this abstraction acutely, as Sophia, a Mexican American woman from Little Village, conveyed in her interview:

> We're not only data. [Mayor Lightfoot] needs to . . . speak to at least one person, . . . so she can understand what's going on. . . . There's so many stories, so many, many people that, like, didn't have enough resources, that had a bad time during COVID, that lost their jobs. . . . She has to sit down with them . . . so she can understand . . . we're just not numbers, we're humans.[62]

By distancing the epistemic effects of racism from its structural causes, the circulation of racial statistics operates as a "racial spectacle."[63] Racial spectacles concentrate the public gaze into a decontextualized and restricted display, completely detached from lived, racial realities. Racial spectacles obfuscate critical debate about the causes of inequality and uphold white supremacist systems of domination.[64] The COVID-19 racial spectacles included surface-level concerns with racial statistics. The circulation of these statistics without social context reified racial group differences *and* pulled attention away from the need to repair the broader "racial design of public health" as a whole.[65]

The circulation of racial statistics during the COVID-19 pandemic sometimes biologized race (by explaining higher death rates in racially marginalized communities via comorbid conditions), but often, it *spatially ontologized racial difference* by targeting parts of the city as high-needs areas without attending to the historical conditions that created the converging slow emergencies people in those neighborhoods were facing. This is the third way in which the city's virus response failed to attend to accumulated vulnerability. Because data are abstracted from people's lived conditions and then circulate for political capital in a spectacular way, racial difference gets naturalized as an inevitable risk. And it treats the *most* racially marginalized communities with policies that are distinct from the rest of the population, thereby enacting a caesura in the administration of health.[66] As such, the city engaged in a practice often referred to as *medical hotspotting*. Typical analyses of medical hotspotting analyze cases in which "high-healthcare-users" are identified and given preventive health care.[67] The same logic applies to Lightfoot's "racial equity" approach. While purportedly addressing racial differences and working against them, these policies subtly insinuate that certain bodies, located in particular neighborhoods, should be treated as social problems, which spatially ontologizes structural racism.[68] Medical hotspotting governs through emergency. Particular people are chosen for exceptional aid, in the midst of an emergency, without attending to broader infrastructural lacks. It is a means of presuming a scarcity of resources and triaging care, and it employs cost-benefit analysis to health care spending. Further, it requires and necessitates the ongoing use of surveillance technologies to track which neighborhoods and census tracts are most vulnerable at any given time. All of these processes not only extract out from people's lived realities, but they ignore endemic emergencies and naturalize racial harm in spatial ways. To be counteracted, these converging emergencies cannot be simply blanketed over with a porous safety net or treated with austerity and medical triaging. In the rest of this chapter, I explain the historical conditions that gave rise to the endemic emergencies I describe throughout the book, provide historical background on the neighborhoods in which I conducted interviews, and discuss the converging "demics" current residents face in Albany Park, Austin, and Little Village.

THE HISTORICAL ORIGINS OF CHICAGO'S ENDEMIC EMERGENCIES

Situating this study in the city of Chicago offers a unique lens into COVID-19 policies and their effects on vulnerable communities. Chicago was one of the first cities in the US to report news about racial disparities in coronavirus infection and death, and like most of the nation, it sustained disproportionate racial inequalities in case, hospitalization, and death rates.[69] Mayor Lightfoot became a household meme because of her strong stance on enforcing the stay-at-home order.[70] Further, Chicago is often used as the paradigmatic sociological model of racial segregation.[71] Chicago is as segregated today as it was fifty years ago.[72] I begin with a history of how this segregation was initiated and maintained, thereby shaping the conditions for the development of endemic emergencies among Chicago's immigrant, Black, and Latinx communities.

Throughout the twentieth century, Black, Latinx, and immigrant laborers fueled the city's industrial growth, yet they were forced to live in substandard, crowded, and segregated housing; were discriminated against in education, housing, and employment; and were overly surveilled and policed—often leading to imprisonment or deportation. In this section, I briefly review the history of how Black and Latinx Chicagoans were segregated into neighborhoods on the Northwest and West Sides of the city, and how they were impacted by deindustrialization. In some ways, these stories are similar, and in other ways, Latinx and Black Chicagoans experienced different forms of exclusionary inclusion.[73]

Chicago attracted a large number of working-class Black people during the Great Migration, who mostly settled on the South Side of the city, and discriminatory housing policies kept them in overcrowded conditions. In the 1950s and 1960s, Black Chicagoans moved into Chicago's West Side, including the neighborhoods of East and West Garfield Park, the Near West Side, and North Lawndale.[74] As such, Chicago's "Black Belt" expanded, but it was consistently shaped by racist housing policies. Residents of these neighborhoods found work in the multiple factories concentrated on Chicago's West Side, including Sears Roebuck, the Brach candy factory, and Western Electric Hawthorne Works.[75] From the 1940s through 1960s, the Chicago Housing Authority (CHA) began constructing large public housing units that were concentrated in neighborhoods with established and growing Black populations, and simultaneously, the federal government subsidized "white flight" to the suburbs by providing tax deductions, federal mortgage guarantees, new highways, and track housing.[76] Further, through redlining, the Federal Housing Authority (FHA) refused to insure housing construction that disrupted community composition (i.e., already existing racial segregation) until 1968.

Before and during World War II (1939–45), the federal government and corporate employers (in agriculture, railroads, and meatpacking) actively recruited Mexican and Puerto Rican workers through the Bracero Program and Operation Bootstrap. Workers were given temporary contracts that were supposed to supply room and board and pay minimum wage; however, conditions were often so poor that workers broke their contracts and moved to cities such as Chicago in search of better wages and conditions.[77] Laborers were sometimes used to keep wages low and break strikes, their jobs were very poorly paid and insecure, and they were not offered opportunities for skill enhancement. As such, Mexican and Puerto Rican workers were often "used as a reserve labor force and as shock absorbers in times of economic dislocation."[78]

As Mike Amezcua explains, Mexican immigrant laborers were both actively recruited and needed to fuel capitalist accumulation, while being simultaneously criminalized and signified as perpetually "alien."[79] Multiple civic and corporate entities were involved in helping to circulate immigrant workers from Mexico through industries where their labor was needed, but Mexican immigrants were simultaneously discriminated against in housing, welfare, and education provisions. From the 1950s onward, Mexican immigrants were also increasingly surveilled and criminalized, and the segregated neighborhoods where they lived were often raided by the US Immigration and Naturalization Service. Mexican immigrants in Chicago lived under a constant threat of deportation. Not only did their construction as an "alien," replenishable workforce keep immigrants in constant fear of deportation, but their segregation into certain neighborhoods facilitated their active exploitation *and* deportation by immigrant enforcement agencies. Clandestine networks helped circulate migrants *as* a labor force, but their forced segregation through racist housing and criminalization policies also made them easier to economically exploit *and* deport by an increasingly xenophobic federal government. As such, Mexican workers were an "ideal expendable labor force" *because* they were perceived as "perpetually deportable" and "permanently controllable."[80]

In the 1940s and 1950s, the West Side of Chicago was home to Jewish, Italian, and Greek immigrants, as well as Latinx immigrants and Black families living often in integrated neighborhoods. In the late 1950s and the 1960s, construction of the Eisenhower Highway, the building of public housing primarily for Black families, and the destruction and urban renewal projects that accompanied the building of the University of Illinois at Chicago caused white residents to flee, and the West Side of Chicago was forcibly segregated into separate neighborhoods for Latinx and Black communities.[81] As a result, Latinx communities were concentrated in Pilsen, South Lawndale (Little Village), and Humboldt Park, and Black communities were concentrated in East and West Garfield Park, North Lawndale, and Austin.[82] But in fact, the removal of racially and socioeconomically marginalized populations from particular neighborhoods targeted for "redevelopment" was a city project enabled by racism, capitalist exploitation (and the shifting logics of city politics), and criminalization. For example, Amezcua explains that heightened federal deportation programs launched during the McCarthy era of the 1950s targeted Mexican immigrants who lived in the exact neighborhoods the city sought to capitalize upon through gentrification, urban renewal, and the construction of highways and schools. Amezcua explains, "For Mexicans, urban renewal and immigration policy were enjoined forms of material dispossession and urban erasure."[83] Incarceration also became an increasingly common strategy to manage growing poverty in Black neighborhoods after deindustrialization, which I return to later in this section.

Chicago has often been depicted as the "paradigmatic industrial metropolis," and then subsequently as the epitome of rust belt deindustrialization, which occurred from the 1970s through the 1990s in Chicago.[84] The economic restructuring that accompanied deindustrialization began with recessions in the 1970s and 1980s, and it entailed three primary processes: (1) a shift from manufacturing to producer and business services (and even within manufacturing, a shift toward the production of scientific instruments and industrial machinery and equipment) as well as a concentration of corporate headquarters in downtown Chicago; (2) the suburbanization of production and the casualization, informalization, and deunionization of employment; and (3) the erosion of middle-income jobs and the polarization of the labor market, marked by growth of highly skilled service and professional jobs, on the one hand, and very low-wage, contingent, insecure jobs, on the other.[85]

After restructuring, workers without educational degrees competed for low-wage service work. Women were employed as home health aides and day care workers, and some men found contingent work in the factories that survived deindustrialization, construction sites, and warehouses. In addition to cutting jobs and moving factories to suburbs, the wages offered in the work that remained were extremely minimal, making it increasingly difficult for workers to support their families, even when they could find work. Wage labor no longer protected workers from poverty.[86] Latinx and Black workers competed for the lowest-wage jobs at the bottom of the segmented labor market, though they were often more likely to work in distinct industries. Latinx workers were further exploited by temporary staffing agencies, often located in Latinx neighborhoods. These agencies recruit local workers for temporary, low-wage positions often in suburban industries. Staffing agencies help industries cut wages, limit hours, avoid worker protections, and exploit racial stereotypes about Latinx workers being compliant and replenishable.[87] Black workers in unionized jobs, or those with a college education, were employed in transportation, postal work, security, and health care, but many lower-income and lower-educated Black workers were forced out of the labor market altogether. Joblessness was highly concentrated in Black communities.[88] Martin Luther King Jr. lived for a few months in Austin in 1966 working on a fair housing campaign. After his assassination in 1968, riots broke out throughout the city. Stores and businesses throughout the West Side were forced out of business or pushed out of the neighborhood by insurance companies.[89] Businesses in North Lawndale and Austin were shuttered.

From the late 1980s through the first decade of the twenty-first century, in response to issues associated with concentrated poverty, many large public housing units were demolished throughout Chicago. They were replaced with subsidized mixed-income housing and voucher systems. These programs displaced families, contributed to Black out-migration from the city, and ultimately failed to desegregate communities, as voucher housing is also spatially clustered in historically disadvantaged communities.[90] As part of a 2010 urban renewal plan, seventy "underperforming" public schools were closed and replaced with charter schools, which contributed to the displacement and disadvantage of racially marginalized Chicagoans.[91] Shifts in housing and education policies often converge to compound social vulnerability among Chicago's Black and Latinx communities.

Toward the end of deindustrialization, welfare and other social provisions were drastically reduced and paternalistically circumscribed. Since the passage of the Personal Responsibility and Work Opportunity

Reconciliation Act (PRWORA) of 1996, the right to public assistance was replaced by "workfare"—that is, people who receive federal welfare provisions must find employment. Further, the aid itself and the wages earned in the low-skill, low-wage jobs available to those on welfare are so minimal that families struggle to survive. Further, there are minimal opportunities for job advancement, no incentives for skills training or education, and a lack of support for caregiving considerations.[92] PRWORA deemed certain immigrants "unqualified" for welfare and barred them from receiving food stamps (SNAP), nonemergency Medicaid or Medicare, Supplemental Security Income (SSI), and Temporary Assistance for Needy Families (TANF).[93] Even "qualified" immigrants who entered the US after 1996 were subject to a five-year ban on accepting public assistance.

During this same period, the federal government cut provisions made to cities, which reduced their capacity to offer social assistance and other programs to the poor. President Ronald Reagan's regressive tax policies reduced federal tax revenues made available to cities, so state taxes were often increased.[94] Cities rolled back municipal social programs and cut funds for schools, libraries, and hospitals to free up money for redevelopment. Therefore, the poor paid higher taxes and had fewer social assistance programs on which to rely.

The cumulative effects of this ongoing restructuring of economic, housing, welfare, and state policies from the 1970s through the early twenty-first century concentrated poverty in racially marginalized neighborhoods, which were also then targeted with oversurveillance and overpolicing. Since the 1980s, Ryan Lugalia-Hollon and Daniel Cooper argue, the criminal justice system has become the primary means of governing poverty, especially among Black Americans. Austin is a site of what Lugalia-Hollon and Cooper call "concentrated incarceration," at least in part because it is also a prime location for the drug trade.[95] Often termed the Heroin Highway, although more recently it has become the conduit for the opioid crisis, the Central Avenue exit off the Eisenhower Expressway allows commuters from all over Chicago to access drugs in the heart of Austin, and then turn around and return to their lives in the suburbs or middle-income areas of the city.[96] Concentrated incarceration occurs when a relatively small number of neighborhoods account for the majority of arrests and convictions. Austin experiences heightened criminalization and surveillance, as well as concentrated incarceration. More than $100 million is spent annually in Chicago to keep Austin residents incarcerated, while only $6 million is spent for services provided to residents by the Illinois Department of Human Services.[97] Chicagoans' tax dollars are spent on incarcerating Austin residents instead of providing them job creation and skills development, education, public transportation, or housing. In this way, Austin residents are punished for their disadvantage. High rates of concentrated incarceration also exacerbate accumulated vulnerability in Austin because those with felony convictions are often barred from certain kinds of employment, from subsidized housing, and from certain kinds of social assistance.

These are the conjunctural origins of the converging "demics" that faced Black, Latinx, and immigrant Chicagoans throughout the city of Chicago at the onset of the COVID-19 pandemic. Although I have focused specifically on Black and Latinx Chicagoans, issues associated with low-wage work, segregated and substandard housing, educational inequalities, and lack of access to social assistance plague most immigrant communities in Chicago. The undocumented population in Chicago has also grown substantially since the 1990s. Many undocumented Chicagoans maintain transnational ties and strong local social networks, especially among migrant civil society organizations, to survive their difficult work and living conditions.[98] Latinx, Black, *and* immigrant workers were already exploited for their labor in low-wage, unprotected jobs and then faced "precarity convergence" during the pandemic.[99] With very minimal wealth or savings, and lack of access to federal welfare programs (if undocumented or previously incarcerated), workers in low-wage industries had no choice but to put themselves at risk of coronavirus infection once the pandemic began. And many of the people I interviewed were dealing with other crises in their lives as well—underemployment or unemployment, drug use, mental health strain, chronic illness, and deaths in their families as a result of police and gun violence, to name just a few. The same communities engulfed in slow emergencies are also subject to sacrificial labor policies and overpolicing. I turn now to providing specific histories of the neighborhoods where I recruited interviewees.

HISTORICAL BACKGROUND OF ALBANY PARK, AUSTIN, AND LITTLE VILLAGE

I chose three Chicago neighborhoods for interview recruitment based on their racial and economic makeup and whether they were targeted by the city for "racial equity" initiatives: Albany Park, Austin, and Little Village.[100] Figure 0.1 illustrates where each neighborhood is located in the city. Table 0.1 lists key demographics for the three neighborhoods as well as for the whole city of Chicago.[101] Austin and Little Village were included in the city's RERRT initiative because Austin had high COVID-19 death rates and Little Village had high positivity rates in April 2020. Although Albany Park also experienced high rates of both positivity and death and has a large population of people who worked as "essential workers," it was never given additional resources from the City of Chicago. Although each of these neighborhoods was initially home to ethnic white populations in the early twentieth century, each went through a dramatic demographic transformation in the 1960s and 1970s. In this section, I provide background on and descriptions of these communities.

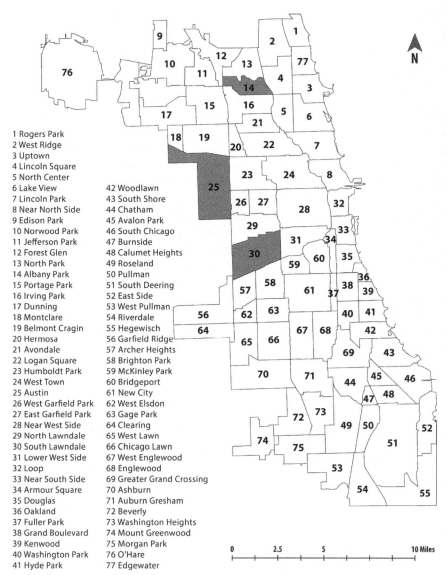

1 Rogers Park
2 West Ridge
3 Uptown
4 Lincoln Square
5 North Center
6 Lake View
7 Lincoln Park
8 Near North Side
9 Edison Park
10 Norwood Park
11 Jefferson Park
12 Forest Glen
13 North Park
14 Albany Park
15 Portage Park
16 Irving Park
17 Dunning
18 Montclare
19 Belmont Cragin
20 Hermosa
21 Avondale
22 Logan Square
23 Humboldt Park
24 West Town
25 Austin
26 West Garfield Park
27 East Garfield Park
28 Near West Side
29 North Lawndale
30 South Lawndale
31 Lower West Side
32 Loop
33 Near South Side
34 Armour Square
35 Douglas
36 Oakland
37 Fuller Park
38 Grand Boulevard
39 Kenwood
40 Washington Park
41 Hyde Park

42 Woodlawn
43 South Shore
44 Chatham
45 Avalon Park
46 South Chicago
47 Burnside
48 Calumet Heights
49 Roseland
50 Pullman
51 South Deering
52 East Side
53 West Pullman
54 Riverdale
55 Hegewisch
56 Garfield Ridge
57 Archer Heights
58 Brighton Park
59 McKinley Park
60 Bridgeport
61 New City
62 West Elsdon
63 Gage Park
64 Clearing
65 West Lawn
66 Chicago Lawn
67 West Englewood
68 Englewood
69 Greater Grand Crossing
70 Ashburn
71 Auburn Gresham
72 Beverly
73 Washington Heights
74 Mount Greenwood
75 Morgan Park
76 O'Hare
77 Edgewater

Figure 0.1 Chicago Community Area Map

Source: Decoteau et al., *Deadly Disparities.*

Table 0.1 Neighborhood Demographics: Albany Park, Austin, and Little Village

	ALBANY PARK	AUSTIN	LITTLE VILLAGE	CHICAGO
2020 Population	48,549	96,753	71,402	2,746,388
Population by race				
Asian	6,133 (12.6%)	496 (0.5%)	313 (0.4%)	185,202 (6.8%)
Black	2,054 (4.2%)	72,863 (75.0%)	8,655 (12.3%)	788,673 (28.9%)
Latinx/Hispanic	22,220 (45.5%)	17,317 (17.8%)	56,840 (81.0%)	787,795 (28.8%)
White	16,968 (34.8%)	5,206 (5.4%)	4,067 (5.8%)	907,499 (33.2%)
Other categories	7 (0.0%)	17 (0.0%)	10 (0.0%)	2,224 (0.1%)
More than one	1,401 (2.9%)	1,290 (1.3%)	282 (0.4%)	61,675 (2.3%)
Foreign-born population	17,041 (35.1%)	6,753 (7.0%)	28,468 (39.9%)	559,714 (20.4%)
Identified as female	23,740 (48.9%)	52,053 (53.8%)	32,488 (45.5%)	1,406,425 (51.2%)
Aged 65 and older (%)	11.4	15.3	13.2	13.8
Below poverty line (%)	13.7	25.4	23.9	17.1
Median annual household income ($)	71,978	43,790	40,359	66,576
Severely rent burdened (%)	17.6	35.9	18.7	25.66
2020 COVID-19 case rate (% of population)	8.0	7.8	11.2	7.8
2021 COVID-19 case rate (% of population)	9.1	9.5	6.3	9.3
2020 COVID-19 death rate (per 100,000 population)	273.1	224.1	268.9	174.6
2021 COVID-19 death rate (per 100,000 population)	86.3	131.5	55.5	83.8
Primary COVID-19 vaccine completion rate (%)	75.2	53.9	68.6	70.8

Sources: Chicago Health Atlas, "Chicago Health Atlas: Access Data for Chicago"; City of Chicago, "COVID-19 Vaccine Coverage by Geography."

Albany Park is situated eight miles northwest of the Loop, the heart of downtown Chicago, and it was initially settled in the early part of the twentieth century by Swedish and German immigrants. Most of the housing, which is exceedingly diverse compared with other Chicago neighborhoods, was built before 1940.[102] Fleeing demographic shifts that took place on the West Side of the city, a large Russian Jewish population settled in Albany Park from the 1930s through the 1950s. This population began to move to the suburbs in the 1960s, and Albany Park became an immigrant destination port for new migrants from Korea, India, Pakistan, the Middle East, the Philippines, Mexico, and Puerto Rico. In the 1960s and 1970s, the population decreased and many homes and stores stood vacant, so the neighborhood was targeted by the city for "urban renewal." The community successfully organized against the city's gentrification plans and established its own community revitalization project that highlighted its diverse makeup.[103] By 1990, 31 percent of residents identified as coming from a "Hispanic origin," 24 percent identified as Asian, and 3 percent identified as Black; however, 47 percent of the population was born outside the US.[104] In fact, census data on racial makeup in Albany Park is likely skewed because it does not allow Arab American communities to be demarcated as a racial group.[105] Another influx of migrants settled into the area in the 1990–2009 period, and migrant civil society organizations in the region worked to help new arrivals access services and provided the missing safety nets that undocumented communities could not access from the government.[106] Part of the reason Albany Park has managed to remain one of the most racially and ethnically diverse neighborhoods in the city is because of the diversity in the kinds of housing units available—from single-family homes, to two-or-three-family and eight-family units, to larger apartment complexes with subsidized units.[107] As Table 0.1 illustrates, in 2023, Albany Park remained extremely diverse, with a large immigrant and undocumented population. The median income of residents, however, was slightly higher than the city average, as was the monthly rental rate. Albany Park has experienced bouts of gentrification, but the diversity of its housing stock has kept some level of socioeconomic and racial diversity intact.

Austin, which is seven miles west of the Loop, is one of the largest of Chicago's seventy-seven neighborhoods, both geographically and in terms of population. Until the 1960s, Austin was a predominantly white neighborhood, home to people of Italian, Irish, English, and Scottish descent, who lived in brick bungalows, two-flats (two-story buildings with each floor comprising a separate apartment), and duplexes (attached single units comprised of two floors with interior stairs connecting them both). In the 1960 census, the population was 99.9 percent white, but by the 1980 census, the Black population made up 73.8 percent of the neighborhood.[108]

Black families began moving to Austin in the 1960s seeking integration and to escape racist housing policies on the South Side. White families began moving out, and racist policies such as redlining and blockbusting drove housing prices in the area down.[109] Though redlining was declared illegal in 1968, there were still subtle mechanisms used to bar Black residents from buying homes in integrated neighborhoods. These processes fueled racial segregation and the concentration of Black communities in particular Chicago neighborhoods.[110] Many Austin residents found work in the Brach's candy factory, Western Electric Hawthorne Works, and Sears Roebuck, but between 1970 and 2000, these factories significantly cut their workforces, contributing to unemployment in the region.[111] In the 1990 census, the population was already 87 percent Black, and 23 percent of the community lived below the poverty line.[112] As Table 0.1 illustrates, in 2023, Austin remained a predominantly Black neighborhood, and about 25 percent of its residents lived below the poverty line. The annual income of residents is far below the city's average.

South Lawndale, which is now referred to as Little Village (or La Villita), is five miles southwest of the Loop. It was also a predominantly white neighborhood until the 1960s. It was initially populated by Czech and German immigrants and their descendants who settled there to work in the Harvester plant and Western Electric factory which border the neighborhood's west side. Between 1960 and 1980, many white residents moved out, and Mexican immigrants moved in—buying property in the region at increasing rates. Whereas in the 1960 census 93.9 percent of Little Village residents were white, by 1980, 74 percent of the residents were Mexican Americans, and the area was home to 20 percent of the Mexican residents in the city.[113] During this same period, the Harvester and Western Electric factories closed, and the 1990 census shows a 14 percent unemployment rate.[114] Factories have moved in and out of the Little Village neighborhood over time. Overcrowding is common because the housing stock has remained largely unchanged since the 1920s.[115] In addition to the residential and industrial regions of Little Village, Cook County Jail and the Criminal Court House and House of Corrections are located in the neighborhood, so 8 percent of its population lives in containment. Little Village is home to the largest concentration of Mexican Chicagoans in the city, and by 2000, nearly half (48.3 percent) of the population was foreign-born.[116] Table 0.1 indicates that in 2023, the population was still predominantly Latinx, and about 24 percent of the population lived below the poverty line. In the next section, I provide an analysis of the accumulated vulnerabilities the people I interviewed experienced as their endemic emergencies were accelerated during the pandemic. Chapters 4 and 5 are also dedicated to elaborating on these points.

CONVERGING "DEMICS"

> What does it mean for people declared disposable by some "new" econ-
> omy to find themselves existing out of place *in* place?
>
> ROB NIXON, *Slow Violence*

Analyzing environmentally degraded sites, Nixon suggests that people often experience a sense of displacement while remaining *in* place as their
"once-sustaining landscapes . . . [have been] gutted of their capacity to sustain by an externalizing, instrumental logic."[117] As well-paying jobs dried
up and local infrastructures withered under neoliberal restructuring and
the gutting of care infrastructure, many people in Austin, Little Village, and
Albany Park found themselves being displaced of their livelihoods while
remaining in place. In this section, I review some of the contemporary
"demics" that residents of these neighborhoods endure, which were compounded by pandemic precarity.

In some ways, residents of these three neighborhoods face unique conditions that are not shared across the sites, and I begin by discussing each of
these. Then I explain how these distinct slow emergencies nonetheless converged into accumulated precarity for many racially and socioeconomically
marginalized groups during the COVID-19 pandemic. Because the city enacted an urgent, medicalized response, it failed to respond to the converging crises many communities experienced. And because slow emergencies
are sustained by barriers to social safety nets, they often exist alongside conditions of labor sacrifice, which was also accelerated during the pandemic.
I end this section by explaining how sacrificial logics and slow emergencies
merged to expose lower-income Black and Brown Chicagoans to premature
death during the pandemic.

Austin residents face unique conditions that are not shared by inhabitants
of Little Village or Albany Park. Bernice, a fifty-six-year-old Black woman, has
lived in Austin most of her life. In her interview, she reflected on some of the
emergencies that arose for the Black community in Austin over time:

> Living on the West Side of Chicago, it's written off by society as a poverty-
> stricken neighborhood. I've never agreed to that. . . . I had a bike. I went
> on vacation. I went to a private school. I don't always agree with how
> they rated my neighborhood . . . [but] it's a pretty rough neighborhood
> now . . . because of the violence and everything with younger people to-
> day. . . . A lot of the young people have gotten conditioned to believe that
> they're nothing, they're not gonna be nothing, they're not gonna have
> nothing. . . . A bunch of things start to occur in the neighborhood when
> everybody's fighting for . . . a piece of place or something that they think

is theirs. With a lot of young people now, a lot of hope has been lost. . . . This neighborhood has become a big drug neighborhood. . . . I think it really started . . . [with] the gentrification of the community—taking over areas and moving people and shifting them is what started a lot of the change. Tearing down the projects and not dealing with those people. . . . A lot of things changed after that.[118]

As Bernice suggests, the tearing down of public housing, gentrification, and disinvestment began what would become a slow decline that has led to contemporary youth having lost hope or needing to fight for a place "that they think is theirs." She went on to explain that COVID-19 sped up a lot of these ongoing emergency conditions.

While many residents noted that drug and alcohol use, as well as violent crime, have been historic features of the Austin neighborhood, loss of jobs and the stress of the pandemic increased incidents of violent crime as well. Derek, a Black man from Austin, told me:

Lotta peoples got job issues. Job issues been the number one thing for peoples in my neighborhood. . . . Sometimes, when you get a group of kids together or young adults like that with nothin' to do, no way of goin' out, enjoyin' their self, sometime it can be bad, and that can lead into some violence. . . . People have a right to be angry. We, as Black peoples, we done been through this here for so many years and years. Every time you kill a Black man, you kill a Black woman, don't too much happen about it. Peoples are angry. Peoples are fed up. Peoples are tired.[119]

Derek links job loss and the stress of quarantine with upticks in violence, but he also suggests that people are justified in feeling angry. Given how difficult life can be for Black residents of Austin, and the high rates of police surveillance and violence, people are often righteously angry and "fed up." These conditions predate the pandemic but were also worsened by its effects.

Austin has extremely high incidences of opioid- and fentanyl-related deaths. As figure 0.2 indicates, drug-related deaths were highest among Black communities in Chicago even before the pandemic.[120]

According to the Cook County Government, opioid-related overdose deaths numbered 1,840 in 2020, 1,936 in 2021, and 2,000 in 2022. Fifty-six percent of these deaths were concentrated among Black residents of Cook County.[121] The concentration of these overdose deaths in Black communities on Chicago's West Side was ignored because of the city's singular focus on the pandemic.[122] Given the fact that the Heroin Highway runs through the heart of Austin, it is perhaps unsurprising that incidences of

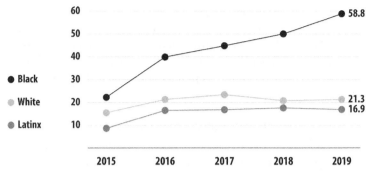

Figure 0.2 Drug-Induced Mortality Rate per 100,000 People in Chicago, by Race,
2015–19
Source: Decoteau et al., *Deadly Disparities,* 59.

drug overdosing were accelerated by pandemic conditions. And instances
of violent crime also rose precipitously in the region. Table 0.2 indicates
reported violent crimes by victims during the pandemic in the three neighborhoods where I conducted interviews, and Austin's victimization counts
are about three to eight times higher than the other two neighborhoods.

In his analysis of the disproportionate impact of the 1995 heat wave
on Black Chicagoans, Eric Klinenberg provides an ecological, social autopsy analysis of North Lawndale, a neighborhood that borders Austin and
shares many of its features.[123] Klinenberg explains that the social abandonment of Black people during the heat wave was facilitated by socio-
ecological conditions in Black neighborhoods, including dilapidated open
spaces (with boarded-up buildings and businesses), lack of robust community organizations, high crime, low employment, high drug use, and
high rates of social isolation. He contrasts these conditions with those of
South Lawndale (Little Village), which is densely populated and has higher
employment, more robust community organizations, and stronger social
networks. Austin and Little Village still epitomize these socioecological
portraits, but slow emergencies are not neighborhood conditions. They
can be bolstered by neighborhood disadvantage, but they are caused by

Table 0.2 Violent Crimes Reported by Victims by Neighborhood

	ALBANY PARK	AUSTIN	LITTLE VILLAGE
2020	320	2,346	603
2021	239	2,001	661
2022	265	1,830	715

Source: Mayor's Office of Violence Reduction, "Violence and Victimization Trends."

racist policies, economic conditions, and the retraction of aid, which can occur in any kind of neighborhood, especially as emergencies compound during crises such as the COVID-19 pandemic. The slow emergencies that led to accelerated disadvantage among residents of Austin may be slightly different from those experienced by lower-income, racially marginalized residents of Little Village and Albany Park—but many of the compounded outcomes are the same.

The precipitating conditions in Little Village include urban redevelopment and hyperexploitation by temporary staffing agencies. The ongoing gentrification of Little Village continues to displace lower-income Mexican residents. For example, a Mexican American alderperson explained:

> We understand that to address the issue of displacement, we have to understand the power dynamics . . . that facilitated the basic takeover by developers of an area that was very working-class and a port of entry for many immigrants for generations. And all of a sudden [it] became the home for luxury housing, luxury restaurants. . . . There was nothing accidental about these trends, but was a very deliberate effort by the City of Chicago. . . . We understood what was at stake here was to protect the investments of big developers . . . that would benefit by this policy. But the effects on the working-class people, the majority of residents that were already struggling with housing costs, property taxes, and maintenance on the properties [were negative]. So it was very clear that the city agenda did not take into account the struggles of the average family in the neighborhood, but was really interested in bringing investment and development without really [any] consideration of the effects, which will fuel displacement.[124]

While Austin has been a site of disinvestment, where abandoned homes and businesses stand empty, Little Village is an ongoing site of "urban renewal," which displaces working-class Mexican American communities as new developments go up and rental and home prices rise.[125] In addition, Little Village residents are preyed on by temporary staffing agencies that recruit laborers from the region to staff industries in the suburbs. These agencies keep wages low and help industries avoid instituting worker protections by replacing workers who are injured, get sick, or demand better work conditions.[126] Local displacement and labor exploitation were the preconditions in Little Village that led to accumulated vulnerability for residents during the pandemic.

In Albany Park, which is home to many lower-income undocumented and immigrant communities, housing affordability is a primary challenge.

Gentrification is driving rent and mortgage prices higher.[127] People often engage in informal housing agreements with landlords (without formal, written leases) to secure affordable housing, which often facilitates housing exploitation because landlords can keep units in substandard condition (lacking heat/air, without ventilation, with bug/rodent infestations), overcrowding is common, and families are subject to informal evictions.[128] When the pandemic began and many workers lost hours or employment, residents fell behind on rent—this left them vulnerable to landlord retaliation and heightened risk of informal eviction. One housing attorney described the situation this way:

> The more immediate problem people have had is a lack of maintenance—landlords saying they're not getting rent, so therefore they're not fixing the apartments. . . . Or more frequently . . . informal evictions where you tell somebody they gotta get out . . . [and] you do things like turn off their water or change the locks . . . in order to get them out.[129]

When rental assistance became available, people who rely on informal housing arrangements were unable to apply for assistance without their landlord's participation. Therefore, housing insecurity was an endemic emergency for many lower-income residents of Albany Park, which was then compounded by pandemic conditions (which I explain in more detail in chapter 5).

Lack of sustainable jobs and infrastructure (in Austin), displacement from urban renewal and hyperexploitation (in Little Village), and lack of affordable housing (in Albany Park) contributed to conditions of converging precarity during the pandemic and often resulted in food insufficiency, which increased for Black and Latinx communities as the pandemic progressed. US Census Bureau Household Pulse Survey data, represented by the bar graph in figure 0.3, indicate that 16.6 percent of Black families in Chicago did not have enough food in the first year of the pandemic, and this percentage *increased* to 17.6 percent in the second year of the pandemic.[130] Latinx families also experienced food insufficiency, with 16.0 percent indicating that they did not have enough food in the first year of the pandemic, and 13.8 percent in the second year of the pandemic. In the Household Pulse Survey, respondents were asked, "In the last 7 days, which of these statements best describes the food eaten in your household?" The answer choices, summarized in figure 0.3, were (1) "Enough of the kinds of food (I/we) wanted to eat," (2) "Enough, but not always the kinds of food (I/we) wanted to eat," or (3) "Sometimes not enough to eat" or "Often not enough to eat."

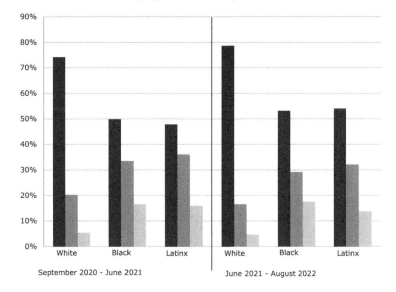

Enough of preferred food ■ Enough, but not preferred food ■ Sometimes or often not enough to eat

Figure 0.3 Food Sufficiency by Race in Chicago, 2020–22
Source: US Census Household Pulse Survey Data Public Use File.

Food insecurity may have increased for some families because of rising inflation. Innumerable Chicagoans commented in their interviews on how difficult it was to stretch food stamps and meager wages with the price of food so high. During the pandemic, federal free lunch programs were expanded, but this expansion ended in May 2022, and income eligibility rates in 2022–23 did not keeping pace with rising food costs.[131] Further, the US Congress authorized states to allow families to access the maximum allotment of SNAP benefits for their household size, but as I explained, this did not always benefit the most vulnerable families who were already receiving the maximum allotment. And the State of Illinois canceled these emergency allotments as of March 1, 2023.[132] Many undocumented or mixed-status families were ineligible for food stamps during the pandemic. Food insecurity may become a lasting legacy of the pandemic for low-income families in the United States.

Tables 0.3 and 0.4 provide indices of vulnerability in each of the three neighborhoods where I conducted interviews to illustrate the shared conditions of many residents living amid converging endemics.[133]

Table 0.3 Neighborhood Housing and Food Measures

	ALBANY PARK	AUSTIN	LITTLE VILLAGE	CHICAGO
2017–2021 Crowded housing (% of occupied housing)	5.2	3.8	7.7	3.5
2018 Eviction filing rate (per 100 renter households)	1.3	5.2	1.7	2.7
2019 Low food access (% of residents)	3.9	32.4	4.8	21.9
2017–2021 Households receiving food stamps (% of households)	15.9	34.4	22.8	19.6
2017–2021 Households in poverty NOT receiving food stamps (% of households in poverty)	55.8	39.0	52.0	50.0

Source: Chicago Health Atlas, "Chicago Health Atlas: Access Data for Chicago."

Table 0.4 Neighborhood Health Measures

	ALBANY PARK	AUSTIN	LITTLE VILLAGE	CHICAGO
2017 Avoidable emergency room (ER) visit rate (per 10,000 population)	287.0	1,253.6	668.7	542.7
2017 Drug-related hospitalization rate (per 10,000 population)	6.5	126.2	48.5	32.1
2017 Asthma ER visit rate (per 10,000 population)	34.7	243.0	112.0	85.8
2017–2021 Uninsured rate (% of population)	14.4	10.5	19.0	9.8

Source: Chicago Health Atlas, "Chicago Health Atlas: Access Data for Chicago."

Many respondents mentioned in interviews that their neighborhoods would feel the impact of COVID-19 far longer than more wealthy or white neighborhoods of Chicago. For example, Miguel, a Mexican immigrant from Albany Park, explained:

I don't think we'll be over this fast. . . . Some people will get better and better and better. Others will be the same, the same, and the same for another twenty years. . . . The social effects will take a few years to repair. Yeah, maybe it will take a lot of time . . . because some of the communities have been hurt, and they're gonna be hurt for long time.[134]

Although the pandemic exposed, to some degree, the invisibilized processes of slow death that vulnerable communities have experienced for decades, there was very little political will to counteract the effects. Both Black and Latinx respondents—for example, Harold and Carlos—explained how they felt as though their communities were ignored, left to wait for aid, while white neighborhoods were protected first:

> There should have been more drastic action taken as far as certain communities. The people in those wealthy areas were getting help and things of that nature ASAP when people . . . in what they consider poverty-stricken neighborhoods were in wait. *They were in wait.*[135]

> [White people] get more attention than Hispanic communities do. I think they get more information, they get better treatment at hospitals. . . . There was more stuff available to them, that the minorities didn't [get]. . . . *They left us for last.*[136]

Harold and Carlos point to the fact that their ongoing suffering, sped up under COVID-19 conditions, facilitated their political abandonment during the pandemic. In fact, recognizing the intractability of structural inequality led many politicians to disavow their responsibility to address it—as if it were an ontological truth, as opposed to a result of political decision-making. Because of structural disadvantage and the fact that certain communities were already living on the edge, state officials "let die" certain racially marginalized communities by not intervening with broader social supports.

In addition, however, slow emergencies converge with sacrificial logics, as the same populations often suffer from both. This is because welfare requires workfare; because people living through slow emergencies often have few accumulated resources on which to rely when disasters strike, forcing them to accept unfair labor conditions; and because low-wage insecure labor has always been racially segmented in Chicago. During the pandemic, the sacrifice of "essential workers" was initially heralded in the media, but the sacrifice lower-income frontline workers made was not compensated—worker protections were nonexistent, remuneration was measly, and sick pay was withheld. Because lower-income frontline workers also faced slow emergencies and often could not access structural safety nets, workers were forced into an impossible choice between feeding their families or being exposed to death. Sharon called this a "double negative." She told me:

> That's the double negatives, because they have to make a living because everybody who's working has a family. . . . They have to pay bills. . . . How

am I gonna feed my kids? Or take care of my elderly mother if y'all forced me out at my job? But then you gonna tell me I have to work in this pandemic. You don't give a fuck. You don't care about my safety. You're not protecting me. So like I say, it's a double negative.[137]

Low-wage, frontline workers are exploited in an immediate way—their lives were literally thrown into emergency each day of the pandemic, to protect the norm from exposure.

In an interview with the chief architect of the city's "racial equity" team, I asked why work protections were not a citywide priority, given that city officials knew that high infection rates were driven by unsafe work conditions. She said that it is not the city's job to impose work restrictions and safety measures and asserted that "there was very little we could do."[138] And yet, other states did provide hazard pay protections for "essential" workers.[139] An activist I interviewed pushed back against the argument that city government could not protect workers, suggesting that the city could have put more stringent workplace protections in place:

The city does technically have some oversight over businesses . . . the Mayor's Office was as much there to support business interest as it was its residents, probably more so. Right, because the business community didn't want to shut down. . . . How does the city not have power to support the rights of workers when they're very much intentionally supporting the business owners?[140]

Epidemiologists were also marveling after a full year of the pandemic at the new risk category of "occupational hazard" that had emerged during the pandemic, suggesting that vulnerability maps were skewed because more working-class neighborhoods were hit hard alongside ones suffering from historic disinvestment. That frontline workers became a new risk group during COVID-19 was well known by city policymakers, yet nothing was done to protect them. In addition to the paradoxes of being called "essential" but being put in harm's way for the sake of the economy and the middle class, the fact that undocumented communities were ineligible for pandemic aid communicated clearly that state officials saw them as disposable.

In this section, I have provided historical context for the development of slow emergencies and sacrificial labor logics, which often overlap to expose the same communities to premature death through multiple mechanisms of exclusionary inclusion. Slow emergencies necessarily take more time to develop and operate via the intransigence of structural reproduction. They are largely invisible and protected by their slow evolution, which facilitates the obfuscation of their causes. But they perhaps have the most lethal, long-term effects. Whereas slow emergencies are largely governed via "letting die" policies and operate at the outskirts of the norm, the emergency of "essential work" is enacted through sacrifice. Certain people's livelihoods are exploited for the protection and profit of others. Frontline workers are included in the social imaginary but are disposed of as a sacrifice for the sake of the nation and the economy. Both of these endemic emergencies were ignored *and* exacerbated by the policies enacted to govern the emergency of COVID-19, which presumed scarcity and triaged care. Governing through emergency is anticipatory in nature—policies are put in place for a delimited amount of time to govern the immediate emergency, until the system as usual regains its stability and the norm is ensured protection. Bounding these emergencies temporally necessarily involves obfuscating the links to more sustained, protracted, and converging emergencies that the racially marginalized have been facing for decades. For those enduring slow emergencies, sacrificial exploitation, or both, the urgent/immediate and the everyday/mundane are intimately linked. For people experiencing these conditions, the protracted crisis of slow violence is often disrupted by more acute and immediate emergencies, such as death, eviction, or political protest. Constant anxiety and trauma and the gnawing boredom of quarantine take place amid more immediate crises of pandemic times.

BRIEF OUTLINE OF THE BOOK

Chapter 1 analyzes the convergence of crises that befell racially marginalized communities in the summer of 2020. From the beginning of the pandemic in March 2020, Black and Latinx Chicagoans experienced the severe impact of years of disinvestment in their communities as they were overcome by illness and death and felt they were made to wait for any relief or aid. Their slow emergencies turned into acute crises and were being ignored by governmental actors. Then, with the murder of George Floyd and the violent state repression of uprisings that occurred in its aftermath, these communities felt the double assault of prolonged neglect (letting die) and hypersurveillance and police violence (making die) at the same time. The chapter revisits Foucault's theories of racial biopolitics to analyze the enduring legacy of this historically specific convergence of emergencies for Black and Brown Chicagoans, and it explores the ways in which their racial devaluation was often experienced as ontological and temporal insecurity.

Existing scholarship suggests that slow death arises from capitalist work relations and environmental toxicity, but in chapter 2 I illustrate how the historical disinvestment in health infrastructures (health care, public health, and mental health care) helps explain the disproportionate racial toll COVID-19 took. I analyze why and with what effect structures and pathways of care are continually obscured and fragmented by neoliberal governance and structural racism, leading to conditions of health apartheid. I theorize this as *uneven* investment in infrastructure, wherein certain infrastructures are highlighted and prioritized (in this case, epistemic) and others are rendered invisible or intransigent.

Chapter 3 focuses on the City of Chicago's "racial equity" response to the pandemic. It analyzes how such an approach marks a departure from neoliberal colorblind racism toward more race-conscious discourses that nonetheless support neoliberal orthodoxy and white supremacy. The chapter provides four mechanisms by which COVID-19 was managed: (1) public health interventions were economized based on a presumption of scarcity; (2) the city built a robust epistemic infrastructure to triage resources; (3) it outsourced the provision of triaged resources to private and nonprofit sectors, and (4) it enacted means-tested strategies to deliver minimal aid, resulting in bureaucratic barriers to access.

Slow emergencies fade into the background and make attributing blame difficult. Chapter 4 renders visible the converging endemic emergencies that Black and Latinx Chicagoans have faced historically and illustrates how they were compounded by pandemic conditions. In the face of political obfuscation and willful ignorance, it is important to *highlight* the causes of structural inequality and their accumulative impact on marginalized communities. This chapter illustrates how a focus on the pandemic as a *medical* crisis could not possibly address the entangled "demics" certain communities face, which made their experience with COVID-19 so different from that of more protected communities.

Chapter 5 focuses on how workers in precarious, front-facing jobs in agriculture, meat production, delivery, food preparation, and public transit were sacrificed to salvage the US economy. It analyzes the paradoxes and strains put on the families of those who continued to work in "essential" jobs. While slow emergencies and sacrificial exploitation happen to the same communities, this chapter also illustrates how the logic of sacrifice operates differently from letting die.

During the pandemic, social media were impugned for fomenting distrust and conspiracy theories among the racially marginalized, who were then blamed for not getting vaccinated. Chapter 6 provides evidence that Black and Brown people's distrust of vaccines and COVID-19 policies were often situated in direct experiences of racial devaluation by state actors and health professionals. The chapter then illustrates how one mutual aid organization in Austin countered the fear associated with racial devaluation and provided the social safety net that the state failed to deliver. This organization provided a powerful example of how racially and socioeconomically marginalized communities survive endemic emergencies and counter the thanatopolitical strategies of a white supremacist society.

The coda cautions against forgetting the lessons learned from this and past pandemics. As a society, we are too quick to declare emergencies over, and we leave behind the people still suffering their worst impacts. It also suggests that the US missed an opportunity to reckon with our racist history and the ongoing legacy of structural inequality and examines moments in the pandemic when a different outcome could have been seized.

1: EXPOSING AND GOVERNING RACISM

By the end of May 2020, Black Americans accounted for 60 percent of the deaths from COVID-19 in Chicago and had the highest infection rates in Illinois.[1] Black Chicagoans felt the acute and immediate impact of their long-term structural disadvantage as they experienced the relentless deaths of their family and friends. In the Austin neighborhood, Shirley spoke to me as she prepared to attend her aunt's funeral, just weeks after losing her fiancé. She whispered, "COVID took a lot of people. *A lot* of people."[2] Marlin told me he had "been to so many funerals, right? . . . Everybody walking around in trauma."[3] Walter, whose wife suffers from chronic obstructive pulmonary disease, described the first few weeks of the pandemic:

> It was scary. . . . I didn't know how I was goin' to be able to feed my wife. I didn't know how I was goin' be able to support her. . . . When you see all these peoples every day, like in March . . . when you turn the TV on, that's all you was seeing, peoples just dying all the time, and not just one or two. It was a hundred a day, you know what I'm sayin'? . . . It was hard for us, especially for Black people. . . . Peoples dying every day. . . . It was hard for us to even try an' wrap our mind around.[4]

Not only were Black communities suffering from the immediate effect of decades of slow emergencies, but state actors were not responding to the mounting deaths with immediate action. Rather, communities felt as if they were made to wait for services. Austin resident Anthony echoed this perspective:

> The government was not handling it fast enough. . . . It's too many people dying before they even do anything about it. It's like they turned a blind eye to the statistics out here. . . . How [do] they wait so long before they come up with anything?[5]

And then on May 25, a Black man named George Floyd was murdered by the Minneapolis police, and protests immediately erupted all over the country. They were incendiary in Chicago. Not only were Black Chicagoans trying to make sense of the violent police murder of Floyd, but they were met with brutal police repression in Chicago as they tried to express their righteous anger at racial devaluation. The city government called in the National Guard to protect the prosperous Magnificent Mile in the tourist area of downtown Chicago, the police arrested and terrorized protesters, and riots spread throughout the South and West Sides of the city.[6] Black Chicagoans felt abandoned and violently targeted at the same time. The double assault of neglect (*letting die*) and violence (*making die*) came to a head, as the emergencies of structural abandonment and police brutality converged.

During the summer of 2020 in Chicago and across the nation, people protested against the devaluation of Black and Brown lives evident in both the disproportionate impact of COVID-19 and in police brutality. Although letting die and making die are constant means by which state actors manage the paradoxes of white supremacy, racialized others (and their allies) demanded recognition of US state racism during the widespread unrest that spread throughout the nation in May and June 2020. Everyday Americans forced the underlying crisis tendencies associated with the paradoxes of racial biocapitalism to a breaking point, calling attention to the brutal and structural violence of white supremacy, and the state had no choice but to respond. City, state, and federal officials governed the converging crises of police murders and COVID-19 deaths through emergency operations. Declarations of emergency were made, official juridical proceedings were suspended, and some additional services and policies were rolled out in response. The point of these declarations of emergency was to momentarily recognize state racism, govern *through* it, until racism could, once again, fade into America's structural background. The American people who took to the streets in the summer of 2020 did force a reckoning and recognition, but once the emergency was governed, it was declared "through"—the immediate crisis was over, and the everyday business of racial devaluation could return to "normal."

Sholanda, a Black woman from Austin, explained that crises like COVID-19 or Hurricane Katrina momentarily expose to the public the everyday, structural racism that people of color endure all the time. Americans who benefit from racism only glimpse white supremacy and its impact during moments of crisis, and then this knowledge once again fades into indifference. But Black and Brown Americans are not afforded this ignorance. Sholanda said:

Yeah, they swept racism right under the rug like they do [after the crisis is over] . . . like America always do. Anything that blemishes America, they cover it up. But now they done pulled the cover off again. . . . [Racism] never went nowhere. It just changed the look. It took off the hoods and put on judge robes, police officer uniforms. . . . That's all it did. . . . I'da rather you kept on the white and the hood. Least I know what I'm dealing with.[7]

Today, Sholanda explains, agents of white supremacy wear police uniforms and black judges' robes, as opposed to the white robes and hoods of the Ku Klux Klan, but the racism is the same, just differently authorized and legitimated.

In her analysis of the events of the summer of 2020, Robin Wagner-Pacifici suggests that the racial uprisings of that summer dislodged conventional categories and forced a "double exposure"—not only were Americans exposed to COVID-19 and police violence, but the demonstrations brought systemic racism to light.[8] And yet, as I will show, whether state actors rearticulated new policies based on this momentary revelation depended on their political orientation. For Donald Trump and his supporters, the exposure of racism associated with COVID-19 facilitated an epistemology of refusal, excusing ongoing structural neglect and inciting everyday Americans to take part in acts of racial violence. For liberal leaders, such as JB Pritzker, the governor of Illinois, and Lori Lightfoot, the mayor of Chicago, the "exposure" of structural racism required governing *through* the emergencies of COVID-19 and police brutality. As such, liberal actors made efforts to minimally redress inequalities while they were highlighted, but with policies that left structural neglect and violence intact. And then, once these crises were no longer exposed through daily demonstrations or media attention—once the immediate crisis faded into the mundane—the emergency was declared resolved. As a result, people who were experiencing the convergence of letting die and making die policies were often faced with profound senses of disjuncture, compounding their ontological insecurity.

In what follows, I take up each of these arguments in greater detail. First, I explain how political orientation determined whether the racism on display in the summer of 2020 was ignored or governed. I provide quotes from residents about their experiences with racial neglect and violence during the pandemic and illustrate how racism is only met with state recognition in moments of immediate crisis. I also provide theoretical insight into Foucauldian theories of *letting die* and *making die*. Finally, I provide a narrative of how COVID-19 policies in Chicago often created disjunctures for those experiencing them, illustrating how governing *through* emergencies fails to redress racial harm on the ground. To do so, I provide some details of how COVID-19 unfolded over time in Chicago. Disjunctures between policy and everyday experience compounded the ontological precarity Black and Brown Chicagoans endured.

LETTING DIE THROUGH STRUCTURAL NEGLECT

President Trump's mishandling of the pandemic and his downplaying of its seriousness were experienced by Black Americans as a violent distortion of reality—what Charles Mills refers to as a racist "epistemology of ignorance" that purposefully misrepresents the world to sustain white supremacy.[9] This epistemology of ignorance was used to support systemic, structural neglect, as Black and Brown Americans were bearing the brunt of the economic and mortal impacts of COVID-19. Becky, a white woman from Albany Park, contended that Trump's inaction amounted to genocide: "Trump essentially committed genocide by not doing anything, mostly of Black and Brown people. I mean, I literally think he committed genocide. It feels like a big war crime, to be honest, through doing absolutely nothin'."[10] And in fact, this blatant disregard and devaluation of Black and Brown lives left many observers to speculate about whether Trump knew more than he admitted, or whether he could have done more to control the coronavirus's spread. Sholanda, for example, countered conspiracy claims that COVID-19 was not real, but she wholeheartedly believed Trump could have done more. She told me, "Do I think COVID exists? Absolutely. Do I think Trump could have controlled it better? Absolutely. . . . Too many people died from something that could have been prevented and controlled."[11] Keisha, a Black woman from Austin, told me quite plainly, "Trump's been lying and lying and lying. . . . He didn't give a damn about all these people going to go die."[12] These quotes express the frustration and indignation felt by Black Chicagoans that thousands and thousands of people were let die because of inattention and disregard among government officials, especially those in the Trump administration.

Kelly, a young Black woman from Albany Park, explained how neglect and violent white supremacist attacks converged under Trump's leadership:

> Trump could have *done something*, so we all didn't go into, like, our mad panic. . . . It just seemed like he was just inciting violence and the tension that was already there, he was making it ten times worse. . . . I just don't feel like he cared that so many people were losing their jobs and losing their lives and family members. I really don't think he gave a shit. . . . I feel like him aligning himself with white supremacists, while at the same time telling people that masks are stupid . . . I think that goes hand in hand.[13]

Kelly explains how two racially thanatopolitical tactics—medical neglect and racist violence—go "hand in hand." For Trump and his supporters, the recognition that COVID-19 was having a disproportionate impact on Black and Brown Americans enabled medical and structural neglect. If the virus was mostly killing Black and Brown Americans, then its impact was unimportant to him. Such a recognition facilitated the white supremacist backlash that Trump willingly supported.

Anthony Hatch argues that the widespread publication of racial disparities in coronavirus infections *precipitated* Trump's "malignant indifference," "structural inattention," and the withdrawal of "federal public health infrastructure that would have mitigated the loss of Black lives."[14] Hatch specifically points to Trump's often inconsistent support of widespread COVID-19 testing.[15] And in fact, the disproportionate impact on Black and Brown communities often made it seem to middle-class white populations that the pandemic was *not* an emergency *for them* and was therefore isolated in its impact. Allison Harell and Evan Lieberman conducted an experimental survey in which they gave respondents information on COVID-19 racial disparities and then asked what kinds of public health interventions they preferred.[16] The study found that when white respondents were presented with evidence that COVID-19 risks were highly concentrated in Black and Brown communities, white respondents felt less at risk themselves and indicated preferences for lifting mask and vaccine mandates. This survey illustrates how the circulation of racial statistics about the impact of COVID-19 bolstered white supremacist attitudes among certain political conservatives, which in turn led to political barriers to implementing extensive support for those most impacted.

Beyond blaming Trump personally for sustaining racialized structural neglect, Black and Brown Chicagoans were experiencing tremendous inattention from city government officials. Although liberal actors did recognize the disproportionate toll COVID-19 was taking on Black and Brown lives and instituted various emergency measures that were touted as racially equitable, many Chicagoans of color experienced these policies as delayed and insufficient. As I will discuss further in chapter 3, testing and vaccine resources were initially extremely limited in resource-poor neighborhoods and then were triaged to only those with the highest death and infection rates. This approach left many residents of racially marginalized neighborhoods scrambling to access even the most basic medical services. In addition, rental assistance was delayed and minimal, and when it finally was given sufficient attention, there were tremendous bureaucratic barriers associated with accessing it. People also experienced delays and disruptions to unemployment payouts. Respondents pointed to the uneven rollout of aid as factors that illustrated the devaluation of Black and Brown lives.

Rodrigo, a Mexican American man from Little Village, discussed how undocumented people were forgotten and abandoned:

> The government never gave us the adequate warnings, and since the government didn't give us the warnings, the undocumented communities here in Little Village were not even talked about. We were disenfranchised. We were not included. They didn't send face masks to Little Village. They didn't send sanitizers to Little Village or instructions in Spanish. . . . We noticed that our community was not being treated equally.[17]

Many respondents explained that communities of color were made to wait while white communities were given more resources and support. Delay and the imposition of "waiting for help" can be an important feature of letting die during a pandemic. For example, Ben, a Black man from Austin, explained:

> People were scared. . . . There's this pandemic out here, but you guys . . . got nothing here in place for us. People got scared. 'Cause I knew I did. I was, like, where's all the test sites? Where's all the things? Where's the stuff that we need?![18]

Charles, a Black man from Austin, talked extensively about how despite claims that the federal government was doling out extensive financial support, there were delays and interruptions to accessing it at the state and city levels, which compounded people's sense of vulnerability and uncertainty. He told me:

> They're not giving the people the help that they really need immediately. Some people waited months to get unemployment and public assistance. I don't know what they're doing. . . . They should've moved in action quicker . . . for individuals who are impacted from unemployment . . . and needed assistance. . . . Because the federal government did not move fast enough.[19]

The slow pace of aid and the neglect to act quickly when the statistics were illustrating a disproportionate racial impact are forms of structural inattention that let die Black and Brown communities. *Making people wait* constitutes profound devaluation during a pandemic.[20]

When George Floyd was killed in late May 2020, this sense of inattention and devaluation converged with the eruption of another kind of endemic emergency: police violence. And in fact, Trump's exoneration and indulgence of white supremacist violence continued to stoke Black and Brown Americans' sense of being racially devalued throughout the pandemic. Although the murder of Floyd and the City of Chicago's response to the protests that followed were a temporally bounded emergency, governed in a particular way by state agents, the feeling respondents had of being doubly assaulted by structural neglect and violence endured.

POLICE VIOLENCE AND *MAKING DIE*

After Floyd's murder by Minneapolis police, demonstrations erupted throughout Chicago. The crisis tendencies of liberal white supremacy came to a head, and people protested the converging emergencies of structural neglect and police brutality. On May 30, the first planned demonstration took place. Media accounts suggest that protesters turned violent and began destroying property in downtown Chicago. In response, Mayor Lightfoot raised the drawbridges over the Chicago River, weaponizing this iconic Chicago infrastructure and effectively cutting off downtown from the West and South Sides of the city. Some people were trapped downtown, and others were unable to join them in support. Lightfoot also imposed a citywide curfew and suspended public transit, and the police used tear gas and arrested 494 people.[21] The drawbridges in downtown Chicago had not been raised in response to public protest since 1855.[22] As Annie, a young Korean American respondent from Albany Park, said, "for the first time in my life, I realized that a bridge also functions as a wall of control."[23] Lightfoot then enlisted Governor Pritzker to call in the National Guard. Pritzker declared Cook County a disaster area and deployed 375 National Guard soldiers and 100 state troopers to downtown Chicago on Sunday, May 31.[24] The National Guard had not been called in for crowd control since the 1968 protests that erupted in Chicago after the murder of Martin Luther King Jr. From May 31 through June 2, riots spread throughout the city but were concentrated on the West and South Sides, as local stores and pharmacies were looted and burned. Violent clashes between protesters and the police continued into the first week of June as communities demonstrated against racial devaluation and police violence.

About Lightfoot's response, Kelly described how she felt:

> When the riots and stuff started to break out downtown, [Lightfoot] pretty much shut off downtown. Everybody got, like, an emergency . . . notice on the phone [to] say that a curfew had been put in place. And she locked up downtown and raised the bridges, and I don't know, that just kind of . . . showed she caters to downtown . . . because that's where most of the more lucrative, more rich people of Chicago kinda live. . . . When

she did that and raised the bridges and then suspended the [transit] lines and stuff like that, it almost seemed like she was cutting the city off from [the] South and West Sides of the city. We know that that's . . . predominantly, like, Black and Brown areas.[25]

Lyla, a young Arab American woman from Albany Park, whom I interviewed twice, was actively involved in the protests surrounding Floyd's death, and she talked about how she felt constantly surveilled and under threat from the police in the summer of 2020. Describing that summer, Lyla said she felt as though "everything evil about the world was popping out. . . . I was so scared, like, all the time." She said, "no matter where you went . . . during this time, there was a police presence. . . . I would go to the grocery store . . . and there would be police people with guns, like five of them, lining the door." None of them wore masks, and she was concerned about her autoimmune disorder. She recounted:

> I was scared because I felt like I was being surveilled all the time. And that . . . all of the power imbalances that . . . I find, like, really horrifying were being leveraged to make the people that I love feel incredibly small, and I was worried that my friends were gonna get killed. And I couldn't do anything about it . . . well, it's just that there was so much militant violence on the streets.[26]

Ebony, a Black woman who has lived in Austin her whole life, bemoaned the uneven way in which wealthy neighborhoods were protected but communities of color, where looting was concentrated, were not:

> I want to say it felt like the purge was going on. . . . We had looters, then rioters . . . you saw firsthand how big businesses . . . and certain city officials only cared about the dollar of certain people. So we're going to protect the Gold Coast.[27] We're going to protect Magnificent Mile. We're going to protect all of these areas because that's where the money comes from. And then to be in the middle of it or to watch everything occur on the West Side of Chicago, there was no protection there, so every man was for himself, which is why so much damage was done . . . [because] all the manpower was downtown protecting that area. . . . It was sad to see how much the city only just cared about their money.[28]

Several residents spoke about how the looting decimated areas that already suffered from disinvestment, and the toll this took on communities on the South and West Sides of the city—mostly inhabited by Black and Brown Chicagoans. Jada, a Black woman from Little Village, explained:

You knockin' out business. Where we gonna go shoppin' at? . . . They take that business, shut everything down. What's gonna be next? It's like a graveyard. I don't think the governor is doin' they job. These politicians is not doin' nothin'. It's all about them, wrap the money up in they pocket, and go and doin' they business. They not lookin' down at people. They lookin' where they goin'. They don't care about people. They messin' up—it's polluted down here. It's polluted all over.[29]

Unlike other residents who felt that the police were unfairly targeting them with violence, Jada articulates a different political position. She suggests that there were not enough police in the areas of town that needed protecting. Whether there should be more or less police presence in Black communities is a political issue that is highly contested in Chicago, and this tension came to a head in the summer of 2020 in response to the widespread looting of local businesses.

In February 2021, it emerged that Mayor Lightfoot spent 60 percent of the city's discretionary funding from the Coronavirus Aid, Relief, and Economic Security (CARES) Act, totaling $281.5 million, on police personnel. She was critiqued by progressive alderpeople for prioritizing policing over rental and cash assistance.[30] Many Chicagoans suggested that Lightfoot's militant response to the protests that erupted after Floyd's murder became justification for expanding police presence in the city.[31] Annie told me:

I feel pretty disappointed in how the city has handled their approach to COVID. Yeah, I think that, like, too much money was spent on policing. . . . I really do think that the protests following George Floyd's murder was a justification of overspending on our already overinflated police budget.[32]

Sholanda said, "Why are you patrolling my neighborhood if you that damned scared of me that you would shoot me first instead of talk to me? If you that scared, get out of my neighborhood!"[33]

In fact, the broader calls for police reform that echoed throughout the nation in the aftermath of the 2020 uprisings were accompanied in Chicago by calls to punish police repression during the protests from May 29 through June 7. In an Office of Inspector General report on the protests, widespread misconduct was reported, from problems with mass arrest and use of force to obstacles in accountability and lack of coordination among police officers.[34] As a member of the American Civil Liberties Union declared, "protests that decried police violence were met with yet more police violence."[35] In response, in February 2021, Governor Pritzker signed into law a police reform bill, which included the elimination of cash bail and a requirement that by 2025, all police officers will wear body cameras. The law also limits police capacity to pursue fleeing subjects, prohibits the use of choke holds, and enhances police training.[36] Yet, only one month after the law came into effect, two young Latinx men were shot by the Chicago police as they fled. In March 2021, a white Chicago police officer killed Adam Toledo, a thirteen-year-old Mexican American boy who had his hands raised, in the middle of the night in Little Village. The officer was cleared of all charges.[37] Anthony Alvarez, a twenty-two-year-old Latinx man, was shot in the back by Chicago police while fleeing just weeks after Toledo was killed.[38] The Illinois police reforms recognize the problem of police brutality while simultaneously failing to contend with its causes—a classic example of governing through emergency. When met with public outcry, state actors enact emergency-type policies that seek to temporarily recognize and contain a much larger structural problem, until it once again fades into the background.

UNVEILING RACISM

Many scholars and journalists have analyzed the ways in which Trump tapped into and condoned feelings of racial resentment among white citizens, many of them working class and poor, who engaged in violent acts to defend white supremacy.[39] These sentiments and actions obviously have deep historical roots in white supremacist America, but Trump used his political platform as president to unleash this underlying "racial backlash" in exceptional ways. Given the high incidence of these thanatopolitical racial acts during the pandemic, many Black and Brown respondents felt as though they lived in a police state and were in imminent danger. And this emergency was compounded by the ongoing social neglect Black and Brown Chicagoans experienced during the pandemic. Some of the events that interviewees frequently mentioned included the police murder of Adam Toledo; the exoneration of gun-toting white teenager Kyle Rittenhouse after his murderous response to protests over the police killing of Jacob Blake, a Black man; the storming of the US Capitol by white supremacists on January 6, 2021, after Trump's unwillingness to accept his 2020 election defeat.

About the Toledo murder, Tomás, an organizer and longtime resident of Little Village, reflected on how he could have been this kid. He explained that violence is handled poorly by policies that fail to address the root causes of street violence.[40] Elena, a Mexican American mother from Little Village, spoke extensively about the Rittenhouse exoneration and the kind of message that sends to her children of color. She asked, "I mean, how do you explain this to your kids? What are you supposed to tell them? . . . You need some type of *degree*, you need some type of *money*, you need some type of *color* in order for you to be okay?!"[41] Elena explained the impossibility of communicating to her children how to navigate a society in which they are judged and devalued based on the color of their skin. She did not know how to be realistic with them but also engender hope and ambition.

Several respondents talked about the racial double standard in how white police officers and rioters are treated versus those against whom they wage racial violence. Sholanda explained that she knew Trump was racist, but "the police officer you called and that you thought was going to help you. He end up shooting you." She scoffed at the irony when she said:

> You remember when all the people went to the Capitol? All those people stormed the Capitol, they tore up stuff and they did all that stuff. Now the honest[-to-]goodness truth is, if those would have been Hispanic and Black [people], they'd've shot us down like dogs. They'd've shot us. The National Guards would've came in. They would have did us terribly. And every person of color knows that.[42]

In events surrounding the storming of the Capitol and the Rittenhouse acquittal, the perpetrators were people who identify as white supremacists defending the whiteness of the nation, and they were let live, while Black and Latinx men, women, and children are daily targets of immediate police violence. Ebony described the event on Capitol Hill as a moment in which "hope went on vacation" because it was so obvious "how America really feels about Black people. This is how you *really* feel about white supremacy. It's really scary."[43]

The acceleration of slow emergencies during COVID-19, which resulted in heightened numbers of deaths and illnesses among Latinx and Black Americans, coupled with the ongoing assault against Black and Brown life through police murders and white supremacist violence, converged into a series of racial uprisings that demanded policy response. As Sholanda explained in the quotation from the introduction to this chapter, white supremacy was unveiled to the general public in particularly salient ways in 2020, demanding state recognition and reckoning.

Racism becomes obvious to the privileged norm when disasters hit, but because racially privileged groups benefit from white supremacist ideologies and logics, they fail to reckon with the way racism structures everyday policies and practices.[44] This is part of the consequence of governing through emergency and using racially conscious discourse to claim political legitimacy. Governing emergencies as temporally bounded events turns racism into a political tool, wherein its effects are delinked from its causes. When racism is discussed only in moments of crisis, in an exceptional, urgent way, it is made to seem like a momentary glitch instead of an enduring structural reality. Governing through emergency allows those who are protected by racial biopower to forget the ongoing and everyday slow emergencies associated with racism.

Phyllis, an older Black woman from Austin, described the perpetual police violence that is continually excused in contemporary society as a new expression of a racist logic that extends back to slavery, and then she immediately switched to the topic of vaccines and explained that "people don't want the shots" because they think that the vaccine is "something that will harm us more than help us."[45] To her, distrusting government-mandated vaccines is logical given the perpetual racial violence Black populations have endured for centuries. I spoke with a considerable number of people who believed that the coronavirus or the vaccines were a form of racist population control. Consider these reflections from Walter and Monique—both from Austin:

> They got to get rid of people. They got to get rid of people, so I feel like if I get the vaccine then, now I'm telling you this out of my mouth, I guarantee you it's gonna be a lot of people that die from it.[46]

> I believe . . . the government came up with this epidemic . . . to kill Black Americans. . . . People have to die in order for other people to live.[47]

Monique could be quoting Michel Foucault's theory of racism directly. Black and Brown lives are devalued *so that* the white norm can be protected and returned to "normalcy." Returning to "normalcy" not only entails no longer being exposed to the coronavirus (and its threat of hospitalization or death) but also being able to safely inhabit a world of ignorance where structural racism fades into the background of everyday reality.

The level of distrust exposed in these quotes about population control stems from an inability to forget and a need to remain vigilant against the racial harms of white supremacy. Many Black and Brown Americans feel they are in immediate risk of dying—directly, from police violence, or indirectly, through lack of employment options, disinvestment in their neighborhoods, financial insecurity, lack of affordable housing options, and poor health care. Reginald from Austin provided the ongoing list of ways in which he feels racial devaluation as he navigates US society as a Black man:

> We already knew America was racist. Because when you go into these hospitals . . . they look at you like you the scum of the earth. Don't go in none of these stores like Gucci or something. They're gonna follow you around. . . . Everywhere you go. They don't follow the white people around, you know what I'm saying? . . . And it was already being revealed before the COVID came out with all these racial shootings and

stuff. Cops killing Black people and . . . getting away with it. You know, right before COVID came out, there was this young boy got shot like sixteen times in the back. . . . Yeah, COVID has really brought [racism] out because you know, these people, most of these people dying are Black. Or foreigners. You know? It's just, it just exposed something that was already there, it just pulled the cover off a little more.[48]

Reginald points out how the unequal patterns of death associated with COVID-19 revealed to white Americans the ongoing reality of racist infrastructure and policies, but for people of color, this racism is always present, always acknowledged, always experienced—in interactions with hospital staff, retail workers, and the police. For Black and Brown Americans, racism is both an ordinary structural reality and an urgent form of violence—both are experienced as emergencies. But they are only treated as emergencies that demand response from state agents when there is symbolic capital to claim from addressing them or the crisis tendencies they expose are so blatant they cannot be ignored. And when the problem of racial violence and neglect is governed through emergency by state actors, it is treated as a temporary and not a structural problem, thus leading to disjunctures between people's experiences and official policies. Before I attend to this sense of disjuncture, I provide an update to Foucault's theories of racial biopower.

RACIAL BIOPOWER: ORDINARY AND SPECTACULAR

> [Racism] establishes a *positive* relation between the right to kill and the assurance of life. It posits that "the more you kill [and] . . . let die, the more you will live."
>
> ANN L. STOLER, *Race and the Education of Desire*

For Foucault, racism justifies the death function in a regime focused on the administration of life, by introducing "a break in the domain of life . . . between what must live and what must die."[49] Given that he analyzes Nazism as the exceptional instance of state racism, Foucault focuses on the need to *make die* certain populations deemed internal national enemies because they are biologically threatening to the health and well-being of the norm.[50] He does consider more mundane cases of letting die, wherein security apparatuses are "installed around the random element inherent in a population of living things" to maintain equilibrium and ensure the maximum health of the normative population.[51] But Foucault never theorizes the relationship *between* making die and letting die, and Giorgio Agamben collapses the distinction altogether.[52] Agamben does so at least in part because he fails to consider the fact that exclusion and death making can be sanctioned *by* the law and are not simply authorized by states of exception when the law is suspended.[53] And yet, how do we make theoretical sense of both ordinary and spectacular state violence, and the link between letting die and making die?

I argue that making die and letting die are both racial tools used in the normal administration of state racism within liberal, white supremacist societies. They often target the same population, but they do not operate through the same mechanisms of exclusion. They are normative but also *crisis-ridden* because they expose the fundamental paradox at the heart of American liberalism: that it is founded on democratic principles of equal access but only protects white wealth and life, and both excludes and exploits racialized others for political and capital gain. At moments when these paradoxes are exposed or come to crisis, the state governs the emergency by newly operationalizing exclusionary inclusion, suspending normative legislative action until the norm can be restored, or providing minimal inclusion or recognition to some racialized others while sustaining structural racism. Letting die occurs when lifesaving infrastructure is fragmentary or absent, and people are abandoned to conditions of protracted, premature death—these are slow emergencies. Making die is a more immediate enactment of state violence, and in recent decades it has been spectacularized by social movement actors seeking to expose the paradoxes of liberalism and normative racial devaluation. The Black Lives Matter movement highlights the *political* processes that have led to *both* neglect and racial devaluation *and* the ongoing onslaught of police violence within communities of color—both are deemed emergency conditions by movement actors.[54] When these slow emergencies are politicized and named, they cannot be ignored as structural fact and must be governed.[55] But the governance is always an effort to get *through it*, until the emergency can, once again, fade into the background.

Foucault argues that the security apparatus is crucial to the functioning of biopower because it links together economic maximization, health optimization, and police securitization—all made possible by the capacity of the state to calculate and measure its population through statistics.[56] For Foucault, security operates through calculations of risks and probabilities, an acknowledgment of scarcity, and a laissez-faire governance of life wherein the protection of the norm occurs at the cost of letting those at the margins die from "natural" occurrences, such as hunger, illness, or disability. For Foucault, policing/surveillance, health/welfare, and statistical knowledge are intimately linked. In this chapter I illustrate that under a racial biocapitalist regime and enabled through robust data collection, racially marginalized subjects are overly targeted by police surveillance and violence *and* neglected and underserved by care infrastructures—these are two caesuras within biopolitics that enact making die and letting die exclusions. When these emergencies are exposed, turned into crisis conditions, or politicized by the racially marginalized, they must be governed—usually by targeting one exceptional problem with a series of technocratic solutions while leaving broader infrastructural disinvestment intact.

In the summer of 2020, *both* the structural inequity exposed by COVID-19 outcomes *and* police violence were declared states of emergency, and exceptional responses were mounted. And yet both were treated as temporally bounded emergencies that eventually were halted. For example, most pandemic social assistance was terminated in the fall of 2021, just as the Delta variant was mounting new assaults on communities of color. Policies continued to signal an "end" to the emergency of COVID-19 as the Omicron variant raged in Chicago, hospitalizing more Black Chicagoans than ever in the pandemic's history. Once vaccine protocols were in place, the government declared their exceptional response over, leaving Black Americans to contend with the worst effects of Omicron without any safety net. Because these emergencies were considered temporary, the impact on racially marginalized communities was disavowed, leading to feelings of incredible abandonment and neglect. Similarly, calls by movement activists to defund police departments and find alternative harm reduction strategies to address community violence lost political resonance as people moved past the George Floyd crisis and returned to their ordinary lives. Governing through emergency presumes scarcity and treats ongoing crises as temporary problems that can be met with triaged resources. And yet, the people who suffer from the double assault of letting die and making die experience them as protracted, convergent, and cumulative, marked by ordinary and extraordinary state racism. The accumulative impact of these entangled emergencies compounds the ontological insecurity that was a major feature of the pandemic. Most Americans experienced the pandemic as temporally unmooring, and uncertainty abounded, but people who were already living with multiple endemic emergencies experienced pandemic precarity in unique ways, often through heightened senses of ontological disjuncture between government response and their own grounded experiences.

ONTOLOGICAL INSECURITY

According to Pierre Bourdieu, temporal disjuncture is a form of domination.[57] The inability to predict one's daily conditions or future life can feel incredibly disempowering. Yet, everyone who lived through the COVID-19 pandemic experienced temporal disjuncture and an inability to predict and to therefore act knowledgeably in the world because uncertainty abounded. Though for Bourdieu, having to wait is a sign of domination, the pandemic imposed a general condition of waiting on us all. The virus ebbed and flowed, with surges and plateaus, and when it surged in one city or state, it abated in another. These fits and starts also disrupted timelines and forecasting. Kevin Grove and colleagues argue that one of the prevailing consequences of the pandemic was the blurring between normalcy and emergency and the inability to determine the pandemic's "end."[58] And yet, the extent to which the pandemic continued to be experienced as temporally disjunctive depended on one's social location.

Scholars of temporality rarely attend to the ways in which state actors can impose multiple, contradictory registers of temporality on the oppressed at the same time.[59] I argue that governing through emergency, which treats problems as temporary, urgent, and fixable with technocratic solutions, leaves broader structural problems intact. Therefore, it is quite common for marginalized people to experience temporal lags and disjunctures between their experiences of crisis and the recognition of emergency by state actors. Even in everyday conditions, slow emergencies become normal and may be interrupted with instances of urgent crisis. During moments of recognized crisis, spectacularized attention is often coupled with government neglect. After emergencies are declared over and new terms of exclusionary inclusion are rearticulated, the constancy of temporal disjunction is often compounded. The pandemic overdetermined already existing fault lines and exacerbated their effects. In addition, when the COVID-19 emergency was declared over and privileged people began to move on, the most vulnerable people continued to face devastating conditions of existence. For some, "emergency" is an ongoing lived condition that can also be intensified and made more acute by exceptional events. In this section, I provide examples of how the people I interviewed experienced temporal disruption and uncertainty by providing a narrative of key moments in the pandemic's timeline in Chicago.[60]

The first case of the coronavirus in Chicago occurred on January 24, 2020, but cases only began to steadily rise in early March. Camila, a Mexican American woman from Little Village, worked at the information desk of a hospital near Little Village, and she spoke about how it felt in that first week in March:

> No one was prepared for this. I'm, like, how is not anyone prepared, especially the hospital? Not having enough masks even for us! I was, like, how is this even possible, and we're going to be in the middle of a pandemic? . . . We don't even have Lysol and the sani-wipes! Do I have COVID, do I not have COVID? It just played a lot with my mind.[61]

Camila's two kids and husband relied on her paycheck because her husband had been fired, and she could not afford to stay home to stay safe. She

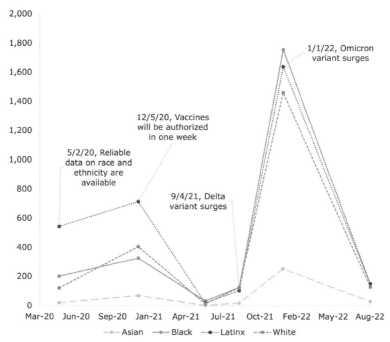

Figure 1.1 Average Daily COVID-19 Cases by Racial Group in Chicago, March 2020–August 2022

Source: City of Chicago, "COVID-19 Dashboard."

ended up contracting COVID-19, and it spread through her entire household and extended family. Figure 1.1 illustrates how disproportionate the rates of COVID-19 infection were in the Latinx community at the start of the pandemic.[62]

The shelter-at-home order was in effect in Chicago from March 18 through May 30. The people I interviewed remembered those early weeks when they thought the pandemic would be short-lived, and many spoke about how its gravity started to really sink in when they began to lose loved ones. Mary, a Black woman from Austin, recalled:

> I thought it was gonna be short term. You know, I thought we'll be in this for a minute. But as time went on, uh, it really got scary. And then I lost a friend of mine. She was diagnosed and she did die. I was like, Lord, this is really, really serious. It has hit home. You know, you read about it. But then it hit home. And then panicking, just really set in.[63]

A doctor I interviewed who works at a Federally Qualified Health Center (FQHC) that serves a predominantly lower-income Latinx community explained that part of the uncertainty also stemmed from the unpredictability of COVID-19 itself—that people did not know whether they would be asymptomatic or affected seriously if they contracted it:

> The specter of COVID and death hung over families. . . . It's such an odd phenomenon . . . [that COVID] might enter your home, and then . . . many of the people in your home just have mild symptoms, right? Then one person might die, or two people might die, right? I feel like it's a very bizarre threat to deal with because the spectrum of disease is so broad. I feel like there were probably very, very few families in our practice that did not have someone die from COVID. Some of those people [who] developed COVID did not wanna go to the hospital because of fear of what was going on in hospitals when people [were] dying alone. . . . For the patients who went to the hospital, right, no one could visit them in the hospital. For the patients who died, there was no funeral. . . . There's a collective grief that goes along with the collective anxiety.[64]

He told me that almost every family in their practice had someone die in that first year of the pandemic, and the collective, unmourned grief also contributed to general anxiety, fear, and depression.

The shelter-at-home order expired in late May, just as the protests against police violence began. Businesses began to reopen that summer, and business interests were buttressed not only by government grants but by lack of oversight from the city on enforcing worker protections. Vaccines were rolled out to health care workers in December 2020, and the Protect Chicago Plus program, which prioritized fifteen neighborhoods for vaccine prioritization, began in February 2021. By April 2021, anyone could get a vaccine, and by July, masks were no longer required in most public settings. Schools reopened in August 2021 (after having been shuttered the entire previous year). In the fall of 2021, most of the pandemic programming and assistance began to wane. The vaccine was the primary end goal of governing through emergency—once it was established and distributed, the state mostly began to fold up emergency operations. Social assistance began to dry up, just as the Delta variant was gaining hold. In September 2021, pandemic unemployment insurance ended; in October 2021, the eviction moratorium expired; in early December 2021, the recommended quarantine period was shortened from a recommended ten days to five; and in late December 2021, child tax credits expired. These policies were out of keeping with the experiences of especially Black Chicagoans, who felt the brunt of the Delta and Omicron variant surges. Kelly told me the withdrawal of support was a "slap in the face" that reminded her "how this country really sees its people . . . as disposable."[65]

Figure 1.2 indicates that deaths were consistently higher among Black Chicagoans throughout the pandemic but were especially severe in the early months and during the Delta and Omicron surges from December 2021 through February 2022. Figure 1.3 also indicates how high hospitalization rates were among Black Chicagoans, and how they also peaked during the Omicron surge. These figures also make it clear that even in the same city, different groups were experiencing the pandemic in drastically different ways.

Many interviewees told me that the variants made the virus more confusing and uncertain. In February 2022, when the Omicron variant was surging in Chicago, there were more infections and hospitalizations concentrated in Black communities than at any other point in the pandemic. Yet, the country had already moved on. In March 2022, President Joe Biden declared: "We're now in a new moment in this pandemic . . . COVID-19 no longer controls

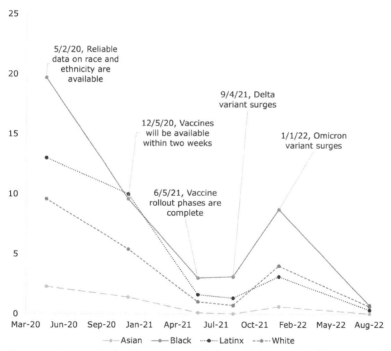

Figure 1.2 Average Daily COVID-19 Deaths by Racial Group in Chicago, March 2020–August 2022

Source: City of Chicago, "COVID-19 Dashboard."

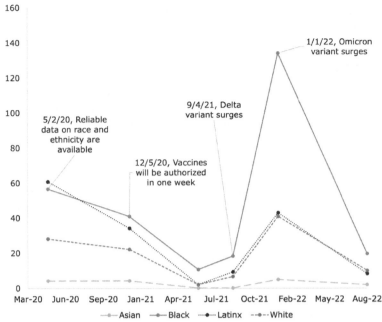

Figure 1.3 Average Daily COVID-19 Hospitalizations by Racial Group in Chicago, March 2020–August 2022

Source: City of Chicago, "COVID-19 Dashboard."

our lives . . . Americans are back to living their lives."[66] Yet, as Shantal exclaimed in an interview at this time, "as long as people are dying, it's still an emergency."[67]

By spring 2022, most federal relief had ended. There was a disconnect between people's experiences with the pandemic and the public discourse on its effects, especially in racially marginalized communities that were disproportionately affected by the Omicron variant. Willie, a Black man from Austin, explained:

> This is terrifying. It's like going from strain to strain to strain. . . . So many people are dying before they finally come up with an antidote. I don't want to be one of [the dead]. . . . Every time I look around, they coming up with a different strain, man, it's getting scarier and scarier by the day.[68]

Ana, a Mexican American woman from Little Village, reflected on the inability to determine when the virus would be "over" and for whom. She explained, "When COVID first hit, my friend read some prediction online that 2022 . . . is when things will start to get better . . . but then 2022 . . . came around . . . and the sickness and stuff isn't getting better."[69]

Many respondents discussed how confusing the expert advice had been throughout the pandemic—that the experts had no idea what to suggest and the official federal guidelines and best practices kept shifting—out of line with the disproportionate effect of the virus on Black and Brown communities. Dolores, a Black woman from Austin, put this quite succinctly in an interview in February 2022:

> We can't wait on our so-called government with this COVID thing. If we sit around and just literally wait on them to come up with a cure, we all gon' be fucking dead. Because they still don't know. They grasping at straws. Right? . . . They still don't know and its going on, what, over two years? And it's 'posed to have went down. But the numbers are back up again. We still wearing masks in 2022. . . . First they was saying you had to quarantine for ten days, now they saying you gotta quarantine for five days, and that was because [of] the economy. . . . That's why I'm, like, with this COVID thing, even the scientists really don't know. . . . At first they was saying get the shot . . . you won't catch it. Right, you will be protected. But now you could have the shot and still catch it. You just won't get as sick. . . . I don't know. . . . How do [you] protect yourself? Right? When you steady getting wrong data. If y'all don't know, y'all don't *know*![70]

Dolores was exasperated that the advice kept shifting. First, vaccines were thought to protect against infection, and then it was discovered in the summer of 2021 that vaccines only protect against hospitalization and death. Then, in December 2021, the required quarantine time after infection was reduced from ten days to five days.[71] Scientists were proven wrong again and again, so whom should the public trust? As Dolores asks, "how do [you] protect yourself" when the experts change best practices, and people are still dying at alarming rates? Dolores exclaimed, "Now what, it's, like, eight hundred thousand people done died from COVID? That's a lot! And y'all still ain't got it right. . . . This is what researchers and doctors and scientists [are] supposed to do . . . especially in this day and age with the technology that we have."[72]

Part of the problem is that because the pandemic was governed as a temporary emergency whose end was in site, policies kept reducing protections, even as the worst effects were still transpiring in communities of color. In September 2022, President Biden declared the pandemic "over" in a *60 Minutes* interview: "The pandemic is over. We still have a problem with COVID. We're still doing a lot of work on it. But the pandemic is over."[73]

This interview occurred when four hundred people per day were still dying from COVID-19, and the state of emergency was not terminated for another eight months. Governing *through* emergency meant that the point was to terminate the exceptional response, but those suffering from the convergence of slow and immediate emergencies experienced expert advice and shifting policies as temporally disjunctive and ontologically unmooring.

Annie pointed out that treating the pandemic as *temporary* and as something we can all *move beyond* is eugenic because such an approach ignores the compounded vulnerabilities the pandemic instigated. She questioned the logic of herd immunity because the premise is that the most vulnerable can be left out of the protective loop:

> I mean, we didn't know enough to imagine that Omicron would happen. We don't fully know what it's doing to people's bodies. And just the attitude that, like, the healthiest among us will walk away unaffected and those who aren't, well, hope they have insurance to deal with the problems but everybody that doesn't is going to suffer, and those who are undocumented, uninsured, don't speak English, distrust of hospitals, whatever, they can, like, suffer and die.[74]

Annie argues that such a policy allows the "weak" to die so that the strong can move on to experience the pandemic's "end." This is an important consequence of governing *through* emergencies.

The broad uncertainty and the blurring of lines between emergency and normalcy affected all who lived through the pandemic, but it was experienced as compounded devaluation by communities who were disproportionately affected—in part because it was lived as part of a longer tradition of disinvestment, precarity, and violence. While the racial inequalities exposed by the pandemic were discussed and highlighted early in the pandemic, the ongoing insecurity exacerbated by the pandemic was never addressed, and the emergency focus on racial equity also waned, especially as safety nets were retracted, even as variants surged.

*   *   *

The acceleration of slow death from COVID-19 and the spectacularization of police murder were turned into emergencies that the state could not ignore by everyday Americans who took to the streets to protest their racial devaluation in the summer of 2020. As such, federal, state, and local governmental actors were forced to contend with structural racism and the devaluation of Black and Brown life. State racism had to be addressed and recognized. State actors declared emergencies and governed *through* them with temporally bounded liberal governance strategies aimed at merely halting the immediate crisis ignited by George Floyd's death and the uneven racial impact of COVID-19. But once these immediately urgent crises were *through*, state actors could return to passively accepting them, allowing them to fade into the structural background. The timing of when the emergencies ebbed depended on one's social location. Those experiencing the compounding effects of converging endemic emergencies experienced the temporality of COVID-19 differently from those governing *through* them—which resulted in temporal disjunctures and ontological uncertainty.

Governing through emergency, wherein state actors institute temporary technocratic policies, fails to contend with the effects of converging endemic emergencies normalized under white supremacy. Samira, a Black woman from Little Village, argued that Mayor Lightfoot's policies were never meant to address these protracted emergencies:

> The crux of all of the problems that exist, like inequality and housing insecurity and all the things that sort of make it hard for people to live . . . [are] problems that, like, can't be fixed . . . [by] the policies. . . . Lori Lightfoot . . . said she did. . . . The problem is actually white supremacy. And if that's not understood, maybe those other problems that people are experiencing, like poverty and stuff, will always be there.[75]

As Samira indicates, the crux of these converging emergencies is the ongoing perpetuation of white supremacist policies that leave the most vulnerable people behind again and again. Until that deeper structural inequality and the ideologies that excuse and obfuscate it are unveiled and confronted in a *permanent* way, the entangled emergencies of letting die and making die will endure.

2: FRAGMENTED HEALTH INFRASTRUCTURE

During the COVID-19 pandemic, political actors in the United States often cited structural inequalities as causes for the disproportionate toll on racially marginalized populations, but they failed to enact policies that would begin to redress historically entrenched disparities. This behavior mimics a broader trend in which journalists, social scientists, government actors, and health scholars repeatedly bemoan the intractability of racial health disparities without explaining the *causal* processes by which structural racism and a market-based approach to the provision of health care sustain and retrench health apartheid. Some of these causal pathways include bodily weathering from experiences of interpersonal and institutional racism, racist structural neglect, and violence; interpersonal discrimination within health care settings; residential segregation that facilitates uneven exposure to environmental toxins and poor housing as well as substandard health care; and barriers to high-quality health care access.[1] Entrenched structural racism and a market-based approach to health provision converge to expose lower-income, racially marginalized populations to unhealthy lives and premature deaths.[2] While critical scholars readily critique the ways in which scientists and health professionals continue to biologize racial difference to explain racial health disparities, it is equally problematic to gloss over the structural determinants and infrastructural lacks that cause slow emergencies and their catastrophic effects during epidemics.[3] When "health disparities" are treated as an unchanging category without structural context or causal explanation, racial difference is accepted not as a biological reality but a fixed historical fact.[4] Failing to *explain* the causes of racial health disparities is another means by which racial difference is naturalized.

This chapter explains the role that fragmented health infrastructure in the US (associated with health care, mental health care, and public health) played in exposing lower-income Black and Brown Americans to COVID-19's worst outcomes. This chapter responds to two primary questions. First, in the midst of a pandemic, why were health care and mental health care not prioritized for reorganization and an infusion of funding? In fact, the structure of our fragmented, inequitable, and market-based approach to health care was accepted as good enough for the poor. Paul Starr argues that US health care suffers from policy entrenchment, making its contours and form exceptionally difficult to challenge, despite the profoundly unequal outcomes it instantiates.[5] This policy entrenchment was revealed during the establishment of the Affordable Care Act (ACA) of 2010 and again during the pandemic. The US's market-based health care system disadvantaged lower-income and racially marginalized Americans, and certain city policies (or lack thereof) exacerbated Chicagoans' unequal access to health care and medications during the pandemic. In addition, major deficits in healthful infrastructures, such as food security, and gross inadequacies in mental health care provision not only disadvantaged vulnerable groups in Chicago but will likely mean a longer-term recovery from the lingering impact of the pandemic.

Second, why did the tremendous federal funding funneled into public health departments not better meet the needs of those most vulnerable? Answering this question requires briefly analyzing the history of public health in the US and how that legacy stymied an approach to COVID-19 that took the structural determinants of poor health into account. I explain how during the pandemic, public health turned its attention to epidemiological responses and the building of big data infrastructures *instead of* addressing core inequalities in housing, occupations, and health care access. While epidemiological data can render visible and actionable certain disparities, political actors can also use population health metrics to obfuscate preexisting infrastructural vulnerability, which can ontologize racial difference. Governing through emergency entails leaving patchwork infrastructures in place *and* triaging technocratic care to only those deemed most vulnerable. Before explaining how this worked during COVID-19, I provide background on theories of infrastructure.

INFRASTRUCTURE

Emergency governance renders certain infrastructure visible and actionable while simultaneously naturalizing longer-term inequalities. *Infrastructure* refers to "systems of substrates" that undergird the everyday functioning of modern states and economies.[6] Infrastructure underlies critical systems and facilitates the distribution of resources, networks people to one another and the state, and integrates spatially dispersed operations. But it also wields tremendous power in often taken-for-granted ways. Most often, the term is used to refer to *material* networks, such as transportation, water, sewage, electricity, and telecommunication systems.[7] *Critical* or *vital infrastructure* denotes those systems that are most crucial for state security and emergency management, and *social infrastructure* signifies spaces that facilitate civic engagement.[8]

Within this literature, there is a failure to theorize *care infrastructure* or consider how disinvestments in health and welfare systems leave the most vulnerable Americans at risk when disasters strike.[9] In this chapter, I focus specifically on the health infrastructure associated with health care, mental health care, and public health. Infrastructure is often theorized as imperceptible and taken for granted, until it breaks, but in fact, political movements and state actors can render certain infrastructures invisible *by making other infrastructure the target of investment*.[10] A spotlight on certain features of how inequality manifests can drive political action in a way that takes existing structural inequality for granted. State actors manipulate the visibility versus intractability of inequality by separating effect from cause and by treating social problems with urgent, technocratic policies. A temporally bounded governing strategy renders deeply entrenched structural inequality natural and politically unactionable.

Given the lack of attention in existing literature to care infrastructure, I analyze why and with what effect structures and pathways of care are continually obscured, fragmented, and corporatized by neoliberal governance and structural racism. The City of Chicago adopted a series of public health measures to respond to COVID-19 vulnerability, such as testing, contact tracing, and vaccine distribution. City officials employed metrics such as positivity and hospitalization rates to direct those resources to certain vulnerable communities. In this way, they sought to render COVID-19 visible via quantification and the activation of epistemic infrastructure. While these efforts are critical during a pandemic, the sole focus on technocratic resources triaged according to COVID-19 metrics also rendered *invisible* other forms of vulnerability associated with work protections, financial precarity, housing insecurity, and even broader health vulnerability. It also concealed the labor that lower-income care workers provided in the interstices of fragmented health infrastructure. The mobilization of one type of infrastructure in an *uneven* way renders other infrastructural needs unseen and unmet.

In fact, as I explain subsequently, while city officials did provide additional resources to local clinics, safety net hospitals, and mobile testing sites, and the federal government expanded Medicaid coverage, these efforts simply bolstered existing care infrastructure and failed to reimagine it. One might legitimately wonder why we should expect state actors in the US to redesign health care provision in the midst of a pandemic. But in fact, the federal government *did* attempt, for a brief moment during the pandemic, to overhaul critical infrastructure by incorporating attention to work conditions, childcare, caregiving, and housing. In March and April 2021, several newspapers ran editorials debating the meaning of the term *infrastructure*, in response to President Joe Biden's American Jobs Plan, which proposed funding to rebuild and strengthen transportation systems (roads and bridges) but also to provide affordable housing, support worker training and research development, and expand access to caregiving for the elderly and those with disabilities.[11] This bill went through several revisions as it met with tremendous opposition in Congress. The eventual 2022 Inflation Reduction Act maintained some material infrastructure investments (roads and railways) and employment and health care protections, but without the enhanced social safety net provisions first discussed as part of the Americans Jobs Plan. Further, even the infrastructure plans that were initiated had to be curtailed because of high rates of inflation in 2022.[12] Therefore, the promise of investment in care infrastructure was short-lived. At the local level, City of Chicago officials admitted that disparities in COVID-19 outcomes stemmed from historic legacies of structural inequality, so adopting a "racial equity" approach should include not just a recognition of the causes of inequality but also efforts to redress them. Therefore, at both the federal and local levels, politicians recognized the fact that fragmented care infrastructure led to pandemic inequalities, but they nonetheless chose mitigation policies that naturalized existing structural inequality.

Within the current system of underresourced and fragmented health infrastructure, lower-income Americans must expend tremendous labor to pull together health and mental health resources. Such toil is disregarded by politicians. People who are poor work hard to stay healthy, relying on illicit health economies, local herbal shops (botanicas), social networks, and local clinics.[13] The work they do to pull together disjointed systems is invisibilized by the state when state actors accept the status quo and discuss historical structural inequalities as simply ontological facts. Although the underresourced and fractured nature of US health care, mental health care, and public health was revealed during the pandemic, it was accepted as a natural part of our social system—rendered invisible and intransigent. When uneven infrastructure is naturalized, racial difference is spatially ontologized. City officials prioritized quick technocratic fixes (e.g., mobile testing, vaccine drives) and invested in data infrastructure in order to claim "success" in redressing immediate harm while slow emergencies accumulated in the background.

MARKET-BASED CARE AND INFRASTRUCTURAL DISINVESTMENT

Since the early 1900s, strong political maneuvering by hospitals, insurance companies, and physicians inaugurated and sustained America's market-based (as opposed to nationalized) approach to health care provision despite the fact that the US spends far more on health care than other wealthy nations do, yet suffers higher disease burdens.[14] Because the US has adopted a profit-driven, market-based health care system—wherein the private insurance industry serves as gatekeeper to health care access, the pharmaceutical industry regulates drug pricing, and citizens are not guaranteed coverage for medical services—vulnerable communities have long struggled to access even basic health care. Although a market-based approach to health care may seem racially colorblind, it works in tandem with structural racism to enact and sustain a system of health apartheid wherein the wealthy enjoy technologically advanced, premium preventive and specialty health care, and the poor experience underresourced, fragmented, and substandard care in often segregated settings.[15] Although the passage of the Affordable Care Act in 2010 was heralded for closing gaps in coverage for the poor, significant health inequities remain for lower-income and racially marginalized Americans.[16] The consequences of this reality were laid bare in dramatic ways by the disproportionate toll the coronavirus took on Black and Brown communities. In what follows, I draw on interviews with doctors who provide health care to lower-income Chicagoans and Chicago residents who utilize Medicaid for their health care needs to illustrate the gaps, frustrations, and poor-quality care that lower-income Americans experience and how this vulnerability was exacerbated during the pandemic.

There are several sources of health care made available to the most vulnerable residents of Chicago. Illinois was one of the states to expand Medicaid coverage under the ACA in 2013, to adults whose earnings were at 138 percent of the federal poverty level or less. Black and Latinx Chicagoans are publicly insured at the highest rates. According to the American Community Survey (ACS), from 2015 to 2019, 51.25 percent of Black and 43.13 percent of Latinx Chicagoans were publicly insured.[17] According to the health care providers I interviewed, ACA expansion significantly cut back on the number of uninsured patients in Chicago. Nevertheless, the ACS reported that 8.30 percent of Black and 17.00 percent of Latinx Chicagoans were still uninsured between 2015 and 2019.[18] As I will illustrate with my interviews in this chapter, Medicaid coverage is patchy and problematic, sustaining historic inequalities in health care access.[19]

When the Health and Human Services Department declared COVID-19 a public health emergency in March 2020, federal law prevented states from requiring citizens to requalify for Medicaid coverage, so vulnerable Americans were "continuously enrolled."[20] As a result, rates of uninsured Americans decreased during the pandemic, but millions of people lost this coverage when the official public health emergency expired on May 11, 2023.[21] Further, people also lost access to free COVID-19 testing, treatment, and vaccines.[22] Undocumented immigrants are not eligible for benefits under the ACA, although undocumented residents of Illinois who are 65 or older can access Medicaid-like benefits.[23] Undocumented Illinoisians in the 42–64 age range could access state-funded health insurance during the pandemic, but this program was terminated in the spring of 2023.[24]

In addition to using Medicaid to access health care at private clinics and hospitals, vulnerable residents in Chicago can access health care through the twenty-two Federally Qualified Health Centers (FQHCs) in Chicago. FQHCs are subsidized by the federal Health Resources and Services Administration, and they accept all patients, regardless of their ability to pay. FQHCs accept Medicaid and Medicare (as well as all private insurances), and there is an income-based sliding fee for those without insurance. FQHC providers also help patients access reduced-copay medications through the 340b federal program and connect patients to specialty and hospital care when needed. The City of Chicago also used CARES Act and American Rescue Plan Act funds to provide personal protective equipment, licenses for telehealth technology, coronavirus tests, and vaccines to safety net hospitals and FQHCs throughout the city. (*Safety net hospitals* are care facilities that serve the uninsured, the underinsured, and people on Medicaid and Medicare.[25])

And yet, receiving care from FQHCs and through public insurance programs such as Medicaid and Medicare can feel disjointed, frustrating, and expensive. First, some people are not even aware that FQHCs exist or offer care on a sliding scale. Often the health infrastructure that is available to the poor is invisible to those who qualify for services. Medicaid access is often poorly understood or declined because of distrust of government programs.[26] Medicaid is managed by private corporations, and each of these managed care programs has different rules and networks.[27] Hospitals, specialty care, or private physician networks may only accept one type of Medicaid managed care and not another.[28] Medicaid does not reimburse clinicians at high rates, so doctors and health systems are not incentivized to accept Medicaid patients. For example, one FQHC administrator told me:

> I think that the Medicaid system in Illinois is racist. I know that's a big word. It's really a perfect example of systemic racism. Because what happens is 54 percent of the people on Medicaid in Illinois are people of color. At the same time, Medicaid pays pennies on the dollar compared to private insurance. People of color in our system, in Illinois, we as a society, pay less for their health care . . . which means that they're gonna get less health care.[29]

As this FQHC administrator argues, systemic racism is buttressed by the market fundamentalism of US health care and the health apartheid it sustains.

Although conservative politicians often suggest that market-based health care provides consumers with more health choices, most patients using these services find the opposite. Ebony, a long-term resident of Austin, lost her job and health insurance during the pandemic and then was diagnosed with cancer. She had Medicaid but talked about how hospital staff treated her poorly and limited her care options because of her insurance. Ebony told me, "The challenging part with Medicaid was selecting a primary care physician. . . . I didn't like the selection you were given based on your zip code. . . . I want to go where *I* want to go. . . . And some places are not the best when it comes to people of color . . . it's almost like they look down at you!"[30] Existing scholarship documents how common it is for people on public insurance to experience stigma from health providers.[31]

In addition, rules of coverage under Medicaid managed care are constantly changing—a procedure or medication that is covered one year may not be covered the next. Medications can be extremely expensive, even with subsidization, especially for those on multiple drugs. An FQHC provider explained: "A ten-dollar, fifteen-dollar, twenty-dollar copay, a lot of people think it's nothing. But if you're taking multiple medications, and for some of our patients twenty dollars a month is a lot of money. It's making them choose between rent, food" and medicine.[32] Other providers told me that costs often delimit which medications they can prescribe because only certain types of drugs will be covered under certain plans—and the medications covered may not be the most effective treatment option.[33]

Referral for specialty care can be exceedingly expensive and difficult to find. The only option for people without insurance is to attend specialty services at Stroger Hospital through the County Health system, but the waiting lists are exceedingly long.[34] People can also wait for day-of outpatient services, and many line up before the sun has risen and may not see anyone before it sets. One FQHC provider told us that she advises her patients to bring their breakfast, lunch, and dinner as well as a backup phone charger when they seek specialty care at Stroger.[35] For those on Medicaid, it is possible to find other options through "charity programs" at safety net hospitals, but there are often hidden fees patients must cover. For example, Barbara, a Black woman from Austin, told me that she is on Medicare and whereas her examination for a sprained ankle was covered, the leg brace cost her $254. "I have to pay some of my income towards paying some of these high medical bills. . . . Then when you don't pay 'em, some of 'em mess up your credit. . . . We need to have a change with the medical care."[36] An FQHC provider explained that sometimes hospitals hire a specialty physician (especially in their emergency rooms, or ERs) who is under contract with a different insurance system than the one that covers the hospital. Therefore, a patient may get a bill after an ER visit because their anesthesiologist, for example, was out of network, even though the anesthesiologist was working in the hospital's ER. The FQHC provider explained, "It is just the fragmented nature of health care, but when we have patients that are getting a big bill and we are working hard to get them the care that they need to live healthier lives, everything is kind of a jigsaw puzzle of trying to make it all work."[37]

Further, when FQHC providers refer their patients to hospitals, they usually choose hospitals with existing arrangements with those FQHCs. If a patient wants to seek care at a different hospital, they cannot be assured that system will accept their Medicaid managed care plan, because each hospital system negotiates these contracts separately.[38] In addition, when people are referred for specialty appointments, they often are required to make their own appointments, may lack knowledge and language skills, or suffer transportation barriers. According to one FQHC provider, "there are barriers upon barriers upon barriers" in seeking services in the fragmented, market-based health system in the US.[39]

Further, an FQHC administrator told me that safety net hospitals that rely on Medicaid and Medicare payments from the state have no financial cushion. They are frequently in danger of closing or cutting services *because* most of their patients are on Medicaid and *because* Medicaid payments are insufficient to cover hospital expenses.[40] Safety net hospitals generally rely on FQHCs to provide primary care. During the COVID-19 pandemic, FQHCs were doing the bulk of the provision of care because safety net hospitals were so understaffed and underresourced.

There is an unequal distribution of preexisting health conditions in populations that are underemployed, living in substandard housing in segregated cities, and provided inferior health care. Many of the residents I interviewed had underlying chronic illnesses, which they knew put them at greater risk for hospitalization if they were to contract the coronavirus. Brenda, a Black woman from Austin, told me, "I already have asthma . . . and I've had walking pneumonia five times and my lungs are damaged from that. . . . I'm being more cautious of things I do and where I go. A lotta times, I make sure I have on two masks, have my hand sanitizer. I try not to go too many places."[41] And Terrance, a Black man from Austin, explained in a late 2020 interview that not only his preexisting conditions but also his lack of access to health care made him especially frightened during the pandemic:

> I have never seen so many people dying from the disease in my life. I'm a diabetic now, you know, and my anxiety is high. . . . I got bronchitis, I'm a perfect candidate. But I wear my mask, and I do what I need to do to not get affected from this stuff. . . . I'm a Black poor man. And it's hard for us as African Americans because when you get sick or something, you don't have the proper medical resources. . . . It's very frightening.

Believe me, I wash my hands on a regular basis. I look so fanatic when it comes to washing hands.[42]

People who already face health access challenges were under tremendous anxiety as the pandemic progressed, and they watched people in their communities get sick and die.

Vulnerable communities also often face the dangers of living in "trauma deserts." Trauma deserts occur when nearby hospitals do not run trauma units, forcing ambulances to travel long distances to find a hospital that can treat traumatic injuries such as gunshot wounds. Marlin, a Black man from Austin, explained, "So many people die trying to make the run. . . . Right now, we've got the busiest trauma units . . . more busy than Pizza Hut."[43] A 2019 study found that 79 percent of Black residents of Chicago live in trauma deserts.[44]

In addition, during COVID-19, there were disruptions to health care coverage as people lost work and signed up for Medicaid. Gabriela, a Mexican American woman from Little Village, and William, a Black man from Austin, conveyed their frustrations:

> Another big thing . . . [was] having to change health care options. That can be such a stressful thing. . . . I have chronic leukemia, and so I have to be constantly going to the doctor. I can't really go without health insurance. I had to immediately try to navigate the Medicaid process and also the unemployment benefits process. . . . For . . . both Medicaid and unemployment, I feel like it took a couple months to get a response.[45]

> You know with the health care, man, they've been . . . cutting me off, man, but then I get back on with my health care. I'm having problems getting my blood pressure medicine on time and all that other stuff. . . . Well you know, when you have to reapply for your benefits, and then when it comes up with an error saying that you didn't pay on time and then it cuts you off, it's just a whole bunch of mess.[46]

Other residents talked about how they made slightly too much money to be able to apply for Medicaid, but they could not afford to pay for private insurance and were not offered insurance from their employers. These people were stuck in what one provider described as "the middle area," and they spent months trying hard not to get COVID-19 because they were uninsured. An FQHC provider explained that many people lost work during COVID-19, but "between unemployment and additional subsidies . . . it was just enough that people weren't eligible for Medicaid."[47]

In addition to lack of insurance, in Chicago and throughout the US, working-class and poorer residents often encountered technological barriers to accessing health care. During most of 2020 and 2021, all clinics were offering telehealth services, which have advantages for people who experience transportation and employment obstacles. However, many FQHC providers discussed how difficult managing new technology was for the elderly, and often people did not have enough data or a strong enough internet connection to support their telehealth needs. Others had a difficult time managing online systems for enrolling in Medicaid and other public aid.

In general, many low-income Chicagoans struggled to find affordable care during the pandemic, and many worried about accruing new costs and debts associated with testing, vaccines, and hospitalizations. Bernice, a Black woman from Austin, explained:

> To me … there's just not enough health care or not enough facilities, free facilities, in our neighborhood for people because a lot of people can't afford the health care. . . . People don't go and get tested 'cause they don't want that bill. 'Cause I had a friend, she was sick. She was like, "Girl, I'm not going to the hospital 'cause all they're gonna do is send me a bill." I said, "But you're sick." She was like, "Girl, look. I'll get over it." Because a lot of people don't have health care.[48]

Marlin told me that safety net hospitals were too understaffed or underresourced to properly serve vulnerable communities at the height of pandemic surges:

> Well, number one, we … don't have the greatest health care system in the Austin area. . . . And I think when it came to health care and COVID … it seemed like … the people in higher places … were just uncompassionate. Because you can understand people were catching COVID. And the hospital didn't know what to tell them. And they were just turning people around, right? You couldn't even get in the hospital.[49]

There were other barriers to healthiness that Chicago residents experienced acutely and that were exacerbated by the actions or inaction of local state actors. For example, residents in Austin mentioned again and again that essential businesses, including grocery stores and pharmacies, were looted and abandoned during the protests in the summer of 2020, after the murder of George Floyd, and the owners were not able to reopen. In some ways, the looting following Floyd's murder was an effort made by residents of poorer neighborhoods to highlight disparities in infrastructural provisioning between Black, Brown, and white areas of the city, but when the city failed to provide aid to struggling businesses, these communities were left further decimated. The city blamed residents for their behavior instead of investing in rebuilding. Many respondents mentioned how far they had to go to get groceries and essentials such as Lysol and cleaning supplies. Others mentioned that they could not get their medications because pharmacies were closed, and they had no means of transportation. The shuttering of local businesses intensified already existing food and health care insecurity in certain communities. Ebony explained:

> One of the only two grocery stores that we had . . . packed up probably in the middle of the night almost and closed without letting anyone know in that community. And it . . . really hurt a lot of people who walked across the street from this high-rise . . . to get their grocery items. . . . COVID . . . highlighted . . . what was always there and . . . we didn't realize it was as bad as it was. It just it pulled the veil off.[50]

Ebony points out that infrastructural decay and fragmentation are not invisible to the people living in these communities, even if this condition was ignored and naturalized by city officials.

Another issue raised by residents throughout my interviews concerned a lack of trust in their local hospitals. Jada, a Black woman from Little Village, exemplified this view: "Then, too, if you do get sick, you scared to go to the hospital 'cause they might tell you, 'Oh, you done caught COVID' . . . People's scared that, 'they gonna put me on that machine. I'm a die.' Peoples got mixed ideas, and they scared. It's scary out here."[51] Miguel, an undocumented Mexican immigrant living in Albany Park, said that early in the pandemic, it was exceedingly common on Spanish-language social media to read stories advising people to stay away from hospitals to avoid death.[52] This fear caused many residents to wait too long to go to the hospital, and by the time they were admitted, it was too late to help them, thereby supporting the misconception that the hospitals were at fault.[53] One FQHC provider explained that the fear really circulated around dying alone: "Initially . . . everybody avoided the hospital at any cost. . . . There's this whole understanding that if you developed COVID and get hospitalized, you will be alone. I do think that that creates some avoidance for better or for worse for people who have symptoms and think they may require hospitalization."[54] Some residents told me that they feared hospitalization because they knew the nurses were overworked and the technology was outdated. Austin resident Walter told me, "There's been people that died in the hospital maybe 'cause their machines are old and . . . the nurses don't have all the equipment."[55]

This fear of hospitalization is not unique to Chicago, but Chicagoans have a long history of skepticism regarding public safety net hospitals. These hospitals are structurally underfunded by the city and state, are often stretched thin, and have reputations for treating patients poorly.[56] Disparities in hospital capacity and resources were exacerbated during the pandemic. During surges, Chicago's safety net hospitals struggled to respond to the needs of vulnerable communities. A local physician told me that most wealthy, private hospitals in Chicago did not accept transfers of uninsured or Medicaid-reliant patients from safety net hospitals that were filled to capacity during the height of the pandemic.[57] In Illinois, there is no state system to facilitate patient transfers or require hospitals to take on patients when emergency rooms or intensive care unit beds are full, so doctors rely on their social networks to find available bed space, which disadvantages patients on public benefits.[58] Because COVID-19 patients often require extensive care for extended stays, hospitals are not incentivized to take on patients who are on Medicaid or without insurance. Several FQHC providers I interviewed suggested that the city should have stepped in to regulate hospital transfers during coronavirus surges.

In addition, several safety net hospitals closed or were in danger of closing under the strains of COVID-19. St. Anthony's Hospital, which serves the primarily Latinx communities of Little Village, was on the brink of closing because the state delayed Medicaid payouts to the hospital.[59] Four community hospitals on the South Side of Chicago, which had planned a merger to save costs, were in danger of closing as a result of pandemic-caused delays in state funding allocations.[60] And one of those four, Mercy Hospital, did end up closing in February 2021.[61] About these closures, Marlin said in indignation, "Just our health care system, at a time like this, how could you possibly think about closing down a hospital? That just goes to show you where they at with us. . . . At a time like this, you pick this time to shut a hospital down. . . . We in a crisis. Hundreds of thousands of people are dyin', and one of the only places we have that could possibly help us, you wanna shut that down?!"[62]

Within the marketized US health care system, healthiness must be bought, and lower-income Americans have to cobble together assistance from extremely fragmented systems of support. The City of Chicago did provide some additional funding to safety net hospitals and FQHCs during the pandemic but avoided even basic policy measures that could have redistributed resources from wealthy hospitals to lower-income residents. For example, one FQHC administrator told me that the mayor refused to require wealthy university hospitals in Chicago to provide free testing to city residents.[63] While the plight of health care workers during the pandemic was momentarily spotlighted in the media, the apartheid health system was just taken for granted, fading into the background of "the way things are." Invisibilized and ignored.

MENTAL HEALTH CARE

Mental health care is even more difficult to access in Chicago. In 2012, then Mayor Rahm Emanuel closed six of twelve community mental health clinics in Chicago. The reasoning offered was that consolidation was necessary because of lost federal funding and a reduction in available psychiatrists. Additionally, the mayor's office argued that the expansion of the Affordable Care Act meant more people could use Medicaid to access mental health care at FQHCs in the city.[64] The closure of these clinics sparked tremendous protests from the Mental Health Movement and the Collaborative for Community Wellness, which claimed that Chicago suffers from a crisis in mental health care access, especially in vulnerable communities on the South and West Sides of the city. According to a citywide survey conducted by the Collaborative for Community Wellness in 2020, demand for affordable mental health services is high, but residents face barriers associated with cost, lack of insurance, too few providers in their neighborhood, and lack of knowledge about access.[65] Further, without local mental health provision, the police are more likely to respond to mental illness events, exacerbating the criminalization of mental illness.[66]

When Emanuel's term ended in 2019, the City Council unanimously passed a resolution to establish a task force to assess mental health coverage.[67] While campaigning for mayor, Lori Lightfoot promised to reopen the six community health clinics, but once in office, she decided on another tactic to address mental health needs, which led to increased tension with the City Council, who wanted the clinics reopened.[68] The City Council even temporarily stalled the appointment of Dr. Allison Arwady as health commissioner, demanding that the mayor reopen the shuttered clinics.[69] Instead, Dr. Arwady and Mayor Lightfoot devoted additional funds for mental health services at the remaining community clinics and twenty "trauma informed centers of care," including FQHCs and community organizations.[70] According to both health providers and the residents I interviewed, these resources all fall short. Furthermore, while there was a mental health crisis before the pandemic began, it was alarmingly exacerbated by COVID-19 as vulnerable Chicagoans struggled to deal with isolation, anxiety, depression, trauma, substance use, violence, and racism.

One psychiatric physician assistant I interviewed explained that to truly treat mental illness, providers need to combine psychiatric medication (for those who require it) with long-term therapy and wraparound services (e.g., housing and food support), and yet only the six remaining community health clinics have such capacity and even they are stretched to their limits.[71] She explained that many people end up just taking the medications without the wraparound support needed to succeed: "Medications cannot fix mental illness. . . . But it's easier to find psychiatry and to get prescribed medications than it is to, say, find a therapist."[72] FQHCs take the overflow of patients who cannot access services at community clinics, but without enough staff and resources. She said that not all FQHCs provide mental health support because insurance reimbursement rates are lower for mental health appointments. Another mental health care provider explained that waiting lists are long and community clinics limit therapy to twelve to twenty sessions, making long-term care difficult to access for lower-income residents.[73]

For those who require immediate or high-needs care, often hospitals do not have psychiatric beds available. For uninsured patients or those using Medicaid, the care provided at hospital psychiatric units is minimal, fragmented, and often completely disconnected from the other mental health care services people may be receiving.[74] Several mental health specialists mentioned that hospitals do not routinely contact a patient's mental health care provider to inform them of the patient's hospitalization, creating a lack of coordination between hospitals and mental health specialists.[75] One provider explained:

> Hospitals just want to discharge someone and . . . they don't put a good follow-up plan in place. They just wanna check some boxes, and sometimes they'll provide, like, three days of medication that they started the patient on and that's it. Then they're just off on their own.[76]

There is, therefore, often a lack of coordination between mental health care institutions.

Several residents I interviewed spoke about the shortage in mental health care created by the closure of the community health clinics. For example, Armando, a Mexican man from Little Village, told me:

> When it comes to mental health, I don't think there are many options, really. . . . I know there have been long wait times . . . because of . . . closing down many mental health clinics that, you know, even before COVID, that now because of COVID, we see, you know, the negative impacts of something like that.[77]

Other residents mentioned that it is practically impossible to find therapists, psychiatrists, and other mental health specialists who are Black or Brown.

"It's not fair," Shantal put it. "We should be able to access quality health care in our communities," and "we shouldn't have to go to the north of the city to get mental health care."[78] In Marlin's view, "We fell into a mental health crisis, and right now, I think we need a structure of the best Hispanic psychiatrists we can find, the best African American psychiatrists we can find. Right? . . . It's not so much a racial issue, but it's the issue of trust."[79]

The FQHC providers I interviewed all mentioned that long-term mental health strain would be a lasting legacy of COVID-19. For example, one provider said, "It's been astounding the need that has presented itself for behavioral and mental health needs during this time. All of the agencies that provide behavioral health throughout the city have really been overwhelmed in this time trying to give the help that patients need."[80] Another FQHC provider explained that vulnerable Chicagoans were facing multiple compounding traumas that all had mental health consequences:

> There's the trauma from the disease and death, and then there's also the trauma from not having money to pay your bills anymore because all of a sudden, you're out of work. It would be hard to overstate how many people had—they talked about the eviction crisis. There was the moratorium on eviction, but it wasn't really necessarily a moratorium. There was still a lot of people who could get kicked out in various ways. Even if they didn't get kicked out, they were living with the stress and anxiety of not being able to pay their rent. . . . You were traumatized if you had to go to work and you were traumatized if you got fired, either way.[81]

Lower-income Chicagoans already struggled to access mental health services before 2020. The pandemic has only widened the gulf between mental health care needs and available services.

Health care and mental health care are two care infrastructures whose deficiencies were woefully exposed during the pandemic. Yet such infrastructure was also largely ignored in local policy responses. Two people I interviewed pointed to a lack of basic infrastructure that was exposed during the pandemic. Ana, a Mexican American woman from Little Village, mentioned disruptions to health care, mail delivery, and public transit in the midst of a national crisis. She contended that the infrastructure that is meant to protect citizens was ignored by state officials:

> Part of the government infrastructure that's supposed to just be there. Like, literally what the government's *for* so that people are protected . . . and their freedoms are protected. Like, that is so so abused and not taken care of at all, and I just don't understand why. . . . And I feel like there should be . . . *public* plans to build sustainable structures or something.[82]

Kelly, a Black woman from Albany Park, made a similar point:

> Like nobody could have seen COVID coming but at the same time . . .
> we have stuff in place for natural disasters . . . like tornadoes or hurri-
> canes. We have stuff like *that*, what the hell is put in place for, you know,
> something like [COVID-19]. . . . I just think with almost any major
> disaster, some of the people who are always going to get hit the worst
> with it are the poor, the people of color, the disenfranchised, all the peo-
> ple at, quote-unquote, the bottom of our social totem pole. Those are the
> people who are going to be hit the hardest. . . . I just feel like if we had
> a government that actually gave a shit about its people who are again,
> quote-unquote, at the bottom of . . . society . . . we damn sure would not
> be in a position that we are right now.[83]

As these two respondents point out, market logics, structural racism, and
decades of federal disinvestment from care infrastructure (e.g., housing,
health care, education) put low-income people of color at greater risk, especially when disaster strikes. Throughout this book, I illustrate how people,
like the women quoted here, were acutely aware that their lives are devalued by the state. COVID-19 made this crystal clear. And yet, fixing sustainable care infrastructure was never considered by most policymakers during
the pandemic. Rather, the pandemic was governed through emergency—
efforts were made to put "Band-Aids" on existing systems and momentarily provide small bursts of funding to already broken systems. In so doing,
the fragmented, dilapidated, underresourced system of care that has always
just been accepted as "good enough" for the poor was left intact. Policies
that fail to attend to infrastructural disinvestment naturalize race and class
inequalities, which are then accepted as ontological features of our social
landscape, outside the reach of political transformation. Yet, "racial equity"
is nonetheless touted as a goal. State actors invested in technocratic devices
and epidemiological infrastructure to buttress "racial equity" discourses
while ignoring the structural origins of racism. In the next section, I provide a brief history of the profession of public health, as it is the care infrastructure tasked with mitigating the spread of infectious disease. Aspects
of its history provide important context for unpacking the choices made by
the Chicago Department of Public Health (CDPH) during the pandemic.

HISTORY OF US PUBLIC HEALTH

Public health's mission is to protect the nation from contagious infection
and to optimize the population's strength by controlling filth, germs, and illness. As such, public health performs a critical disciplinary function under

systems of racial biopower. Foucault traces the origins of public health back to three distinct developments in Germany, France, and England in the late nineteenth century.[84] In Germany, "medical policing" was established to statistically surveil the population and measure its strengths and weaknesses, whereas in France, "urban health" experts focused on building infrastructure (e.g., cemeteries, slaughterhouses, waterways) to control the spread of disease. In response to cholera outbreaks, early public health practitioners in England forcibly segregated the poor from the rich, and only the former were compulsorily medicalized. Statistical surveillance, environmental sanitation, and population segregation merged as major foci of modern public health.

In the US racial biopower system, public health has historically racialized immigrant and nonwhite populations as threats to modern progress. The federal US Public Health Service was established in 1889 to control the nation's ports.[85] Through "objective" scientific methods of the era, public health authorities identified immigrants as a primary source of physical and social ills.[86] As such, contagion was imagined to originate from external and internal racial enemies, thereby instantiating the American body politic as hygienic, modern, and white.[87] Because public health practitioners depicted health and hygiene as standards of "Americanness," they also determined who was included in the US national imaginary.[88] At the city level, although public health departments were not well funded, public health practitioners used their legal authority to regulate people's movement, conduct, and work and housing conditions.[89] As such, city public health workers used "scientific" discourses stereotyping Black and immigrant communities as unsanitary and disease-ridden to promote and sustain segregated housing and health care policies.[90] The institution of public health helped enact racist policies and ordinances but also influenced popular racial opinion. As such, public health was a primary purveyor of racialization in the late nineteenth and early twentieth centuries.[91] This racialization was facilitated by the development and advancement of epidemiology as a means of surveilling the movement of Black and Brown bodies.[92]

For example, during the 1918 influenza outbreak in Chicago, health authorities stoked local racial panic about the Great Migration of Black communities from the South to northern cities such as Chicago through newspaper articles blaming Black residents for the spread of contagious disease.[93] This racist rhetoric buttressed local policies that racially segregated housing, schools, and health care in the city. Despite the fact that infection and death rates from influenza were lower in Black communities than in white communities, segregation was promoted as the solution to contagion. New epidemiological tools were developed to surveil and police Black residents in their homes and in public settings. Further, differential infection rates among Black and white Chicagoans fueled theories of bio-logical racial difference.[94]

At the federal level, in addition to using fears of contagion to promote or justify anti-immigration border policies, the US Public Health Service was a primary purveyor of racial classification and hierarchization. The forty-year (1932–72) untreated syphilis study at the Tuskegee Institute in Alabama provides a particularly poignant example.[95] Treatment was withheld from 439 Black men with syphilis who had signed up for the study because they believed they would be given treatment. Their wives, children, and sexual partners were neither traced nor treated. In this case, the federal Public Health Service actively devalued Black life, engaging in both scientific and government malfeasance.

Although public health's original scope involved sanitation, hygiene, environmental risks, housing, and preventive health care, when germ theory emerged at the turn of the twentieth century, the discipline of public health shifted its attention toward infectious disease epidemiology, quar-antining, and vaccination.[96] Public health's professional scope was estab-lished through jurisdictional battles with the profession of medicine in the early twentieth century. By the 1920s and 1930s, clinical medicine made great strides in professionalizing its field by establishing a national asso-ciation, strong organizational structures, and widespread scientific author-ity.[97] In contrast, public health was decentralized and unfocused.[98] The American Medical Association claimed its jurisdiction over patient care and used its professional and expert authority to avidly oppose the provision of health care through the public sector.[99] As such, public health lost the ca-pacity to provide preventive care, except to those deemed "unworthy" of privatized clinical treatment (e.g., providing services for the indigent). In 1940, the American Public Health Association passed a resolution codifying a standard set of services local public health departments should provide, which was referred to as the "basic six." They included vital statistics, sur-veillance of communicable diseases, environmental sanitation, laboratory services, maternal and infant childcare services, and education on health behaviors.[100] There was great interstate variation in what was prioritized by local departments of health. During this period in the early twentieth cen-tury, public health departments began minimally offering entitlements to communities of color if they adhered to politics of respectability and behav-ioral modification.[101] Racial difference was still an organizing principle of public health work because services were withheld unless racially margin-alized populations could prove their adherence to public health discipline.

In the 1960s, public health departments shifted from a focus on infec-tious disease (because many believed that widespread vaccination and san-itation regimes had vanquished infectious disease in the US) to lifestyle conditions related to consumption, exercise, diet, and drug use.[102] Through large population surveys, public health reformers began to recognize behavioral drivers of chronic illness, such as tobacco use.[103] Local public health departments claimed control over a small field of activities including data collection, disease surveillance, health education, and the promotion of good nutrition and healthy lifestyles.[104] Because of a lack of nationalized health care, public health epidemiologists also helped establish actuarial models to calculate the loss of productivity based on adjusted years of disability to buttress the growing private insurance industry.[105] Actuarial epidemiological models help state actors develop cost-effective health interventions at the population level while presuming gross scarcity of health care resources within a market-based health system.[106]

In an effort to reckon with its racist past, in the period from the 1960s through the 1980s, the discipline of *population health* was established, inaugurating a renewed focus within the public health field on distal, social determinants of poor health. The American Public Health Association adopted a much broader definition of *public health care* including concerns with health disparities and the environment. However, many scholars argue that the professional scope of the field of public health was already too delimited to accommodate these new definitions and concerns. In addition, state departments, for the most part, created new agencies focused on occupational safety, environmental protection, and medical care for the poor instead of expanding the scope of public health.[107] As James Colgrove and colleagues explain, "Though liberal practitioners of public health, and now of population health, have claimed a more sociologically informed and enlightened view of how health outcomes are determined, their political and institutional weakness has prevented them from transforming their vision into reality."[108]

In sum, both federal and local public health departments played a prominent historical role in promoting white supremacist policies that treated racially marginalized Americans as separate, undeserving, and unfit. As such, the discipline of public health helped structure the slow emergencies that lower-income people of color face today. Although the language of "social determinants of health" and the new focus on declaring racism a "public health crisis" attempt to reckon with public health's history of racial violence and neglect, the field is too jurisdictionally and financially delimited to actually extend social safety nets and restructure fragmented infrastructure. One exception is the wraparound social safety net offered to people who are HIV positive or at risk of infection, which includes housing, welfare, preventive health care, addiction services, and treatment support.[109] Like many people throughout sub-Saharan Africa, being HIV positive allows poor Chicagoans to survive their slow emergencies. Yet, this exceptional

HIV policy is an example of governing through emergency because one disadvantaged population group (poor people with HIV) are given robust social services while the broader infrastructural lack that surrounds these groups is left intact. This HIV policy still targets one population in need, carving out a caesura in a broader system of thanatopolitics. When asked, public health practitioners point to HIV services as an exception that cannot be replicated as a broader policy initiative because it is made possible through a very particular federal funding stream.

By the time the COVID-19 pandemic emerged in the United States, the profession of public health was attempting to contend with its racist past, but it had delimited jurisdiction over data collection, vaccination, and behavioral education despite its lofty disciplinary goals of attending to the social determinants of poor health. During the pandemic, the public health practitioners I interviewed expressed a desire to attend to the social determinants of health they knew were driving the uneven racial impact of the pandemic. Yet, they delegated and outsourced food and housing support to nonprofits and focused their attention on building up data infrastructure. As such, they facilitated the invisibilization and naturalization of structural, racial inequalities, even as they claimed to be addressing them.

PUBLIC HEALTH IN CHICAGO DURING COVID-19

When the pandemic began in early 2020, federal, state, and local public health units had been severely underfunded for years. The US Centers for Disease Control and Prevention, as well as most state and local public health departments, were losing funding each year in the decade before the onset of the pandemic.[110] In Chicago, 80 percent of the Department of Public Health's budget stems from federal grants that stipulate precisely how funds must be spent and must be constantly renewed. Only 20 percent of the agency's budget comes from city government and can be used with discretion.[111] The lack of existing public health capacity was readily acknowledged by the people I interviewed. An official from CDPH offered the following perspective:

> Our public health infrastructure and systems were so decimated, prior to COVID, and then, hey, you've got, you know, a whole pandemic that we were expected to run. And I think it has been challenging for public health, and not just CDPH, not just here locally, I mean, across the country, and I think that's well documented.[112]

This official went on to explain that this meant prioritizing community partnerships and relying on other city agencies to provide services where CDPH could not. Instead of prioritizing the extension of social safety nets, CDPH envisioned its task as "visualizing" the impact of the pandemic through data collection. As one epidemiologist who worked on the Racial Equity Rapid Response Team (RERRT) explained, "people wanna see the data" to make sure there are no "communities that are invisible, that we don't see."[113] This focus on using data to *visualize* meant that epistemic infrastructure became prioritized but other forms of infrastructure (missing and fragmented care infrastructures) faded into the background, unseen and unaccounted for as causal determinants. Data became *the* task that CDPH tackled. An epidemiologist at CDPH explained that the health "commissioner, she lives and breathes this data. . . . She's using that information to make decisions," and "policies have been based on what we're seeing in the data."[114] And yet, because of the speed and scope of the pandemic, a new data infrastructure had to be built. A CDPH epidemiologist explained:

> While we have a really adept set of epidemiologists working in communicable diseases, that unit was quickly overwhelmed with the need and the appetite for data around COVID. . . . We have traditionally operated on an annual cadence at best and had to pivot to weekly or even daily reporting for effective COVID response.[115]

Another told me:

> Usually, when we're talking about communicable disease surveillance and outbreak response, it's on a scale that's, for the most part, for most conditions, minuscule compared to what we're dealing with with COVID. . . . The scale is just like orders of magnitude different as far as the volume of information that we're dealing with.[116]

The "appetite" for data to drive policy was voracious, so the "cadence" and "magnitude" of data reporting were escalated but also homed in at the census-tract level, which required investment in building a robust epidemic infrastructure that drew on the expertise and resources from private corporations.

The epidemiologists who worked around the clock to build this infrastructure and use it to help guide resource allocation believed that the data would save lives and promote equity. One CDPH epidemiologist told me that members of his family who "could not pronounce" *epidemiology* were asking him about specific disease surveillance strategies they heard about in the news. He said that during the first year of the pandemic, epidemiologists "command[ed] attention like we never have and maybe never will again," so they wanted to use the investment in data infrastructure to "bring long-lasting focus to some of the issues that we deal with as epidemiologists in Chicago around health equity."[117] The obsession with numbers, as a means of visualizing the threat of COVID-19, brought some semblance of control in those first months of the pandemic when uncertainty and fear were palpable—when experts tasked with controlling infectious disease spread were unclear how this invisible but proficient killer was circulating. And epidemiologists felt poised to help also shine a light on why its impact was so racially uneven. While this visualization was crucial, I argue that it overshadowed the impact endemic emergencies were making—emergencies that could have been ameliorated with more focused attention and funding on housing, work protections, and uneven care infrastructures. Choosing to focus the spotlight on data rendered the causes of inequality shadowy, unknowable, and intransigent.

Although the data were clearly illustrating the uneven racial toll, one epidemiologist explained that CDPH and the Mayor's Office chose *not* to direct COVID-19 public health mandates to specific vulnerabilities or places. Experts wanted to avert unnecessary stigma, even when their hyperlocal spatial data showed clear patterns in infection that were matters of historic inequality and not merely spatial coincidence. One expert explained:

> The next question might be, did we set different thresholds for different communities? We didn't do that. It's always balancing the epidemiological thresholds with the political acceptability thresholds of the community. We did not want to pit communities against each other.[118]

To avoid stigma, they did not impose, for example, mask mandates in certain parts of the city and not others. But city officials did send police to already hypersurveilled neighborhoods to enforce mask mandates, which they did not do in predominantly white communities.[119] Further, city officials *did* purposefully select six racially marginalized communities with the worst statistics on infection, hospitalizations, and deaths to infuse with mobile testing sites and educational campaigns. And they chose fifteen neighborhoods to prioritize for vaccine distribution. So despite not wanting to direct mitigation strategies only toward certain racial groups, officials did carve up the city and treat certain Black and Brown communities differently than others. And this differential treatment was based on what the data told them despite the fact that they *knew* which neighborhoods would be most impacted. Other epidemiologists admitted they were not surprised by the data they collected, but they still waited to collect it to act.[120] One CDPH epidemiologist said, for example, "it wasn't that surprising" which areas were hardest hit. Because "of all the work that's been done around public health in the city, these are familiar places to us. They seem to be vulnerable to COVID, but they're also vulnerable to a lot of other things . . . I think we were expecting it, and the data showed that."[121] But a racial equity officer from the Mayor's Office explained that they did not want to just rely on existing knowledge of vulnerability. They wanted to see the data before acting, even though this slowed down their response.

There was ambivalence, then, among epidemiologists and state actors about whether COVID-19 mitigation should rely on knowledge of existing inequalities, target particular racially marginalized communities and treat them differently, or set the same "threshold" for the city as a whole. This ambivalence likely stems from public health's deep racist history of labeling racially marginalized groups as contagious and treating them with segregationist policies. And yet, city officials nonetheless used the data they were collecting to "hotspot" certain racially disadvantaged neighborhoods for specialized services in order to reduce their rates. A CDPH official explained:

> We've done hot spot / cold spot analyses, and look at those week over week over week over week to see is the hot spot getting cooler? Is it moving? Using information like that, we deploy our community-based COVID testing sites. If we're seeing a community area, or cluster of zip codes, where there are a high number of COVID diagnoses, that's where the testing efforts will go.[122]

"Hotspotting" engages cost-benefit analysis to determine where scarce health resources are to be directed.[123] It is a prime example of governing through emergency. It presumes that resources are scarce and must be triaged, and it spatially ontologizes racial difference. To triage, however, very complex legacies and experiences of racism were boiled down into one metric. A CDPH epidemiologist described the process:

> Taking the data from different sources, including COVID-19 outcomes, information about things like comorbidities or access to health care, different data elements that might be proxies for things that make a neighborhood more vulnerable to the kind of poorer outcomes from COVID-19. We put all of that together into one of the tools that we use. It's like pulling all that into a single index that then you can use, just look at one number to say, this community versus this community, which one is, maybe, more vulnerable.[124]

This index, funneled down from complex indicators of vulnerability and disadvantage, was the deciding factor on which communities received vaccine dosages from the city. It separates the causes of inequality from its epistemic effects by boiling all of history down into one statistical measure, and it literally determined those whose lives were valued and saved versus those who were let die.

Not only were testing and vaccine resources triaged, but instead of investing directly in social service provision, CDPH and state officials relied on already existing nonprofits to buttress the social safety net. A hospital administrator who worked on RERRT explained it this way:

> Our public health system is often underresourced, and so folks might be like, "Well, you know, city government should be able to do this, this, this and this," but that's difficult when your staffing has been cut, your resources and budgets have been cut, so you gotta rely on other providers to be able to help as well, because public health just hasn't been funded as it should.[125]

And yet, public health was awash with funding during the pandemic, as many people at CDPH admitted. And the city government was given billions of dollars in COVID-19 federal funds. As I explain in chapter 3, CDPH and city officials made choices about how to spend that money, and they chose *not* to spend it on expanding the public safety net. They relied on the nonprofit sector to provide a fragmented and minimal safety net, and they justified this choice by suggesting that nonprofits know their communities better. For example, a chief equity officer in the Mayor's Office admitted that she knew that numbers were limited in what they could tell you about a community because it misses the "narratives." But if community members, represented by nonprofits who were asked to join RERRT, could draw on the data, this city official suggested, they could help themselves. But only six nonprofits were given access to this data. She stated:

> Short of constantly surveying a community or something, there's always gonna be a set of information that sits in between what we can capture . . . we call it numbers and narratives. There's just always that in between the numbers [is] where narratives are. . . . It's in a cultural and historical understanding of that community. . . . It's contextual. It's what makes up all of our lives and our experiences. . . . I really value the importance of putting the data on the table with those who are most impacted and creating a table in which they have the ability to name what they think would work. They are the experts in their own experiences.[126]

By offering the data, city officials absolve themselves from having to know and understand the structural causes of inequality or people's lived experiences with endemic emergencies. Offering the data justifies using metrics as stand-ins that delink cause and effect, and thereby enable governing through emergency. Public health agents did not try to reimagine their organizational role during the pandemic when they were given extensive funding. They accepted their limited disciplinary focus on epidemiology and took as a given that the safety net is the responsibility of the federal government and the nonprofit sector. And they did not reexamine or reckon with their own historical responsibility for creating uneven landscapes of care for racially marginalized Americans. Governing through emergency leaves existing structural legacies intact, while creating limited, temporary policy fixes such as building up data coordination to triage testing and vaccines.

Chapter 3 focuses on the city's RERRT approach. Here in chapter 2, I provided insight into why epidemiologists chose to invest so heavily in building a robust epistemic infrastructure and justified *not* enhancing the public safety net. I have done so by providing public health experts' explanations alongside the history of the discipline of public health's role as a key agent of racialization. Public health has historically collected racial statistics to better surveil and segregate racially marginalized communities, justified by the promotion of racialized discourses of contagion. Contemporary epidemiological efforts continue to racially sort and count, without addressing the complex structural landscape that exposes Black and Brown communities to premature death.

INVISIBILIZING STRUCTURAL NEGLECT

State actors rolled out social provisions during the disaster but in fragmented ways that failed to attend to and often obscured existing structural inequalities. In fact, racially marginalized subjects readily acknowledge that their health and well-being are not considered in political battles over public spending. For example, when asked to reflect on the federal response to COVID-19, Isaiah, a Black man from Austin, expressed his frustration:

> Money rules the world. If you're a billionaire, you can buy your way to anything. I'm not a billionaire. I want to be able to be financially stable. I need somebody to help me get a good job and give me an opportunity.... We poor and they take the food stamps [away]. They take all the medical stuff from us that people with a chronic illness need. How are we gonna get well [if] we can't get no medication? If I don't get the insulin, I'll die. You take it away from me as you try to be a politician. You want to get in the office and you decide to say okay, I'm cutting Barack O-care. Or I'm taking out Cook County care. Y'all gotta buy your own insurance. How can we buy it when we got no job and they ain't hiring? I got too many strikes against me. I'm Black on Black on Black. That's a lot of strikes.[127]

Isaiah explains that as politicians debate policies associated with care infrastructure, they fail to consider the most basic needs of people who are poor and racially marginalized. By invisibilizing basic care infrastructures, state actors ignore people's grounded experiences of racial neglect and harm.

The building up of epistemic infrastructure allowed the state to render COVID-19 racial disparities visible in certain ways, but the letting die and making die of populations of color were also enabled by prioritizing medicalized, technocratic interventions *over* direct service provision. The failures and fissures in care infrastructure for the poor were furnished with policy "Band-Aids" or ignored altogether. Vulnerable communities were made acutely aware that the government does not, as Kelly argued, give "a shit about its people" or else Black and Brown Chicagoans would not have been exposed to premature death via COVID-19 inequalities.

3: QUANTIFYING RACIAL EMERGENCIES

In early April 2020, Mayor Lori Lightfoot sounded a "public health red alarm" in response to reports of high COVID-19 cases and deaths concentrated in Chicago's Black communities.[1] She immediately launched a "racial equity" plan, which started with a "non-negotiable" requirement to fix racial data so that the city can "understand the magnitude" of the problem.[2] Lightfoot initiated her Racial Equity Rapid Response Team (RERRT) in partnership with a local nonprofit health group that has long focused on collecting population data to chart racial disparities in health outcomes. City officials name racism a *public health* crisis because epidemiologists can "quantify structural racism" in ways that are "resonant" with the public.[3] Data are important tools when governing emergencies, especially when they can be used to convince the public that policies are successful if statistical differences are reduced.

Chicago officials took racial disparities in COVID-19 outcomes seriously. The Chicago Department of Public Health (CDPH) invested in building epidemiological infrastructure to track disparities at the "hyperlocal" level, and city officials immediately provided testing and later vaccines to vulnerable communities. These are laudable responses to an emerging pandemic. Yet, as the empirical evidence throughout this book will attest, Chicago's initiatives failed to address core vulnerabilities of racially marginalized communities throughout the city. Why? This chapter answers this question by analyzing the "racial equity" initiatives the city implemented.

I argue that the city's efforts to highlight racial inequality constitutes a shift away from colorblind racism toward more race-conscious politics. When neoliberal economics became hegemonic in the 1970s and 1980s, market fundamentalism was used as an excuse to dismantle existing social safety nets, and colorblind ideologies buttressed the notion that the market alone would dictate state policy. Yet, the state continued to intervene to support capital accumulation among the white elite. As Omi and Winant explain, "the hegemony of neoliberal economics is matched and underwritten by the racial hegemony of colorblindness."[4] More recently, however, liberal politicians have shifted their strategies toward *naming* racism and *claiming* an equity approach to garner political capital, and quantification plays a key role in these administrative tactics. The amelioration of racial disparities in *numbers* conceals the ongoing institutional racism that is sustained through colorblind policies.[5] Racial quantification is, therefore, politically useful because data can be fixed to illustrate progress in advancing "equity," while simultaneously drawing attention away from ongoing colorblind rollbacks, a failure to provide direct services, and the reification of structural racism.

Numbers can be wielded as political tools by multiple social actors. Data are immediately palpable and digestible by the public, so metrics can illustrate the failure *or* prove the success of policy initiatives. For example, when Black and Brown Chicagoans were becoming infected and dying at startling rates, the spectacle of "bad numbers" mobilized city politicians to take action. Sholanda, a Black resident of Austin, asserted:

> Only till people from the West Side and people from the South Side [sections of Chicago inhabited by primarily Black residents], and people from poor neighborhoods like, uh, Pilsen and Little Village [predominantly Latinx neighborhoods]—not until those people start *complaining*: "Hey, we're dying at an alarming rate, where's our help? Where's our aid?"... [City officials] probably never would have helped us if we hadn't got on the news and made them look bad. Shoot [*chuckles*]... People are dying at alarming rates. There's no help. So now they look bad, so now here they come to save the day. You and your white horse can keep riding [*chuckles*]. Because it was all crap and bull.[6]

Once the racial disparities became a political embarrassment and made city officials "look bad," only then did the mayor initiate her "rapid response."

A community organizer from Austin who took part in the RERRT task force pointed out how the city's attention was focused on the urgent deaths from COVID-19 because these were difficult to ignore, compared to the slow emergencies already confronting racially marginalized Chicagoans:

> So if the data shows that there's heightened cases of COVID, there's heightened amount of deaths... it tells a story that's much more detrimental to... a government... that is responsible for resources being allocated for the well-being of those constituents. Right. It's a lot different than, oh, they didn't get that home. No, they died.... Because it's more instantaneous than the slower death of being strained on getting access

to jobs or being strained on getting access to healthy food. . . . That's a slower death. . . . So the narrative is different when the death is more instantaneous. COVID was instant. . . . That's harder to spin.[7]

Ignoring deaths from COVID-19 was not politically excusable, this organizer explains, but the political ramifications of ignoring "slower deaths" from housing and food insecurity are negligible. The rate and immediacy of deaths from COVID-19 and the closer causal link between disparity and outcome prompted Chicago politicians to respond with urgent, "data-driven" policies.

Numbers are malleable as political tools because they conceal their own manufacturing. Ensuring that policies are "data-driven" gives them a sheen of objectivity while erasing the processes that yield the production of such metrics and disguising the political authority required to produce and circulate them.[8] Numbers can also exclude certain people or things from enumeration, and they often invisibilize lived realities that defy quantification.[9] But numbers are especially useful tools for liberal politicians seeking to "prove" their "racial equity" credentials. In fact, racial statistics have long been used in racial projects that support white supremacy.[10] In statistical representation, race is a discrete, individualized variable and not a dynamic, relational outcome of social processes. As such, racial statistics constitute and stratify groups according to purportedly objective racial differences, thereby naturalizing race through its decontextualization.[11] Similarly, racial health disparities that are represented numerically without context can spatially ontologize racial difference and reify racial stereotypes about behavior, leading to stigmatization and neglect.[12]

Quantification allows for zooming out—population statistics detach people from their conditions of existence and divorce the *causes* of racial inequality (e.g., segregation, privatized health care, neoliberal restructuring) from their epistemic effects (e.g., high COVID-19 death rates). But quantification can also overdetermine and reify structural racism by presuming that one individualized racial variable can serve as proxy for broader historical and spatial processes. For example, when race/ethnicity variables were missing from the city's COVID-19 positivity and death rates, CDPH epidemiologists "fixed" the data by imputing zip code data.[13] Within the data, people are epistemically "fixed" in place, but the structures that caused this fixation are not the focus of policy changes. Therefore, the data can be "fixed," but the problem of structural racism is left intact.[14] Anthony Hatch challenges the reliance on racial health disparities data during COVID-19 for precisely this reason:

The assumption that collecting data on racial health disparities in the COVID-19 pandemic will lead to the reduction or elimination of those disparities [is an] assumption that keeps scientists in an endless search for more and more refined measurements of racism's harms, while the political and economic systems that comprise the fundamental causes of those harms are given a pass until all the data are counted.[15]

Discourses that claim "racial equity" or that name racism a "public health crisis" are utilized by state actors as forms of political capital. According to Pierre Bourdieu, states impose classificatory systems that obscure their own construction and are misrecognized as natural.[16] Racial statistics are used in precisely this way. In the long-standing Democratic stronghold of a majority-minority city such as Chicago, proving one's "racial equity" credentials are key for success in the polls. Data allow the mayor and other city officials to prove their success in curbing racial disparities related to COVID-19 while simultaneously naturalizing structural inequality by failing to invest in direct services that could better alleviate social suffering. For example, in January 2021, when vaccines first became available and health care workers and the elderly were eligible, 67 percent of those first vaccinated were white and Asian, and only 15 percent were Black and 17 percent Latinx.[17] Later, city officials claimed they had achieved racial equity when 50 percent of first-dose vaccines were going to Black and Latinx residents. And yet, 66 percent of the city is Black and Latinx, so if 50 percent of Black and Latinx residents receive the first dose of a vaccine, the city is still not achieving equity despite how it was presented.[18] Further, city officials only highlighted vaccine uptake; they ignored Black and Brown Chicagoans' experiences with mounting rental debt, food insecurity, work precarity, and underemployment—all of which were exacerbated by pandemic conditions. Using data as a political tool linked to "racial equity" performs a symbolic magic trick: the public is presented the success of administering vaccine doses to racially marginalized Chicagoans while the city's complete failure in addressing inadequate worker protections, lack of health care access, or food and housing insecurity is invisibilized.

Governing through emergency also relies on enumeration. According to Elizabeth Povinelli, in the current neoliberal moment, subjects' biopolitical needs must be measurable and profitable to secure recognition by the state.[19] Cal Garrett and I argue that Chicago city officials enacted "data citizenship" because only residents whose exceptional needs were rendered visible by certain epidemiological data were given tests and vaccines.[20] The CDPH created simplified metrics that hierarchically ranked census tracts by need, thereby triaging testing and vaccine resources. Once rates abated, those resources were retracted and repurposed elsewhere. In this way, data were operationalized as part of an emergency governing strategy to manage austerity. City officials presumed scarcity, collected population statistics to stratify populations by exceptional need, provided technocratic resources, and then moved on, patting themselves on the back for achieving "racial equity"—all while ignoring deeply entrenched structural inequalities.

Scarcity is a core feature of neoliberalism. Government authorities presume austerity in state resources and reward market competitiveness. For public spending on health, welfare, and education to be supported in a neoliberal economy, market-based policies with quantifiable results are employed. Inequalities remain entrenched, people become self-entrepreneurs, and social problems are quantified, triaged, and treated with efficient, replicable, technocratic solutions. Testing and vaccines are technocratic solutions because they are efficient, cost-effective, and scientifically proven. They are essential tools during a pandemic. Epidemiological modeling that attends to racial differences in cases, hospitalizations, and deaths renders inequalities visible and actionable. But the promotion of testing, vaccines, and epidemiological data is not sufficient for addressing core vulnerabilities or entrenched racial inequalities. Further, these tools were often deployed by City of Chicago officials in ways that naturalized racial differences, were reactive as opposed to diagnostic, and were prioritized over other kinds of resource distribution.

I do not mean to imply that the mayor, CDPH epidemiologists, or city, state, and federal officials purposefully neglected lower-income or racially marginalized Americans in their COVID-19 mitigation response. However, in framing the pandemic as *only* an infectious disease crisis that could be governed through temporary mitigation strategies and minimal aid distribution doled out through existing bureaucratic systems, the administrative apparatus that was built to respond to COVID-19 failed to address the exacerbation of existing vulnerabilities among lower-income and racially marginalized Chicagoans. The use of epidemiological modeling to track the virus and the "success" of state efforts in halting its spread contributed to the detachment of the infectious disease response from its more enduring, structural implications. Because COVID-19 was treated as *only* a viral crisis, housing and food support were not prioritized as key components of "racially equitable" initiatives. This approach resulted in the prioritization of epidemiological infrastructure *over* direct social service provision. The hierarchization of governmental priorities was facilitated by the patchwork nature of America's social safety net, by Chicago's administrative structure, and by neoliberal budgeting and outsourcing. This was true in Chicago, which I use as my case, but it was equally true in many other cities throughout the nation.

In this chapter, I provide four mechanisms by which the "racial equity" approach taken by the City of Chicago failed to meet the needs of vulnerable residents. First, public health interventions under COVID-19 presumed a *scarcity* of funding and existing infrastructure (despite federal investments unseen in decades), and officials failed to reimagine how to direct resources. Second, the city built a robust *epistemic infrastructure* to determine how to triage "scarce" resources, and this ultimately detached the epistemic effects of racism from its structural causes, leading to accumulated vulnerability among the poor. The city provided members of RERRT with census-tract-level data to triage testing and vaccine provision in a reactive fashion. Housing, occupational safety, and financial support were never prioritized. Third, this model relied on the *outsourcing* of service provision to community, mutual aid, and philanthropic organizations. Finally, when unemployment and rental assistance were rolled out, paternalistic, means-tested systems were employed, creating immense *bureaucratic barriers* to access. These are the mechanisms through which the city's neoliberal commitments to "racial equity" failed to address the fundamental causes of structural inequalities that were exacerbated by pandemic conditions. Before explaining the city's pandemic policy, background on Chicago's political infrastructure is essential.

CITY STRUCTURE

Chicago's legacy of racial segregation is well documented. Indeed, it has become the model case for analyzing racial urban inequality in the United States.[21] Chicago remains one of the most segregated cities in the US.[22] Therefore, claiming "racial equity" is a major political priority for many leaders in the city.

Chicago's representative government is based on fifty wards, each led by an elected alderperson who represents community interests and sits on the City Council, the legislative body. Officially, the City Council approves the annual city budget, but political experts often refer to the City Council as a "rubber stamp" because of its tendency to bend to political pressure from the mayor.[23] Under emergency orders during 2020, Mayor Lightfoot completely bypassed the City Council and held "discretionary" power over federal Coronavirus Aid, Relief, and Economic Security (CARES) Act funding, for which she was harshly critiqued by progressive alderpeople and activists, and to which I return in the next section.

In fact, Mayor Lightfoot had a tendency (like previous mayoral administrations) to bypass alderpeople as political voices for their wards, especially those who disagreed with her. Her choice of working with nonprofit and for-profit health entities *over* alderpeople in the wards with the highest rates of infection was politically driven. As one alderperson who does not work closely with the mayor observed, Lightfoot's preference was "because of her lack of collaboration with aldermen, particularly aldermen she does not see eye to eye with. . . . When you don't communicate with the people in the communities who are actually driving community work, it's very hard to ensure that you are acting with equity."[24]

In addition, as one community organizer explained, some nonprofit and for-profit organizations also have close ties to alderpeople who are in the pocket of the mayor. He explained why community organizations would not have an incentive to push back against the mayor's initiatives:

> It's political. I mean, a lot of these aldermen are very close to a local non-profit in the community. . . . And some of these aldermen also very close to the mayor's office or are trying to vie for political power. And, you know, that means kind of aligning yourself with business interests. . . . So as a result, there's a kind of a very inherent conflict of interest that the nonprofit sector tends to have when it comes to pushing for policies that better represent community residents that counter the mayor's position. There's a very, very strong reluctance to do so.[25]

The mayor also appoints leadership of CDPH; therefore, epidemiologists and public health officials work directly *for* the mayor and are dependent on the mayor for funding decisions. This leaves them without political will to push back on the mayor's initiatives.

SCARCITY

When Chicago was suffering the deleterious effects of deindustrialization in the 1980s and 1990s, local officials made decisions to prioritize attracting corporate headquarters and elite redevelopment to the city, as factories moved to the suburbs.[26] Tax-free incentives were offered to corporations and wealthy business elites to keep their business in Chicago. Meanwhile, President Ronald Reagan's regressive tax policies led to reductions in government tax revenue, so cities such as Chicago cut funding to schools, social services, and housing.[27] The local social safety net was already decimated long before the COVID-19 pandemic hit. When federal funds were made available to cities through various legislative acts during the pandemic, some were earmarked for particular purposes (e.g., emergency rental assistance), but cities (and states) were also given discretion over certain funding decisions. This administrative devolution allowed Chicago officials to prioritize business and corporate interests, data infrastructure, and policing *instead of* buttressing its social safety net for the poor.

Out of the City of Chicago's CARES Act allocation, $470 million was discretionary, and Mayor Lightfoot bypassed the City Council to determine the allocation of these funds. The mayor spent $281.5 million on police personnel expenses and left another $68 million unspent.[28] The city did not prioritize direct services such as food and rental assistance. Although the city claimed and presumed scarcity in meeting the robust needs of vulnerable Chicagoans, its 2020 allocation was not even used in its entirety. The City Council pushed back on the mayor's use of the emergency power ordinance to take full control of CARES Act spending, but it lost the vote.[29] In the view of a progressive alderperson, "the way that the CARES funding was managed through the pandemic . . . it's criminal, right? [About] $281 million went to police when people were scared of being evicted. That is just so unconscionable. . . . Why didn't we put more money into housing and make sure that at least people's rents were covered? . . . [Housing] was sort of an afterthought."[30] This alderperson is referring to the fact that in 2020, the Chicago Department of Housing created an emergency rental assistance (ERA) lottery with $2 million from its own existing budget (not through CARES Act funds). This program provided 2,000 households with $1,000 in back rent payments in 2020. But the city received 83,000 applications, illustrating how greatly the need outweighed the allotment.[31] The Consolidated Appropriations Act of December 2020 directly allocated funding from the federal government for emergency rental assistance, Supplemental Nutrition Assistance Program benefits, and federal unemployment benefits. This funding allowed cities to make up for early shortcomings in housing support by providing robust rental assistance programs in 2021 and 2022. But this funding was only made available to residents eleven months into the pandemic after many had already accrued tremendous debt to their landlords, which I return to later in the chapter.

The American Rescue Plan Act (ARPA) was passed in March 2021 and allocated federal funding to state and local governments to assist with pandemic recovery. It "gave municipal recipients broad latitude to use funds for the provision of government services to the extent of reduction in revenue."[32] In other words, local governments could use the funds to balance municipal budgets through revenue replacement, which meant paying down existing debt to improve investment rankings. The City of Chicago has a history of taking on high-interest debt to balance its budget. City administrators have used city revenue to refund the principal on loans from prior budget years and then engage new loans to cover expenses for the upcoming budget year.[33] This practice is referred to as "scoop and toss" borrowing, a strategy that relies on continued borrowing to pay down existing debts.[34] In anticipation of ARPA funds that would replace city revenue and cover "essential city services," in 2021, city officials diverted existing city revenues to pay back previous loan principals.[35] For example, in 2021, they used $1.32 billion of ARPA funding to bridge the 2021 and 2022 budget gap in paying for services from the Chicago Fire Department, a department that would have otherwise been funded with city revenue.[36] Out of the $2.56 billion recovery effort made possible through ARPA to the City of Chicago, 69 percent was spent on revenue replacement—more than any other major US city. The City of Chicago used ARPA funds as an opportunity to pay down debts instead of funding direct services and expanding the social safety net. The same progressive alderperson quoted earlier bemoaned the budget priorities the mayor made: "[Lightfoot's] using [federal] money to pay interest to fricking commercial banks. Why are we using money from COVID relief to pay interest?"[37]

Many other US cities also prioritized revenue replacement with ARPA funds, but some cities invested more heavily and earlier in housing resources (e.g., Philadelphia, Seattle), and others used federal allotments to create hazard pay programs for workers.[38] The City of Chicago prioritized corporate and business investment and relied heavily on the nonprofit and for-profit sectors to provide housing, food, and basic services support. Therefore, city officials *prioritized* the city's financial health and corporate and business interests *over* an investment in direct services for its most vulnerable residents. Further, their funding decisions *created* the scarcity framework officials presumed when triaging resources.

The mayor and city officials continuously projected the view that there were scant available resources, and they had to make judicious decisions on how to stretch minimal funding. Data were key to this scarcity management plan. Again and again in interviews with CDPH and city officials, I was told that resources were scarce and there was only so much city governments could do, and yet, what I will show in the next sections is that the city chose to reinforce the neoliberal structures already in place—they outsourced service provision to private entities and communities and employed means-tested bureaucratic requirements for welfare and housing distribution. In other words, the pandemic, which decimated Black and Brown communities and revealed existing infrastructural inequality with breathtaking detail, was treated as business as usual.

In the three subsections that follow, I explain how RERRT was designed and implemented, and I illustrate how frequently officials presumed scarcity in their approach to the pandemic. Next, I argue that city officials and epidemiologists treated COVID-19 as an infectious disease crisis, when it was experienced by vulnerable communities as a much broader emergency, leading to financial, housing, health care, and food insecurity. Finally, I discuss how the city's policy on testing played out on the ground, as an illustration of the constraints involved even when city officials did directly roll out services.

RERRT

In April 2020, RERRT was convened by the mayor's office and a prominent nonprofit working with hospitals on the West Side of Chicago. RERRT provided resources to six (out of seventy-seven) neighborhoods. Three predominantly Black communities were chosen because their death rates were the highest: Austin, South Shore, and Auburn Gresham. A few weeks later, three primarily Latinx neighborhoods with the highest case rates were added: Little Village, Belmont Cragin, and Pilsen. The task force brought together city officials, CDPH epidemiologists, hospital administrators, health care providers, and one chosen community-based organization (CBO) in each neighborhood that already had ties to the city. When asked how the CBOs were selected, a Mayor's Office representative responded that "we know them to be a collaborator" and "team player."[39] Together, RERRT team members designed testing and contact tracing efforts, held community education events, and organized relief efforts in these six priority neighborhoods. One of the main leaders of RERRT explained that the idea was to work together "to figure out where to deploy resources, to look at data on who was being impacted . . . in these communities."[40]

When asked why the city waited to "see" the data to respond to the inequality officials knew would emerge during the pandemic, a Mayor's Office RERRT official replied, "I think there's a danger in constantly seeing that map and just [saying], 'oh, that's just structural inequity that exists in Chicago' and being sort of inactive."[41] In other words, instead of presuming they knew what kinds of inequalities would emerge during the pandemic, RERRT officials waited to design policies until new data were collected. But officials imputed zip code data when race/ethnicity variables were missing from hospital reporting. Zip codes are only reliable proxies for race/ethnicity because of entrenched segregation in the city. So, while officials claimed to be designing policies based on new pandemic data, they were relying on historical inequities to create it. Further, data were not used in a *diagnostic* fashion to prevent emergencies as they transpired. Rather, they were used to *reactively* respond with technocratic solutions in a triaged fashion. This approach delayed the allocation of resources to vulnerable communities.

CDPH also drew on the RERRT model to design vaccine rollout. CDPH epidemiologists created the COVID Community Vulnerability Index (CCVI), which merged social vulnerability matrices from the American Community Survey with COVID-19 positivity, hospitalization, and death rates. In February 2021, the CCVI was used to launch Protect Chicago Plus, an initiative that prioritized the fifteen most vulnerable communities in Chicago for vaccine promotion and rollout.

The city's RERRT approach is a primary example of *governing through emergency*. City officials used epidemiological data to hierarchically rank neighborhoods (and even areas within the same neighborhood) for scarce resource distribution. Neighborhoods were pitted against one another for resource allocation. Such an approach also presumed that case and death rates were a valid metric of vulnerability. City officials deployed cost-benefit analyses to direct health care spending, triaged technocratic resources, and left broader infrastructural needs unmet. A community organizer who did not participate in RERRT put it this way: "In the scarcity mindset, we have to find the limited resources, quote-unquote, we have, and spread them out thinly over these fifteen communities that we just selected."[42] This presumption of scarcity was repeatedly mentioned by officials involved in RERRT. For example, one CDPH infectious disease expert involved in RERRT stated:

> There aren't enough resources, it seems, to be able to meet such a large need. I think what we have done, and what most jurisdictions have done, is very targeted and focused work in a hyperlocal way. That tries to meet the needs of individuals that are having, in this case, the worst health outcomes associated with COVID. We know that COVID is impacting every community area in the city, but it's impacting certain community areas much, much worse.[43]

Hyperlocal was a word used by RERRT experts to highlight how data were driving the community-engaged work of the task force. But the city's scarcity triaging was facilitated by their "hyperlocal" approach. This expert went on to explain the "hot spot / cold spot" maps they provided community ambassadors to direct their outreach. Using these "hyperlocal" data allowed experts to direct resources to only *the most vulnerable* residents at any given time and then retract and repurpose them elsewhere. Resources were, then, moved around even within the same neighborhood on a weekly basis.

Communities that were benefiting from these "scarce" testing resources, in this case, were often confused when those resources were reallocated elsewhere, especially if they had become accustomed to using those services. A Mayor's Office RERRT official described this problem:

> Because CDPH . . . whether it's vaccines or testing, they traditionally don't do, but because of the crisis that we were in, they start offering some of these resources outright. The city had procured resources to provide . . . city-run testing, but it was limited. We were only able to do, I think, six . . . across the city. There were six community groups as part

of RERRT, but the data had showed us that not all of our communities were still the most in need. . . . A number of the community members were, like, "We have been with you since the beginning . . . and so you're telling us that there's a resource . . . you can't provide to our community areas." . . . We were trying to communicate back that [the decision to move the resource was] based off where we see the need in the data.[44]

This official explained that when the data indicated a community no longer had a need because the positive COVID-19 rates declined, then resources were withdrawn and allocated elsewhere. An equity official at the Illinois state level said she was contacted by several organizations on the South and West Sides of Chicago to request testing because the city was not prioritizing their neighborhoods. She said Chicago residents were claiming that "our communities are being left behind."[45]

Within the communities that *were* allocated resources, there were still limitations in access. One community organizer on RERRT told us that neighborhood boundaries were often differently defined by residents than by city officials—the "maps didn't match." The city required people to show proof of residence to receive vaccines, but as the community organizer explained, "it was very, very difficult to have to turn those people away and tell them, 'We can't provide you with a vaccine here.'"[46] The way the Mayor's Office used data to carve up the city and distribute resources left people clamoring for scraps and competing with one another, but it also failed to attend to the real insecurities that the pandemic initiated for most residents because the city *only* responded with testing, contact tracing, minimal personal protective equipment, and vaccine distribution.

More Than a Viral Crisis

> Well, in my eyes I feel like the city, they care to a certain extent . . . because, yeah, they handed out free masks and free gloves. But what about people that's not working? . . . I feel like the city can do so much more than what they're doing right now.
>
> DAVID, resident of Austin, interviewed on October 12, 2020

> [The city] could've focused on . . . making sure that workplaces are safe where people continue to work.
>
> GABRIELA, resident of Little Village, interviewed on March 8, 2021

David and Gabriela point to deficiencies in the city's mitigation efforts because officials failed to provide extensive cash or rental assistance to those who lost work and refused to implement work protections and paid leave to frontline workers. These oversights led to concentrated vulnerability among lower-income residents, many of whom are also racially marginalized.

As previously mentioned, the Chicago Department of Housing provided $2 million in rental assistance to 2,000 families in the summer of 2020, but these funds were limited to $1,000 per household and 83,000 people applied.[47] Then, the State of Illinois provided two rounds of rental assistance from late 2020 through 2021. In the first phase, the Illinois Housing Development Authority (IHDA) distributed approximately $153 million to more than 30,000 applicants in Cook County at a flat payment rate of $5,000 to each applicant.[48] The second round of rental assistance funding was administered by IHDA in 2021 and dispersed $584 million in rental assistance by the end of 2021, with 70.8 percent of these funds going to Cook County residents.[49] The delay in housing support was at least partially a function of how CARES Act funding was allocated, causing most cities to wait eleven months after the pandemic began to offer rental assistance.[50] When emergency rental assistance was finally made available, the support did not meet existing need, and millions of lower-income households throughout the nation faced the risk of informal eviction, food insecurity, and medical disruptions as people scrambled to pay their rents.[51] Later in this chapter I explain how bureaucratic constraints kept many vulnerable Chicago residents from accessing rental assistance even when it became available. Therefore, despite substantial federal investment, rental assistance was often insufficient, came too late, or involved too many bureaucratic barriers to meet the need.

In addition, the City of Chicago failed to require citywide work protections or offer hazard pay for frontline workers. In meetings with both city officials and CDPH experts, I asked why work protections were not a priority for the administration. City officials told me this was outside of their purview and there was little they could do as a city.[52] A community organizer who was not associated with RERRT was very uncompromising in his critique of how little the city did to impose work restrictions and safety precautions on businesses. The city could have partnered with the Occupational Safety and Health Organization, the Department of Labor, and the Department of Business Affairs, he argued, "but that takes a very intentional coordinated effort."[53] He suggested that it was because the city was more interested in protecting its relationship with businesses than in safeguarding worker rights.

Rodrigo, a Mexican American man from Little Village, said that failing to provide housing support or work protections fell hardest on undocumented people, whom he thought the city ignored:

> The City of Chicago has a lot of smart people that works for them. You know, some of these people have PhDs, and they can't even figure out basic stuff. And what we're saying is for the undocumented people, like

they did in other states, like in California and Texas, was that they gave a lot of the essential workers money, you know, they gave them assistance. So even though you're not working, your rent's paid, you don't need to worry about that. In case you do get sick, don't worry, you can stay home. . . . The city has learned to ignore the undocumented community, especially Mayor Lori Lightfoot.[54]

In alluding to "California and Texas," Rodrigo refers to a policy in the State of California that secured hotel and motel rooms to house homeless people in the early months of the pandemic.[55] The city council in Austin, Texas, paid six local hotels for rooms to house frontline workers who needed to quarantine in the early months of the pandemic.[56] By contrast, Chicago residents who faced housing insecurity and work precarity felt they were not a priority for Mayor Lightfoot, and that their needs were ignored in her COVID-19 policies.

Testing Resources in Little Village and Austin

In this subsection, I explore how testing was rolled out in two RERRT communities. Even in communities where resources were allocated based on epidemiological metrics, there were barriers to who could access them, illustrating how the scarcity framework created fractures even within neighborhoods participating in RERRT. City officials were ambivalent about whether the city should provide its own testing, but they eventually determined that testing would help them grasp the scope of the problem they faced.[57] They deployed mobile testing to the six key areas identified by RERRT. Mobile testing was limited because residents were not connected to primary care providers for follow-up, and they could not depend on testing sites that were there one day and gone the next. A CDPH official explained this problem:

> It's complex to make that decision because if you only do static sites, you can only serve a certain number of communities. If you do mobile sites, you can spread the wealth a little bit more. . . . There is a little bit of a trade-off there because everybody wants a permanent site all the time, and there's just not enough resources to really do that.[58]

Despite being targeted by RERRT, many residents of Chicago's Austin community found it impossible to find testing. A community organizer who worked with RERRT explained that part of the problem was simply scale. Austin is one of the geographically largest and most spread-out neighborhoods in Chicago (represented by four zip codes), and finding locations to situate testing sites became politicized. The organizer explained that the mayor did not want to ask the Chicago Teachers Union to use empty schools because of political tensions between them, and she did not feel comfortable asking the Park District for use of community centers.[59] There were few remaining sites where testing could be provided. The organizer said:

> For a community as large as Austin is geographically, for as many residents actually are saturated here, there is very few places where it is intentionally designed . . . for disaster or emergencies that can now be easily converted. . . . The school is closed, but . . . it's shrouded in union labor issues. . . . It's like almost . . . sovereign countries within a community . . . it's like these no-cross zones and so because, again, you need to do things quickly. Right. And so there's all this, like, legality and minutia that you had to go through to do something as simple as setting up a testing site so that people could get tested. . . . It was a mix of structurally not having the spaces and the spaces we did have being shrouded in bureaucracy that was not easily navigated through.[60]

Testing was so difficult to access in Austin that one man, whom I refer to as Marlin, made a deal with a local laboratory and opened his own testing site out of a storefront on Cicero and Madison. Marlin added testing to the services his mutual aid organization provided. Marlin relayed the direness of the need in Austin: "The first testing sites they came up with, they hit the suburbs. . . . In order for somebody [from Austin] to get a test, they had to ride west to the suburbs where they had the drive-through testing for months. For about two months, we couldn't buy a test. We got tested last. Ain't no question about that."[61]

Marlin described the urgency he felt in providing testing services to his community because the city failed to deliver on its promises: "I had one politician tell me that I couldn't even open up a testing site, 'you need to go to the hospital to do that.' I say, 'We'll die waiting on the hospital.' . . . If we hadn't've took the initiative to operate on our own, we would still be a part of the systemic racism that exists, right today."[62] He continued:

> Because the city did not do what they were supposed to do. And Mayor Lightfoot came on that corner one day, and I had to literally walk out there to keep [back] the crowd—they was cussing her out . . . because they was real upset at that woman. Right? Because she didn't do what [she was] supposed to do for these people, she let the people down. . . . With this COVID thing, they let the people down. . . . I know they got a lot of monies to distribute for COVID right. But it never made it to the community.

In Little Village, the problems were of a different sort. First, the out-reach to communities was "politicized," according to local organizers, be-cause city officials did not want to work with local alderpeople.[63] Then, city officials insisted that all communication about testing sites include the city logo. Because many residents fear surveillance by city officials, some people avoided testing sites advertised with the city logo.[64] In addi-tion, residents had to sign up for testing online. A testing provider in Little Village explained why online sign-up could be a barrier: "Knowing that a lot of people don't have smartphones or don't have internet at home . . . we saw how communities of color, Latino communities a little bit even more so, did not have internet access at home, how a lot of people don't have smartphones. And even if they do have a smartphone, some-times they don't have data."[65]

Another organizer who worked in Little Village mentioned that language barriers were paramount. Organizers kept telling the city to translate educa-tional materials, public briefings, and testing information into Spanish, and city officials delayed complying, so local community organizations trans-lated for residents. The organizer in Little Village recalled:

> The information that was coming out about COVID-19 resources, it was coming out in one language . . . And for our community, the one language we speak is not the language the information was coming out in. So I had to translate all of the things that were coming out by the city and by CDPH . . . [and] a lot of our suggestions [to RERRT] were not taken.[66]

Even once the city started translating materials, it was done in a way that was difficult for local populations to understand.

*   *   *

In this section, I illustrated how even when communities were identified by city officials as vulnerable and given valuable, scarce resources, those resources did not always reach the people who needed them most because of political barriers and lack of attention to people's grounded realities. Despite claiming a "hyperlocal approach," city officials did not always heed the advice of community organizers. City officials also used "hyperlocal" data to triage resources under a scarcity framework. Governing through emergency presumes broad infrastructural lack and only infuses excep-tional technocratic aid to *the most* vulnerable subjects in a crisis-driven manner. Next I turn to how epistemic infrastructure was prioritized to make this crisis governance possible.

EPISTEMIC INFRASTRUCTURE

As I explained in chapter 2, over the course of the twentieth century, the profession of public health suffered from a steady narrowing of its scope and function. Despite recognition within the discipline that poor health is caused by "social determinants," public health departments outsourced housing, environmental protection, and occupational safety matters to other governmental entities, limiting their ability to actually address social determinants. By the end of the twentieth century, public health departments had developed a strong emphasis on epidemiological data collection and modeling. When COVID-19 emerged, data infrastructure fit within the public health department's already existing portfolio, and Chicago officials used federal dollars to magnify this capacity. This section explains how the city justified building up epistemic infrastructure *over* directly investing in communities. City officials required "hyperlocal" data to engage in cost-benefit health care provision. For communities to receive resources, they had to be considered the "most vulnerable" by exemplifying metrics that were recognized by CDPH. People could only claim "data citizenship" and access rights to services during COVID-19 if they were able to make themselves seen in epidemiological data.[67]

City officials pointed to the primary need for data from the outset. One of the administrators of RERRT told me that "data was always at the heart of it."[68] In the introduction to this book, I quoted a university epidemiologist who consulted on RERRT who explained that "what gets measured is what gets done."[69] He suggested that inequality remains invisible if it is not quantified. He told me policymakers could not "fix" problems they could not see in the data. And yet, when asked, he admitted that city officials knew where inequalities were likely to emerge and could have planned ahead. Instead, they waited until the inequality was registered in the data. Cal Garrett and I refer to this as "data drag"—delaying resources until knowledge of disparities is newly generated.[70] Data collection, then, is not diagnostic but a reactive process essential to scarcity management. Waiting to see the numbers before allocating resources also wasted valuable time. Further, relying on data to direct policies meant that the numbers became the sole focus, necessitating the building of a robust epistemic infrastructure *instead of* investing in direct services that might have ameliorated preexisting structural inequalities that contributed to the disproportionate racial impact of the pandemic.

As I mentioned in chapter 2, CDPH epidemiologists were quickly overwhelmed by what one called the "need and appetite" for data at increasing speeds and volumes, and they struggled to keep up with the data necessary to enact city policy.[71] Epidemiologists at CDPH partnered with a diverse array of corporations, universities, and other government entities to build new data systems, share data across systems, and develop new capacities for modeling. For example, a corporation shared cell phone "check-in" data so CDPH epidemiologists "were able to estimate what community areas were most compliant with the behavioral guidance of stay-at-home orders."[72] They partnered with corporations providing risk assessments based on flights coming from areas with outbreaks, and they partnered with private entities to expand their capacity to store and model big data at the level necessary for their growth in demand for output.[73] This effort also included partnering with private health providers to share testing and vaccine data. The CCVI metric the CDPH designed for vaccine provision was also developed by a private corporation.[74]

In some ways, this partnering with private entities and across jurisdictions to build a massive surveillant, epistemic infrastructure during COVID-19 is a success that other municipalities and states failed to accomplish. In 2022, reflecting on public health failures revealed by the COVID-19 and mpox outbreaks, several *New York Times* articles blamed incompatible, fragmented, and out-of-date data systems as a "deep fissure in the nation's framework for containing epidemics."[75] These articles blamed decades of disinvestment in public health. Obviously, the efficient and effective sharing of data is crucial for a successful public health response to any outbreak. Yet, this focus on our failing "vital infrastructure," which proved to be a weak spot in a country of riches, obscures a deeper focus on the legacy of disinvestment in *all* care infrastructures and the broader social safety net.[76] Here, data become *the* problem in need of solving, rather than a marketized health and welfare system, unaffordable housing, lack of universal childcare, and poor worker wages in essential industries. "Hyperlocal" epidemiological modeling helped track the spatial patterns of outbreaks as they moved throughout the city but precluded efforts to invest in ameliorating social determinants that caused vulnerability in the first place.

In addition, vulnerable populations had to show up in the data in particular ways to receive resources. For example, an Illinois state equity officer told me that migrant and refugee populations who work in industries such as meatpacking and agriculture were often not captured in public health data, yet were obviously at high risk for infection.[77] Tomás, an organizer who works closely with undocumented groups in Little Village, mentioned that undocumented people often wanted to remain unseen by the state, and so the localized efforts to collect census-tract-level data were interpreted as violent exposure: "The undocumented . . . oftentimes are in the shadows . . . because they would prefer it that way . . . but now with this pandemic . . . they were going to be kind of forced to step outside of the shadows."[78] In addition, the unhoused and people with disabilities were lacking in existing data counts and were not targeted for testing and vaccine allocation in a calculated way.[79] These constituencies are likely less important to politicians who seek to fix and mobilize data for political capital, so their needs were unseen and unmet. And the response by undocumented communities illustrates a contestation over the "value" of being "seen" in the data.

Further, city epidemiologists indicated repeatedly that occupational hazards became a "new harm" during the pandemic. One epidemiologist told me:

> We hadn't, as a department, really used occupation as a risk factor. I think going forward, one of the big paradigm changes we are going to implement is not just talking about race as a proxy for vulnerability but also occupation. . . . When you think about vulnerability in the most traditional sense of economic vulnerability or poverty . . . in most other outcomes . . . you tend to see the poorer a community gets . . . the worse the outcomes are. . . . Then, when you shift over to COVID, you see that it's—while that does play out—there's a bit more of an emphasis towards communities where there's actually high employment rates, and communities where there is a lot of social cohesion . . . that we saw as suffering the brunt of a lot of the COVID transmission in the city.[80]

This epidemiologist, who designed key components of the city's data infrastructure, noted that high employment and strong social cohesion are usually considered buffers against poor health outcomes, especially during disasters.[81] Yet, with COVID-19, this presumption was overturned. Despite this recognition, the city did not design policies targeting occupational safety, work leave, or cash assistance. Even when new risks were recognized within the data, policies that may have mitigated them were not necessarily prioritized.

The city built an immense epistemic infrastructure, and its daily dashboard tracked race and ethnicity data on cases, hospitalizations, and deaths throughout the pandemic.[82] However, these data were collected at the level of zip code, and zip codes in Chicago do not map precisely onto neighborhoods or wards. The city *did* collect census tract data but only shared those data with the six community organizations invited to join RERRT. Organizers were given maps with "hot spots," which they used to target education, testing, and vaccine drives in their neighborhoods. One RERRT community organizer explained:

> They would provide us with these . . . color-coded maps . . . It was like red and blue, and blue areas of the city [symbolized] . . . good vaccine

uptake, or they had low case and low death counts. Whereas like the red areas of the map were high death and high case counts, and low vaccine uptake. So we were just, like, able to use that to determine how we were gonna address those specific areas that were more red.[83]

This "hot spot" approach to tracking COVID-19 was always reactive and never diagnostic, and it facilitated the management of scarcity. As I have discussed in both the introduction and chapter 2, it also constitutes medical "hotspotting," which spatially ontologizes racial difference.[84] Such an approach also creates caesuras even within the same neighborhoods. As "hot spots" shift from one census tract to another, those who are "most vulnerable" and worthy of support also shift, generating divisions between and within neighborhoods and fragmenting "data citizenship."

Further, census-tract-level data were not shared with communities that did not participate in RERRT despite being collected by CDPH. Some organizers considered this lack of data sharing to be a means of gatekeeping information and only supplying it to allies who could be counted on to follow the mayor's agenda. One community organizer not affiliated with RERRT stated:

> Local-level data that analyzed by census track where vaccinations are happening . . . was . . . not made public. It was handed exclusively directly to those organizations [that were] . . . part of the mayor's rapid response team . . . so then that reinforces gatekeepers' space.[85]

In addition, the mayor often overlooked challenges associated with interpreting these data. For example, Lightfoot insisted that local organizations that used CDPH data get 77 percent of their communities vaccinated to improve racial equity numbers. And yet, one organizer said that population statistics were difficult to calculate because the denominator kept changing—for example, as children became newly eligible for vaccination.[86] Another organizer told me that the mayor's insistence on metrics was often "skewed." She explained, "We vaccinated, like, our older folks, but we had not really vaccinated people who were, like, fortyish . . . [and] we know a lot of our community members are young kids. It skews the data so much when we're just told *X* amount have been vaccinated, but . . . What does that technically mean in our community?"[87]

Vaccine drives were offered to the fifteen neighborhoods deemed "most vulnerable" based on CCVI data. One CDPH representative explained:

> With the vaccine initiative, they find out which neighborhoods have high positivity rates and direct vaccines there. Vaccines were a scarce

resource in the beginning, so everyone was fighting for scraps. They had to pick fifteen communities, but communities number 16 and 17 really needed the vaccine too. They took a big gamble on this approach, and they are still barely equal in uptake.[88]

Some of the earliest deaths and outbreaks in Chicago occurred in the South Shore neighborhood, and a community organization there was invited to join RERRT. However, South Shore was not among the top fifteen CCVI neighborhoods and did not receive vaccine resources from the city. The director of the South Shore organization told me:

> According to the city's COVID Vulnerability Index, South Shore was a high-needs community. And because we were doing such a good job with bringing that number down, we worked our way into a medium-needs community. So, while on paper that looks good, the sense of urgency is the same in the neighborhood. You know, the residents don't know that. You know, they just know that, "Hey . . . we want to get vaccinated."[89]

As this South Shore organizer explains, communities had to remain "most vulnerable" to continue to receive support and be "seen" by the state's data infrastructure. As soon as South Shore was no longer considered a "high-needs community" according to the CCVI rank, the resources that residents had been relying on to navigate the pandemic were reallocated elsewhere in the city.

The fact that numbers were key to the mayor's initiative was not lost on residents. People frequently mentioned in interviews that the city only cared about numbers and not residents' real needs. Sophia, the Mexican American woman from Little Village whom I quoted in the introduction, protested the imposition of data citizenship when she told me that residents are not just numbers—"We're human."[90] When asked what they would tell Mayor Lightfoot if they met her, Austin residents Charles and Joseph responded:

> Yep, they going by statistics . . . but they're not out here, reaching out to, touching, sitting down with [us], trying to find out what can they do to help us personally. You know, not looking at stats and statistics and stuff like that. You got people dying out here every day.[91]

> If they came and talked with these individuals, they'd probably get a better insight on what's really going on. . . . We can look at a lot of things that's done on paper, done in the labs, you know, day in and day out. . . . Talk to them in person, instead of looking at graphs.[92]

The residents quoted here, and many others, insisted that their needs were not captured by the statistics driving policy within the city of Chicago. Residents were not benefiting from the mayor's data citizenship model and felt their needs were invisible within the city's epistemic infrastructure. Though the residents may be incorporated into racial statistics, residents' everyday experiences of racial harm and neglect were erased. Data-driven policy is attractive because it is presumed to be objective, which obscures the backstage politics exposed in this chapter. And numbers are very useful for "racial equity" initiatives because they can "prove" success, even when structural inequalities remain unchanged. Quantification is necessary for governing through emergencies because it delinks the structural causes of racism from its epistemic effects, therefore enabling scarcity management and the obfuscation of slow emergencies.

NEOLIBERAL OUTSOURCING

According to Kimberly Morgan and Andrea Louise Campbell, Americans want public services but distrust "big government."[93] Therefore, since the inauguration of Medicare and Medicaid in 1965, the federal government has devolved federally funded initiatives to state and local governments and delegated the administration and delivery of services to nonprofit and for-profit entities. Delegation allows policymakers to respond to pressing demands without seeming to expand the size of the government, to channel government dollars to nongovernmental agencies and private corporations, and to shift conflict away from public arenas. These processes predate the neoliberalization of the state, but once neoliberalism became hegemonic in the 1970s and 1980s, administering federal programs became a for-profit industry.[94] This shift to a for-profit model has resulted in fragmented, bureaucratic, and inefficient services that are often run at high costs. Fraud among private entities charged with this administration is often excessive. Further, "authority over the management of public programs is delegated to actors who are not only not elected but indirectly accountable to the mass public."[95]

Many pandemic social safety net programs were funded by the federal government but administered through state and local governments, which further outsourced provisions to nonprofit and for-profit entities. There are a variety of challenges that accompanied these processes during the pandemic. First, this delegated approach to service provision blurs the lines between public and private oversight, which ultimately yields power to organizations that are not accountable to the publics they serve. A State of Illinois human services official expressed frustration over this process:

> Do you provide more and more funding to community-based organizations that are not state employees, or do you try to improve the state

system? . . . The government cannot relinquish its responsibility. Tax-payers pay the government, so the government can do its job. If the government just subcontracted out, then we've seen what happens, right?[96]

Because the safety net is managed by a patchwork of nonprofits, who are not answerable to public oversight, people are often caught up in corporate logics as they try to access "public" benefits.

One community organizer said that private companies sit on the Board of Health, which gives them tremendous power over policymaking: "Some of the FQHCs that are running the vaccine distribution are also represented in the Board of Health. So there starts being this neoliberal kind of shift, right, where the private sector is also infiltrated in the public sector representation of what the public health department should do . . . [but] they're not accountable to the public."[97] Private actors, then, design state policy but are not held responsible by the electorate.

In a city such as Chicago, with aldermanic representation of each of the fifty wards, the mayor could have used alderpeople to help develop health policy during the pandemic, instead of working with community organizations. But she purposefully sidelined these publicly elected representatives. In city neighborhoods not chosen to participate in RERRT, alderpeople had to find their own vaccine and testing resources, often by partnering with big corporations. One alderperson expressed her frustration about the situation:

I am absolutely enraged about the rollout for the vaccine and how little government was involved with the delivery of vaccines and the execution. They relied on big stores like Jewel [a grocery chain with pharmacy services] . . . and it became *The Hunger Games*. . . . There was no way to get a vaccination clinic in your ward. . . . I am relying on some staff member from Jewel to help me coordinate a vaccination clinic without any support from the health department.[98]

Another unintended consequence of the delegation of the administration of public aid through community organizations is that many residents came to see community organizers associated with RERRT as city workers. One community organizer from a predominantly Black neighborhood explained that residents interpreted their organization's health ambassadors as government agents policing people's behaviors.[99] In this instance, publicly elected officials were distrusted for failing to protect the public, and the private organization was perceived as a government collaborator.

Shantal, a long-term resident and organizer in Austin, explained that when the city chose only six organizations that would receive RERRT representation and COVID-19 resources, it chose organizations that are known to work well with the city and not those trusted by the community. She felt as though these chosen organizations did not represent the robust needs of local groups.[100] She also suggested that the money allocated to these organizations was not being spent in a meaningful way:

> The city gives the money to the same people all the time. And the same people do nothing. . . . If you come in my neighborhood, and you asked about the money . . . that's been spent on contact tracing . . . the success rate is less than 10 percent. . . . The mayor puts the money out there but she don't have, uh, anybody to go behind to make sure this money is being spent correctly. They just dish out the money so they could say, "Well, we gave the money." Okay, you gave it. What was done with it?[101]

One of the main problems in Chicago was that the city delegated the administration of services, but it also failed to provide direct services beyond testing and vaccination throughout most of the pandemic. Instead, it invested in a contact tracing system that also relied on private partnerships. Contact tracers were then tasked with connecting people to resources made available in their neighborhoods by nonprofit and mutual aid organizations. But this system never operated in the way it was envisioned and illustrates the problem with delegating as opposed to providing services outright.

In 2020, Chicago awarded $56 million to establish a contact tracing corps of 850 to 900 people.[102] In addition to tracing recent contacts and providing health advice, these health ambassadors were supposed to respond to urgent need among residents. A CDPH official explained the system to me:

> [Contact tracing] includes reaching out to individuals diagnosed with COVID to gather data, to provide public health guidance, *to help them navigate to resources* if they have needs that compromise their ability to follow our public health guidance, to elicit contacts who may have been exposed to COVID.[103]

With the help of a private corporation that collects data on existing local services and resources, CDPH developed a resource coordination hub. Health ambassadors would plug the zip code of the contact who expressed need for services into the hub, and they would receive a list of existing resources being provided by neighborhood and citywide organizations. This model created a range of problems for the health ambassadors employed by the city. According to one CDPH official:

> One of the struggles . . . [that] we've experienced through this entire process is there's not enough resources. . . . If I was to refer someone to

a particular organization, we didn't know exactly the full range of services that they had. So, for example, an organization is offering diapers. But there are limitations on how much of those diapers they have, right? How long are these services available?[104]

Not only were the resources limited, but the capacity to stay up-to-date on information was lacking. Rather than relying on a patchwork of mutual aid groups, the city could have invested in more direct services. One CBO leader explained why his organization chose not to submit proposals for Chicago's contact tracing funds: "So, when people ask you, 'Okay, well, how am I gonna pay my rent, groceries and the rest?' we're gonna provide them a sheet? A list of food pantries? Those pieces [housing/cash assistance] were not part of the plan."[105] As this community organizer articulates, the expectation was that people who needed housing and food support, people who might still be sick, must shop around for the free resources that might be available in their communities.

The City of Chicago was required to invest in contact tracing to track infectious disease spread, but relying on this core of health ambassadors to connect desperate people to a patchwork of mutual aid and nonprofit organizations in their neighborhood did not work. Further, it illustrates the problems with city officials delegating social service provision to the private and nonprofit sector instead of investing in direct services. The safety net, then, is privately managed and operationalized, which creates bureaucratic barriers and introduces corporate logics into the delivery of care. Governing through emergency leaves existing infrastructural inequality intact because it detaches current crises from ongoing structural racism. The colorblind rollback and privatization of welfare provision that accompanied the neoliberalization of the economy helped create and sustain ongoing slow emergencies for communities of color, and during the pandemic, the city decided to rely on existing patchwork care infrastructure. But this privatized, disjointed system failed to meet the needs of Chicago's most vulnerable residents.

BUREAUCRATIC BARRIERS

Federal, state, and local governments developed multiple social assistance strategies during the pandemic, but these largely offered minimal harm reduction when more extensive resource allocation was necessary to offset existing structural inequalities and their exacerbation by pandemic precarity. Further, financial and housing support were offered in a *reactive* fashion *after* residents had already experienced mounting debt, job loss, and financial insecurity. Although certain CARES Act provisions—such as stimulus payouts, unemployment insurance, and eviction moratoria—went into effect quickly, the way emergency rental assistance (ERA) programs were administered created delays in payouts. Most renters in the US had to wait at least eleven months to begin receiving rental assistance through local programs funded by the CARES Act.[106] Further, residents often faced bureaucratic barriers in receiving this support. This meant that rather than treating financial and housing vulnerability as a public health risk for the poor, policies offered meager repayments, after residents faced arrears and debt. Such an approach pushed people to continue to work and be housed in vulnerable conditions. Providing policies on paid sick leave and work protections, offering cash and rental assistance, and providing free medical treatment at the outset of the pandemic would have better protected Chicago's most vulnerable residents. Because such benefits were unavailable, marginalized residents were forced to expose themselves to dangerous infectious situations—at work, in public spaces, and at home.

Further, ERA programs, while certainly helpful to those who received payouts, did not address the already existing crisis in affordable housing. In 2018, nearly half of all renters in the US paid more than 30 percent of their incomes in rent.[107] In 2019 in Chicago, almost 80 percent of lower-income renting households spent at least 30 percent of their income on rent.[108] Therefore, lower-income Chicagoans (and Americans) were already struggling to keep up with rental payments even before the pandemic struck. Being unable to pay one's rent leads to intense anxiety and poor mental health, and many households prioritize rent payments over food and medical expenses.[109] This means that vulnerable people often reduce their food consumption or disrupt medical care to secure enough money to pay their rent.

Further, pandemic social benefits were *means-tested*, meaning that the burden rested on residents to prove their eligibility. Part of a decades-long tradition in the US, this way of implementing social benefits presumes that people will defraud the system and defensively punishes those who do.[110] Intensive bureaucratic proof is required to access benefits, which creates tremendous barriers for vulnerable people. Obstacles include busy work schedules; childcare, language, and technology barriers; lack of trust; and the ability to produce proof of eligibility in short windows of time. In a crisis, such requirements meant that vulnerable communities could not access resources quickly or at all. In addition, the social assistance programs introduced were only made available *after* the vulnerability had occurred, as opposed to proactively being implemented to prevent vulnerability in the first place.

I begin by detailing struggles residents faced in accessing unemployment benefits, and then move on to discussing rental assistance challenges. Pandemic Unemployment Assistance was inaugurated with the passage of the CARES Act in late March 2020 to cover US citizens who were fired because of the pandemic, and it included a $600 supplemental payment; these funds were administered by states.[111] The Illinois Department of Employment Security (IDES) was quickly overwhelmed by the number of applications, and Illinois residents spent hours trying to get through to staff on the phone to verify their claims. Many were kept waiting for months.[112] Several people I interviewed experienced delays in accessing their unemployment benefits. Sholanda recounted her struggle:

> It was a *fight* to get on unemployment. Because there was no one in the offices. No one around. It was *hard* . . . I mean, it was, like, two months before I even got to *talk* to anybody. And I was, like, oh my God, this is ridiculous. I mean, there's no offices to go to. . . . You would call the phone number . . . I remember one time I held on for three hours . . . for a lady to tell me, uh, "Well, we're looking at your application." That's all she said. And then told me to have a great day.[113]

Kelly had managed to get on unemployment easily, but then in March 2021, unemployment benefits in Illinois halted because IDES changed its online application system and information had to be manually inputted. She explained, "So a lot of people, their unemployment, like, completely stopped for *months*. I know, I was one of them. Like, I didn't receive unemployment from April through . . . June." She explained the amount of labor it took just to get back on unemployment, and meanwhile, she had no income. "I didn't end up getting the majority of the money that was owed to me in one lump sum," she said. "This is what pissed me off with this whole unemployment situation and how it was handled was because it put a strain on the relationship between me and my landlord."[114] She also explained that to keep her unemployment, she had to certify her incoming funds every two weeks and continue to search online for jobs through the web-based Illinois Job Link system. Therefore, she was required to complete ongoing bureaucratic assessments, while the system itself broke down.

Rodrigo said that the process of applying for food stamps was onerous and disadvantaged people in his neighborhood:

> So [even] as a person with a Social Security number, it was very hard for us to get any benefits. You had to . . . pass through a lot of bureaucracy. . . . But the public aid office was closed. You couldn't go there. They didn't even answer the phones. . . . They'll tell you [to] do it through online. I've never even used online.[115]

Although such benefits are means-tested and require ongoing proof of eligibility from residents, during the pandemic, many systems failed—they were overwhelmed and broke down on multiple occasions, leaving already vulnerable people further exposed.

ERA was a hallmark public policy innovation and helped a lot of people during the pandemic. Nonetheless, many tenants struggled with accessing the information required to complete applications. The application process was modified between each round of funding as a result of changes in federal stipulations on the use of funds and concerns with fraudulent applications, which meant that applicants had to effectively relearn how to apply for ERA funds each time.[116] According to Household Pulse Survey Data, there are obvious racial disparities between which populations were behind on rent and those that received rental assistance. Figure 3.1 shows that Black and Latinx tenants in Chicago were two or three times more likely to be behind on rent than white tenants.[117] Yet, 70 percent of Black renters and more than 80 percent of Latinx renters *did not apply* for assistance at all according to HPS data.[118] Figure 3.2 also indicates that white applicants were greenlighted to receive assistance more often, whereas Black and Latinx renters were more likely to be stuck in the "waiting" category.

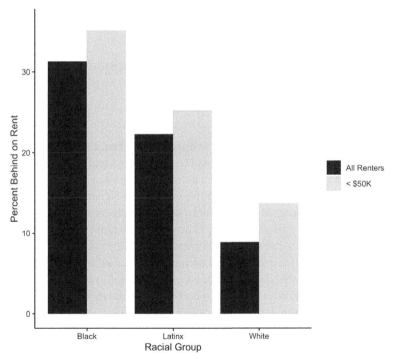

Figure 3.1 Percentage of Renters Behind on Rental Payments, September 2020–June 2021

Source: US Census Household Pulse Survey Data Public Use File.

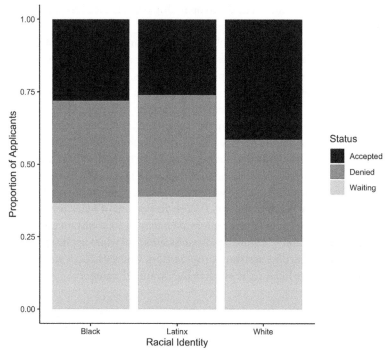

Figure 3.2 Status of Emergency Rental Assistance Applications, June 2021–August 2022

Source: US Census Household Pulse Survey Data Public Use File.

There are several reasons for these disparities. At first, ERA applications required that a formal lease be provided by the landlord, and this meant that tenants who rent informally (without a written lease) were ineligible to apply. Tenants often expressed difficulties in getting their landlord to participate in the ERA program. For example, Luis, an undocumented Mexican man from Albany Park, explained, "The problem is that the homeowner then doesn't want to provide the information that they ask for on the W-9 form because they have to give their tax number or something."[119] Because Luis is undocumented, he and his landlord have an informal rental agreement and the landlord is likely not reporting the rental income as taxable. When receiving rental assistance required a formally documented relationship between tenant and landlord, this interviewee was unable to benefit from that program. Luis relied on personal relationships to survive:

> Well, he [the landlord] doesn't really [help us]. . . . And the truth is . . . my son has been loaning money to me to pay the rent. So, I already owe my

son, like, $4,000. And I wanted to see a way to be able to get that money back to return that money.[120]

Housing programs are designed to assist residents who lost income during the COVID-19 pandemic, but Luis's experience of housing insecurity was incommensurable with formal programs. A human services representative explained the insurmountable problems that the undocumented often encounter:

> So, the landlords themselves didn't want to participate . . . [because] they don't want to receive any money from the federal government and have to deal with it later. And then of course there's lots and lots of landlords who just were unresponsive. . . . The reality is, if you're undocumented, and your landlord says "Get the *F* out," you get out. You don't get a day notice, you don't get ten days' notice, you don't get a month's notice, you're out. And if you're not out, they will call the police, who will call ICE [US Immigration and Customs Enforcement]. They'll threaten to call ICE, or they'll just change the locks on you because what are you going to do?[121]

For many undocumented Chicagoans, the stakes of not paying one's rent are too extreme, so like Luis, people borrow from their family members. But rental assistance programs also do not provide a means of paying back such loans, leading to compounded housing insecurity and compromised social networks.

In addition, many residents, such as Tomás, related difficulties in accessing the documentation and applying online in the time frame allotted by each program:

> You know, with a lot of different deadlines with a lot of documentation, again, when it comes to even, you know, housing assistance for rent, right? . . . Getting certain documents and getting them in a short period of time before the money ran out or before the application period quit. Then it was a barrier.[122]

Extensive bureaucratic requirements to prove eligibility for ERA programs and short windows for applying made these programs feel inaccessible to many residents. A community organizer explained that even when successful, often ERA payments were insufficient: "When tenants did get relief, sometimes they didn't get the full ten months or eleven months or . . . they would get [only] four months of relief and so they're still behind on their rent."[123]

A RERRT community organizer from Little Village listed a series of issues that kept people from even applying for the programs, though they may have been eligible:

> We have people that don't have IDs. We have . . . families that are
> technically couch-surfing and live with other families. We have folks
> that . . . because of their residency status, the bills had to be under their
> neighbor's or the landlord's or [a] cousin's name, because they couldn't
> activate, like, a utility line. . . . We have people that don't apply because
> they think that they're going to have to pay back this money. . . . They
> don't trust the government. . . . [Participants] tell us, "It's like [gov-
> ernment representatives] don't believe us. It's like, what else do they
> need to see? To know that we need the money, and we need to like
> sign with our blood so that we get money. . . . The city and the state
> don't believe that we're struggling? And we need to give you guys all
> of this documentation so that we can get funded to survive a couple
> more months?"[124]

As this organizer explains, not only were there multiple barriers to applying, but people felt as though they had to "sign with our blood" to prove to the city and state that they were struggling. This situation points to the difficulty with paternalistic, means-tested welfare distribution and how it can feel to those who face extensive vulnerabilities. People believe the state has some hidden agenda and formula of worthiness, which they fail to meet. And these experiences compound distrust of government agencies and programs.

The fact that housing and financial assistance programs were means-tested, and only made available in a reactive fashion, not only created tremendous barriers but also increased health risks for those who continued to work in dangerous jobs or for those who had to reduce their food intake or disrupt their medications to prioritize rental payments. These challenges were compounded as the pandemic stretched on, especially as inflation rates rose in 2022 and 2023. Rental rates outpaced wages, and rental pricing soared once the official public health emergency was terminated.[125] Although federal, state, and local governments extended social assistance during the pandemic, they employed neoliberal dispersal systems that placed the onus on the recipients to prove their worthiness. Existing systems of support are porous and ineffective in addressing the precarity caused by converging endemic emergencies. Governing through emergency enacts temporary, scarce provisions when longer-term solutions are required to meet the needs of the most vulnerable Americans.

GOVERNING COVID-19 EMERGENCIES IN CHICAGO

In May 2021, I interviewed a progressive alderperson about the city's response to the pandemic, and she told me a story about a woman who had seven children and had lost her job and her home. In the dead of winter in 2020, her family was found squatting in an abandoned building without heat or water. The mother had gone out to look for food and left the six youngest children with the eldest, her fourteen-year-old daughter. The owner of the building found the kids huddled up together and called the police. The children were taken to the hospital and the woman was taken into custody and eventually charged with seven counts of misdemeanor child endangerment.[126] The alderperson exclaimed, "How do you punish somebody for not having a place to live? . . . You would think that at least the basic measures would be put into place so that a mother with seven children didn't have to go through that, but no, no. Those measures are not in place. There is no safety net."[127]

This story haunted me as I conducted interviews for this project. Why were basic, direct services for Chicago's most vulnerable residents not prioritized in a city that proclaimed a "racial equity" approach? Rent cancellation, cash and rental assistance from the earliest months, and work protections and paid leave in essential industries would have gone a long way toward protecting lower-income Latinx and Black Chicagoans from suffering the brunt of pandemic precarity. Instead, the city prioritized data collection over direct services and employed existing neoliberal mechanisms to administer aid. The RERRT initiative was reactive as opposed to diagnostic, relied on data to triage scarce aid, and pitted neighborhoods and residents against one another in a battle to secure supplies. Chicago city officials prioritized the fiscal health of the city, protected industry, invested in data infrastructure, and triaged technocratic supports *instead of* expanding the social safety net.

Once, when I presented this research, a colleague asked, "But didn't Chicago do better by its citizens than cities in conservative, southern states?" My first impulse was to question whether conservative political responses in the US should be the standard against which we measure success, but this book attempts to uncover the mechanisms by which a city that claims it cares about racial disparities still fails to meet the basic needs of those marginalized by race, class, and nationality during a pandemic.

In this chapter, I identified four mechanisms that help explicate these failures. First, city officials presumed scarcity of basic resources despite the windfall of federal dollars pouring into city infrastructure. Rather than attempt to build care infrastructure decimated by years of market fundamentalism, city officials governed through emergency, triaging technocratic resources (testing, contact tracing, and vaccines) throughout the city as infection and death rates ebbed and flowed. This approach required the building of a robust and "hyperlocal" epistemic infrastructure, the second mechanism that I discussed, because it allowed officials to track the virus as it circulated throughout the city, but only through very specific metrics of "vulnerability." To be given "data citizenship" and receive resources, residents had to be "seen" within this data infrastructure.[128] Vulnerability that fell outside COVID-19 positivity, hospitalization, and death rates remained invisible. Third, the city enlisted a group of community organizations, who were given access to "hyperlocal" data, in order to administer these technocratic resources. This outsourcing of provision made political accountability circumspect and carried a series of barriers for those doing the providing and those receiving the resources. Fourth, when rental assistance was finally rolled out in the city, it used decades-old means-tested bureaucratic systems to deflect fraudulent claims, which kept many people from even applying for aid.

These four features of Chicago's pandemic response enabled city officials to claim the political capital of "racial equity." Through data, the city advertised its success through numbers. It lauded its ability to vaccinate and lower infections in racially marginalized communities while simultaneously employing scarcity management and ignoring pernicious infrastructural disinvestment. This is what Austin resident Marlin labels the "dog and pony show" whereby city officials declare they have achieved "racial equity" without addressing the slow emergencies of Chicago's residents.[129]

4: SLOW EMERGENCIES

What kind of issues have you observed in your community since
COVID-19 began?

Health issues, of course. Mental health. Drug abuse, alcohol abuse.
Domestic violence, crime. . . . Just like the very mask I wear and you
wear, that's what's happening. Everything is being masked, masked,
masked. . . . Racism, of course. It's intensified. . . . It is still an issue
undiscussed, again, hidden.

JUAN, Mexican American resident of Austin,
interviewed on February 8, 2021

In his response to my question, Juan explains that the converging emergencies that many Black and Brown communities experience have been
masked during the COVID-19 pandemic—remaining undiscussed and
hidden.[1] Because federal, state, and local officials governed through emergency and treated the pandemic as a temporary crisis and a purely viral
threat, already existing slow emergencies were ignored and exacerbated.
The causes of slow emergencies are difficult to pinpoint because they are
historical and structural in nature, and the people suffering from them often feel devalued and unseen. This chapter seeks to unveil the invisible and
compounding "demics" that lower-income, racially marginalized people
suffered during COVID-19.

Marlin, the man I described in the previous chapter who opened a testing site in Austin when the city failed to deliver, spoke extensively about
how the state's pandemic response obscured the ongoing crises of Austin
residents. Most notably, he mentioned that fentanyl overdoses had risen as
steadily as COVID-19 deaths. Opioid-related deaths skyrocketed in 2021
and 2022 in Chicago, and they were concentrated on the West Side of the
city, where Austin is located.[2] As Marlin saw it:

They started sweeping stuff up under the rug. They'll call an overdose
COVID-related. . . . I mean, I don't know how much money a hospital

generates when a person come in with COVID. But I'm quite sure it's more than what a hospital generates when a person come in for an overdose [*laughs*]. . . . Now they made everything COVID . . . I mean, COVID took precedent over everything.[3]

Citing posts that circulated on social media during the pandemic, Marlin insisted that hospitals were making money for each COVID-19 death reported. In fact, under the federal Coronavirus Aid, Relief, and Economic Security (CARES) Act, hospitals were given a 20 percent increase in their Medicare payouts for treating elderly people with COVID-19.[4] Hospitals were not "paid" to treat people with COVID-19. Nonetheless, Marlin's general point is important and valid. The way the government only attended to the *viral* threat COVID-19 posed exacerbated the converging crises and slow death that lower-income Black and Brown Americans experience. That fentanyl deaths rose during the pandemic speaks to the trauma, isolation, and misery people suffered as a result of financial, housing, and food precarity.

Shantal, a Black woman from Austin who was quoted in earlier chapters, explained that people who suffer from converging "demics" experience trauma that they cannot process because there is no accessible mental health care in neighborhoods like Austin:

> In my neighborhood, there's no mental health help. I mean, mental health care here is a three- to six-month waiting period. You don't have resources, you don't have people to talk to. . . . People don't have insurance. It's just horrific. If they had been really looking, they should have anticipated violence, an uptick in violence. . . . Here in Austin, as I said, there's no real access to mental health care. None. Especially no therapists that are Black and Brown.[5]

The escalation of deaths, quarantine conditions, and stress from heightened financial precarity created new and prolonged mental health strains that remained invisible to local stakeholders because there are no mental health resources in many lower-income communities.

Marlin explained that the toll the pandemic took on people's lives will be long-term—not simply because of the precarity it aggravated but because of the trauma from loss. Like Shantal, he said this points to a serious need for commitment to mental health support:

> So many people are traumatized. I've been to so many funerals, right? COVID-related funerals. People are traumatized. . . . This is the time when people really need to be serviced for mental health. Mental health

should be a big thing going forward because we in a mental health crisis. Everybody walking around in trauma.[6]

As I explained in chapter 1, COVID-19 mitigation policies did not heed the acceleration of deaths or trauma to survivors that mounted in Black communities over the course of the pandemic.

Attending to slow emergencies is not a political priority for state actors. As Elizabeth Povinelli explains, suffering must be enumerated or given political or economic value to warrant state resources. Those whose trauma is devalued are suspended in the "mundanity of everyday [structural] violence."[7] Politicians often explain slow emergencies away as intransigent legacies of past racist policies and fail to attend to them with current initiatives. Slow violence is concealed, unspectacular, and socially distanced from the corporate and state actors who are responsible for instigating it. As Rob Nixon argues, in his work on environmental toxicity, harmful substances are hidden in a shadow kingdom behind a harmless facade which makes laying blame difficult.[8] Racism operates in a similar way—its effects are deeply embedded in environmental landscapes, segregated housing, fractured infrastructures, and people's bodies.[9] As I explained in chapter 1, COVID-19 momentarily exposed state and institutional racism in stark relief, but it was treated with temporary, urgent emergency governance that focused only on a viral threat. Therefore, this recognition was short-lived, and racism's more enduring forms and effects quickly faded back into the background. People's experiences with racist policies and institutions, racist state actors (e.g., welfare providers, health care workers), and racist ideologies promulgated through the media can accumulate in the body. Linda Villarosa explains that racism gets "under the skin," weathering the body and mind, causing chronic pain and debilitation.[10] My point is that suffering the entangled emergencies caused by repeated interactions with racist institutions, policies, and state actors leads to accumulated and embodied vulnerability that is completely ignored by emergency governance.

Often the literature on slow death or violence suggests that people inertly accept the tense of suspension (the *slowness* of emergency conditions) to which they are abandoned and do not engage in intentional agency that is goal oriented because they are so fully invested in simply getting by.[11] And yet, I illustrate that people who face slow emergencies must constantly hustle to piece together the fragmented forms of welfare they are extended. States do not simply abandon racially marginalized people but extend them aid in patchwork, exceptional ways. In fact, the extension of aid through disjointed systems further obscures the embedded nature of infrastructural racism. Fractured welfare/health care is part of how racial biocapitalism functions to include racially marginalized subjects through exclusionary policies. Racism is concealed in the extension of private, paternalistic, and meager aid and exhausts those who must hustle to access it. The piecemeal and means-tested pandemic aid that was extended to vulnerable communities constitutes another example of exclusionary inclusion.

Lauren Berlant defines *slow death* as a "condition of being worn out by the activity of reproducing life" that results in the "physical wearing out of a population" from the vagaries of laboring in demeaning and exhausting jobs in a neoliberal capitalist system.[12] Berlant critiques existing theories of agency that emphasize conscious, intentional, and self-expansive action.[13] In instances of slow death, Berlant argues, people are often suspended in the inaction of the ordinary reproduction of life—they are not goal oriented but engage in the "lateral agency" of simply surviving. And yet, the people I interviewed did not just give up or get by—they pushed back in multiple ways. The exceptional governance of COVID-19 caused many people to reimagine their relationships to welfare systems and work, and others came together in new social formations to fill in where the state lacked. They sought to take care of one another, in the shadow of state devaluation. People's quiet taking care of one another is an important political act—it violates the logic of letting die.

In this chapter, I provide empirical evidence of the three arguments I have just described: (1) the exacerbation and compounding of emergency conditions during the pandemic were embodied by racially marginalized communities as accumulated vulnerability, and this vulnerability was ignored by COVID-19 policies that were designed to be urgent, temporary, and focused on a viral threat; (2) the extension of aid to lower-income, racially marginalized communities helps conceal how racism subtly operates in the infrastructural background, and people have to pull together these fractured systems and successfully navigate them to survive; and (3) this hustling and taking care constitutes a political act that is often ignored in theories of slow violence and death. I take up each of these points in the empirical sections that follow.

RACISM CONCEALED IN INFRASTRUCTURE AND BODIES

Racism fades into the institutional background and the bodies of those who endure multiple, converging "demics." In policy debates, people are often blamed for these emergencies, even though they are caused by historical and systemic logics and policies. Reginald, a Black man who grew up in Austin, has been living in a slow emergency most of his life. His trajectory through prisons and homelessness illustrates how ongoing interactions with racist institutions can accumulate in the body and mind. Reginald spoke to me from his new recovery home, which he entered after a monthlong detoxification treatment program, after having overdosed on fentanyl twice. He is currently in his fifties and has led a hard life—he was in a street gang in his youth, did several stints in jail, which ended with a thirteen-year sentence, for which he was released after he contested the case with a new lawyer. He was then unhoused and using drugs for years. Reginald barely registered the pandemic because he was using opioids when it began. He explained, "I was heavily on drugs, and I was in denial. I was running the streets. And I was gone weeks at a time. I wouldn't even take showers or nothing, and I just had the same clothes on. And it didn't even bother me because I was like, 'I'm homeless, I don't care about nothing.' . . . And you know, it's pills in fentanyl and that stuff just knocks you out. And I was like, man, eventually all my friends started dying on me."[14]

The last time he overdosed on fentanyl, he passed out. When he woke, he realized he had lost his bicycle, along with his backpack which contained his license, Social Security card, and dentures. He tried to gain entry to his sister's house but then suddenly realized he was on the wrong block. He told me this really freaked him out because he felt he could have been murdered for trying to burglarize a home in Austin.

Reginald spoke extensively about his experiences with the police and the prison system. When he was sentenced to thirteen years in jail, it was because the friend who committed the crime blamed Reginald for stealing a car. Reginald believes the police falsified evidence to convict him. When he was able to request a better lawyer from prison, he got his sentence lifted. In Reginald's view:

> The police is very manipulative. They go out there and they know what they doing. They be lying on people. They . . . rehearse they li'l statements and stuff. And go in the courtroom and they lie and everything. They dirty—it's a lot of dirty cops out there. . . . They manipulate especially foreigners and Black people. . . . This, uh, judicial system is so corrupt.[15]

Reginald went on to assert that there are insufficient services for people who transition out of prison into everyday life. Rather than provide for people, he said, the government "turns a blind eye." This is how state devaluation operates—people are rendered invisible within existing infrastructure. But the effects of racism are incorporated into the bodies of those who travel through punitive institutions. The chronic physical and mental health conditions that result are ignored by welfare systems and other state programs. Reginald told me:

> And then when you come home, it's like they really don't have no good programs for people that [are] coming home or people that's in the

streets that need help. You know, housing and stuff like that. They need
to give people housing, they really do. And if they do that, a lot of crime
would be cut down so low because people will be glad they have places
to stay. Somewhere to lay they head. *The government they just, they turn a
blind eye, that's all that is. They just turn a blind eye. They don't even see you.*
You really like, uh, the dirt under they shoes or something. And that's
how they treat you. For real.[16]

Reginald also spoke extensively about his time being unhoused. Many
of his friends had legs amputated from frostbite and then needed help
applying for disability support because they could not navigate the system.
He also spoke about being treated poorly by hospital staff:

> I think the government should help people because there's a lot of people
> out here that really need help. And they being ignored on an everyday
> basis. They being looked down upon. It's people that don't even want
> to go to the hospital because they treat 'em like shit, you know, when
> they see a person that is homeless and they need medical attention, they
> make them wait all day and they talk to 'em and treat 'em like they ain't
> shit. Because I done experienced it myself. I done been to the hospital
> where, you know, they just look down upon me and everything. I'm like,
> you shouldn't judge nobody because they homeless. I mean, it's some
> good people out there that's homeless. And you know, who are you to
> judge someone.[17]

Reginald feels as though he has been mistreated by the criminal-legal and
health care systems. His acute experiences of racist devaluation permeated
his interview as he retold his life story. Although he is currently trying to
rebuild his life through recovery and has some dedicated resources to do
it, it took almost dying from fentanyl overdose to get the support he could
have used throughout his life. And he will soon lose the room in the recovery home. He will be given housing in a subsidized unit, but he must remain
sober and retain employment to keep it. He is currently (and has regularly
been) employed as a forklift operator in a warehouse, but he does not earn
enough to save money. He will continue to hustle to survive.

Having been through the criminal justice system was a common experience for the Austin residents I interviewed, which reflects how concentrated imprisonment is in Austin.[18] Thirteen out of forty-nine interviewees
from Austin discussed their time being incarcerated, without this being a
formal question in the interview guide. Rather than invest in jobs and skills
development, education, housing, and business opportunities, the state
largely responds to the poverty in Austin through policing, imprisonment,

and coerced and punitive recovery programs. Of the forty-nine interviews conducted in Austin, eighteen people mentioned being in recovery, though this subject was also not included in the interview guide. Through recovery programs, people can get adult education, skills training in computers, employment literacy, legal advice on debt, and housing support. But there are very stringent behavioral and work restrictions imposed, and even with this support, people struggle to survive.[19]

Several interviewees explained that they turned to drugs to mask the trauma and pain that came from constantly living in slow emergency. Reginald was one of them:

> When you get to that point in life . . . you get depressed, you cover up all your feelings. And you know, you don't want to deal with things. So you get high, to mask, to mask it up, you know, in reality because it's a lot of things. Life . . . can be a bitch, eh? You just don't want to deal with it. So you start getting high, and be like, "Fuck everything"—that's, that's the dope fiend prayer: Fuck everything.[20]

Clayton, another Black man from Austin, who was in recovery at the time of our interview, told me:

> I started using drugs, mainly because of a lot of deaths in the family. And I was doing what I could, you know, for my mother, and my little brother at the same time had cancer. And my mother-in-law, she had cancer, and then my grandmother was just getting up in age and she had a heart attack and fell, and she passed. . . . I was working in maintenance at night . . . so that I would have days free, you know, to take them to doctor's appointments, to pay bills and get their medicine, whatever they needed. You know, I mean, I was the one who was doing everything.[21]

Clayton noted that chronic illness is very concentrated among his family members because of the occupational risks they experienced. His brother was exposed to asbestos, and his mother worked with toxic substances in a factory making television sets. This story illustrates the concentrated illnesses that also accumulate in conditions of slow emergency. Clayton described how the trauma of loss and the stress of being a primary support member for his family led him to drug use:

> Mostly the stress and I couldn't sleep. And, you know, I was drinking. . . . And I used to see the guys, the older guys, you know, getting high. . . . It was just the powder that they were doing, sniffing it, you know? And so that's what I started doing . . . after the deaths in the family and me doing

so much. . . . It was a lot on me, you know. . . . Everybody that I was really loving and that love me, were leaving me, you know, and left me, you know, to do everything and take care of everything.[22]

He started doing harder and harder drugs and then overdosed on fentanyl several times and was finally referred to a recovery program.

Mandatory treatment programs (like the one Clayton was required to attend, through court order) begin in a confined, institutionalized space. When people complete that program, they go into a recovery home where their housing is covered, but they must pay for meals. They are given legal advice, housing and work referrals, job skills development, and other forms of support. They are not allowed to have their children or romantic partners stay with them, and they must go through daily urine testing, attend Narcotics Anonymous meetings, and be in therapy. They are required to find supportive housing and work. Even as they leave these homes, they will stay in touch with caseworkers who drop by to administer urine tests and follow up on work conditions, and they must meet these requirements to keep their housing. Andre, a fifty-seven-year-old Black man from Austin, said that he was grateful for the help and support but found it really difficult to make ends meet, even with this assistance:

> I just took a wrong turn somewhere because my life really been hard for me. You know, 'cause I lived with drugs . . . I had pressure from the gangs and stuff like that. So I had to survive by any means necessary. . . . I've been in prison about six or seven times, different times. And it wasn't no long times, like a year here, a year there, eighteen months there, two years there, a year there, year and a half there. Until '03. In '03 I got nine years. Came home in '05. And I said I'll never get locked up again and I haven't been to prison since then. . . . When I came home from prison in '05 I was on parole. . . . But you know when you don't have keys to your place, you considered homeless, right? . . . I had places to go, places to sleep. But I felt like I was homeless . . . one couch to another. . . . Now I slept in my car, you know, a few times. . . . The things I was doing, I was messing with drugs, and I was ashamed for anybody in my family to see me. . . . I'm in recovery now at this moment. . . . And so, today, I got forty-six days clean.[23]

Andre had also been shot multiple times, one time in his spine, which damaged his leg mobility, giving him a lifelong disability. He is supposed to be eligible for Supplemental Security Income (SSI), but for reasons he has tried to fight in court, he is only receiving half of what he believes he is owed. His monthly SSI equals $400, he gets $47 a month in food stamps, and his housing is currently free. Even so, he can barely survive. "For the month, man, it's just, it's crazy. You know, but hey, I'm not gonna give up. I'm not gonna quit. But I mean, it makes you feel that way. Like, you know, 'Hey, well, I really don't have nothing to keep going for.' But, you know, I'm not giving up."[24]

Reginald, Clayton, and Andre have suffered multiple, compounding slow emergencies across the arc of their lives, and they were treated with racist logics, policies, and ideologies in the prison, recovery, and hospital systems. These experiences of racism accumulate in the body, resulting in mental and physical challenges, and in the mind, leading to profound feelings of distrust and devaluation. As Villarosa explains, "from birth to death the impact on the bodies of Black Americans of living in communities that have been harmed by long-standing racial discrimination, of a deeply rooted and dangerous racial bias in our health-care system, and of the insidious consequences of present-day racism affects who lives and who dies . . . and contributes to poor health outcomes . . . in all oppressed people."[25] And yet, people in these conditions are often blamed for their "life choices" and are subject to self-entrepreneurial logics, often in recovery or workfare programs. They are asked to adopt adages of self-management and blame to receive minimal state aid.[26] Reginald, Andre, and Clayton narrated the overt and subtle ways in which racism operated in their lives, accumulating across experiences of entangled slow emergencies, leading to distrust of state and medical establishments and chronic physical and mental health conditions. During the pandemic, scientific experts blamed chronic health conditions for the disproportionate rates of hospitalizations and deaths in Black and Latinx communities, and medical distrust was cited as a core reason these same populations may resist vaccination. Distrust and chronic health conditions stem from repeated instances of institutional racism and structural neglect, which were completely ignored in COVID-19 policies. State agents sought to address racial disparities in COVID-19 outcomes without attending to the conditions that caused them, which are starkly illustrated in the narratives Reginald, Clayton, and Andre provided.

HUSTLING TO PIECE TOGETHER FRACTURED AID

One of the paradoxes of experiencing a slow emergency is the intense labor it requires to survive, even while receiving state aid. This paradox occurs in part because receiving social welfare not only requires laboring in extremely low-income jobs with little opportunity for education or promotion but also because social safety nets are negligible to begin with and require constant upkeep to maintain.[27] Wages are not keeping pace with inflation, and people struggle to patch together various forms of formal and informal support to survive. As Nixon notes, the poor often operate in "now o'clock" because survival requires constant, immediate attention.[28] Slow emergencies may not feel slow to those who must constantly hustle to survive.

Phyllis is a sixty-year-old Black woman who lives alone in Austin. After more than seven years on multiple waiting lists, she received a Section 8 housing voucher, which significantly reduced her monthly rent to less than $500 per month.[29] She has been in substance use recovery since 2002. Since 2007, she has worked as the night manager in the same recovery home where she lived when she was getting clean. She works forty hours a week at minimum wage and still has a difficult time making it from month to month. She said, "It is so hard. . . . Even working full-time, it's hard to make enough to . . . be able to pay rent." Even though she receives a very coveted Section 8 voucher, she struggles to piece together enough to pay her rent:

> I'm so grateful to go home and have a home to go to. You know, it might not be the warmest, but it is warm. . . . If I had to pay market rent, even me working full-time. . . . I wouldn't be able to do it by myself. I wouldn't be able to afford it because rent is so high, let alone utilities and food and all the other necessities. Household items and things like transportation . . . It would be way out of my reach.[30]

The year before our interview, Phyllis was diagnosed with uterine cancer. She could not afford to take sick leave at work because her hours and pay would be reduced, so she worked full-time while she had a hysterectomy and pursued chemotherapy, with no familial support. She engaged in treatment during the first year of the pandemic, continuing to expose herself to risks of coronavirus infection at work despite being immunocompromised from chemotherapy because she could not survive without a paycheck. She recounted:

> I was coming from work going straight to my chemo . . . I would get off of work. They would give me a ride. And I would go to my chemo and then I would be off for two days because the chemo was so strong. . . . And this went on for months . . . because the bills don't stop.[31]

Phyllis then explained why she could not afford to take sick leave from work:

> A lot of times, it's like you're between a rock and a hard place. . . . I already only make minimum wage, and then you're not gonna . . . give me the hours and the amount that I would get if I was working. You would compensate me [on sick leave], but it wouldn't be for the whole amount. So it's already hard from paycheck to paycheck, and you have to balance that out.[32]

In addition, although she has health insurance and the hospital gave her a reduced rate based on her income and put her on a payment plan, she is now paying off her debt to the hospital for her treatment. She had to cover copays and out-of-pocket expenses for CAT scans, x-rays, and blood work, not to mention her chemotherapy and the surgery. And yet, she remained grateful for her ongoing ability to work during the pandemic, without which she would not have survived financially, even with the housing support she gets from both the city and federal governments. In 2020, the Federal Reserve found that about 25 percent of adults were unable to pay their monthly bills or were one modest setback away from being unable to pay their bills, and among workers who were laid off, 45 percent were unable to pay their monthly bills. Further, 40 percent of adults went without medical care because of an inability to pay.[33] Hustling like Phyllis had to do, while sick, is a common experience for those without a safety net or familial network.

Dolores is also a Black woman in her sixties who lives in Austin. Her parents worked in sanitation and for the City of Chicago while she was growing up, and she went to private Catholic school. She and her daughters live in a three-flat house that has been in her family for more than twenty years. Though they nearly lost the house a few times, they have managed to hold onto it. She had several working-class jobs throughout her life—she worked in transportation and loading, and before the pandemic, she was working on the cleaning staff at a small hotel in a nearby suburb. In March 2020, she lost her job and went on pandemic unemployment, but it was not enough to cover her expenses. She also applied for food stamps and rental assistance, and she receives Medicare. She was able to take care of her grandchildren when they were out of school during the first year of the pandemic, and her daughters paid her for this work.

After the first year of the pandemic, she started working part-time at her previous hotel job, but she also started working part-time on the cleaning staff at a local stadium because she was unable to make ends meet. She told me:

> When they gave us the stimulus check, what did we do with it? We spent it right back. . . . We gave it right back to 'em to bring the economy back up. So what did you actually give me? Nothing. For real! Like, did you wipe away some of my debt? (*Laughs.*) Heck naw. Absolutely not. People still in debt and probably more so now than ever, because now people went and stopped working. I mean, that shit changed a whole bunch of people lives forreal. Right, like COVID was—is something else. It changed a lot of people, like, people literally stopped working, and that's your livelihood. So, I mean, if you didn't have no money saved up (*scoffs*), you was basically outta there.[34]

Dolores mentions the fact that many lower-income families not only have no savings or wealth to buffer job loss, but they often have extensive debt, including student loans, credit cards, mortgages, and traffic and parking violation debt.[35] The Federal Reserve Bank of New York found in 2021 that the pandemic caused many lower-income families of color to take on extensive debt, which they will have a difficult time paying back because debt obligations often outpace earnings.[36] Dolores, for example, had to sell her car because she had such a high rate of unpaid traffic and parking violations, she could no longer afford her car. People without existing safety nets and high debt then faced rent and utility cutoffs when they lost work during the COVID-19 pandemic. Dolores told me:

> You either gone swim or you gone drown. And I choose to swim. You know what I'm saying? No matter what. I just can't drown. 'Cause I have other lives in my life that [are] depending on me, right? So I can't let COVID stop me. You know what I mean? We can't let COVID stop us because we still have to pay bills. We still have to eat. We still have to send kids to college. We still have bills. We still have life. Right? So we have to adapt to situations. Because it 'posed to have gotten better. But how? How did it get better? And when the economy is steady going up … the price of food is steady going up, the price of gas is steady going up. And those are the things we need. Not the things that we want. But the things that we need to survive. 'Cause it's like to me now, it's all about survival. *People are not living life, they surviving through this pandemic.*[37]

Dolores makes several important points in this quote. She explains that when the economy began to recover in 2021, inflation ensued, which has further constrained lower-income families. But the bills never stop. She has to find a way to keep fighting through it. When she says COVID won't stop her, she means the economic fallout it has caused her and her family. But she has to keep surviving even if it means she is not really *living*.

Although pandemic aid, like stimulus payments, child tax credits, and pandemic unemployment insurance, helped many lower-income Americans, it was not enough to meet the needs of those suffering from entangled slow emergencies. The administration of welfare contributes to and conceals structural racism. Marlin explained that pandemic aid, which was inconsistent and minimal, did not make much of a dent for people suffering from deeper systemic violence and vulnerability. He explained that he did not expect the city to "take care of people for the rest of they lives," but he did argue that social assistance needed to be more extensive and longer-term, given the lack of opportunities for people to earn a living wage. About pandemic aid, Marlin observed:

> It'd go for a while, then it'd stop. . . . I think it should have stayed consistent. Because if a person can't pay his rent, can't get properly fed, his chances of being sick and making it to the hospital is less than average (*scoffs*). How could he make it to the doctor? He can't even put food on his table. He have nowhere to live, right? And the people that do have somewhere to live, it's, do I get some food? Or do I go to the hospital? . . . That's a hell of a choice to have to make.[38]

In addition to its piecemeal distribution and meager payouts, pandemic aid was not universal. Undocumented Americans were unable to access most forms of aid throughout the pandemic, yet they continued to labor in jobs that were "essential" to economic recovery and that allowed middle-class Americans to work from home. Luis, whom I first introduced in chapter 3, is in his fifties. I interviewed Luis twice, first in April 2021 and then in November 2021. Luis migrated from Veracruz, Mexico, in 1998, and he lives in Albany Park with his wife and younger son, who was in college when the pandemic began. Luis's older son lives nearby with his own family. Luis and his wife both worked in metal factories but were let go at the beginning of the pandemic. Luis told me that all undocumented staff were fired from his factory when the pandemic began. Because he is undocumented, he was unable to collect unemployment, stimulus checks, or food stamps. In the incredibly insightful quote that follows, he lambastes the shortsighted policy of not providing aid for undocumented workers because it created risks that could have been assuaged if everyone were treated equally. In other words, he argues that inequalities in the provision of welfare created COVID-19 risks:

> The only thing that I can observe or that is more noticeable in these six months is how complicated it is for people who do not have documents . . . to obtain economic support. I'm going to say it again, I'm going to say it as many times as necessary. I think it would be healthy to find other ways to support the undocumented community for the simple reason that we are here. We are also working. We are also generating taxes, but we can also be transmitters of the virus. We are not taken care of as we should be . . . like the people who have money are. Maybe I don't have insurance, or I don't have access to medical services . . . and I go [to work] contaminating other people who do have insurance, who can have other types of care, but even if I am not fully protected, I can be like a source

of infection for other people. And if we are all cared for in the same way, I think we are going to end the pandemic sooner.[39]

Eventually, Luis did go back to work in another factory, but he earns half his previous salary. Luis rents from his landlord through a verbal lease, and his landlord would not help him apply for rental assistance because he did not want to pay taxes for the rental property. Luis began getting into deeper and deeper debt. He began borrowing money from his older son, and by the time of our second interview, Luis owed his son $6,000, and it was beginning to strain their relationship. His younger son dropped out of college to work to help support the family financially.

> Really, it's stressful to see the end of the month. You don't have the money available to make rent payments, pay bills, and even sometimes for food. . . . I would really like to receive some type of economic help to reimburse the money to my children. . . . Immigration status is a determinant. Because people who have documents have more access to different kinds of economic and moral support in terms of health and everything. But a lot of us were fine before the pandemic. . . . Now it's complicated to be living on a daily basis—paycheck to paycheck. . . . We pay taxes. [They] take taxes off every week especially because we work. We pay taxes. Now that we are in this type of pandemic, in this type of need, we don't have any type of support.[40]

Lorenzo is also an undocumented migrant from Mexico. He is fifty-three years old and has lived in Little Village since 1996, though he migrated to the US from Mexico in 1986. Lorenzo has children but does not live with or support them, yet he faced similar struggles when he lost work during the pandemic. Lorenzo was working as a bartender and waiter for a company that provides catering for large events, and he paid dues for a union through which he received health insurance. But he lost his job and his insurance at the start of the pandemic, and he burned through his minimal savings of $2,000 quickly. Lorenzo has phone, car, and rental debt. He could not get stimulus or unemployment support, but he was able to receive some support from local organizations. However, he accrued a $5,000 debt to his sisters. He tried to get work as a day laborer with limited success. He protested his exclusion from governmental programs: "You pay taxes. You work, and they take taxes from you. . . . They don't see what color you are. Where you're from. What would have been fair is that it would have been equal for everybody."[41] Because he pays taxes, Lorenzo believes he should have been given the opportunity to receive state support when he lost work during the pandemic.

Lorenzo said that his housing conditions are deplorable. He and his landlord have a verbal agreement for rent, but his landlord engaged in retaliatory behavior as Lorenzo fell behind on rent. According to Lorenzo:

> The manager of the apartment harasses a lot. And he nags a lot. But he never fixes anything. . . . There's no window, not even one. And there's no alarm. There's not even one, for the smoke or anything. I mean, it's more illegal than me. . . . In summertime, I don't have air conditioning. And in wintertime, I don't have a heater.[42]

He even tried sleeping in his car, but running his heater ruined his thermostat and then the car would no longer start. The landlord covered the broken window in the attic with paper, which caused smoke to circulate in Lorenzo's apartment, and he developed breathing problems. Lorenzo's health deteriorated. He was diagnosed with diabetes during the pandemic, and he blames the stress he was under, but he could not afford health insurance. He also began to struggle with depression: "I see it as normal that we feel depressed . . . I sometimes get so depressed that I sleep for two or three days. I sleep, I'm lying down, and I don't feel like getting up."[43]

Undocumented Americans were unable to access most forms of pandemic aid, which, as Luis explained, was shortsighted because it facilitated coronavirus transmission. Not providing aid to a large population whose labor salvaged the economy is an expression of racial devaluation. Undocumented people are treated as a disposable industrial reserve army in the United States. Both Luis and Lorenzo nonetheless attempted to piece together help from their families and local mutual aid organizations, but this effort created tremendous stress and failed to meet their mounting needs. It is not simply that welfare provision is means-tested, paternalistic, and meager; it also obscures the mechanisms of exclusionary inclusion. The pitfalls and piecemeal structure of welfare provision in the US conceal infrastructural racism in two ways. First, undocumented Americans are valued participants in the capitalist system but are excluded from receiving aid. Documented but racially marginalized Americans are given state aid in a fractured system in order that politicians can claim political capital in redressing racial disparities, but not in a fashion that facilitates surviving commingled slow emergencies. In the introduction to this book, I quoted Candice, a Black woman from Austin who questioned why it took a pandemic to dole out stimulus packages or livable unemployment insurance when lower-income people of color need that kind of support all the time. She questioned the exceptional way in which people were governed through emergency, but only in a temporary way. Since the ending of pandemic aid, and with rising inflation, poverty rates began, once again, to soar.

The poverty rate in 2022 rose to 12.4 percent from the rate of 7.8 percent in 2021—the largest one-year jump on record.[44] Governing emergencies through temporary and piecemeal relief conceals and exacerbates the ongoing racist devaluation of those living in slow emergencies.

RESISTING DEVALUATION

In Berlant's analysis of slow death, she argues that people whose lives are consumed with barely surviving and whose bodies weather the accumulation of capitalist exploitation are often most troubled by having to abandon fantasies of the good life—their ideological belief that the future could be different, that their children could achieve upward mobility, that they could ever work their way "out" of slow death.[45] For Berlant, affective attachments to fantasies of the good life constitute "cruel optimism" because they undermine flourishing in the present. Berlant's point is that people who experience slow death are affectively attached to false fantasies of upward mobility, which can keep them in limbo, unable to locate themselves in the social landscape and navigate their current realities.

And yet, I found two profoundly important ways that people challenged their devaluation within the racial biocapitalist system: by reframing their relationship to welfare and work (and therefore abandoning their fantasies of the good life) *and* by providing one another the care that the state withheld. Navigating the racist, fractured systems of care that constitute structural neglect in the US, in some ways, yields a critical form of agency that often goes unnoticed. It does not take the form of a vocal, political uprising. Rather, people quietly push back against processes of devaluation and letting die, thereby resisting their emergency conditions.

Reimagining Work and Welfare

Samira's parents are refugees from Somalia. They were resettled in St. Louis in 1994 and divorced soon thereafter. Out of seven children spread over fifteen years, Samira is the youngest. Her mother raised her as a single parent and relied on various forms of social welfare—refugee assistance, food stamps, unemployment, and Medicaid. Samira grew up trying to help her mother meet the technological and bureaucratic requirements to remain qualified for this social assistance. She explained to me that keeping up with social assistance can be very arduous:

> My mom has been using food stamps for a while. And it's always, like, very tedious, the application process and if something is off . . . it's not super easy. . . . I called the office for her . . . and then I explained that I

was her daughter. And they were asking a bunch of questions. And it was something that my mom definitely couldn't have done on her own. And the questions were, like . . . sort of *interrogative*. They were asking how she was paying rent, and how much her rent was . . . and I was, like, well, my siblings pay the rent. And then we had to have a written . . . document saying [my siblings] paid this much amount, and sign it and just dumb shit like that.[46]

Samira moved to Chicago after college because one of her sisters lived in town, and she started working in a part-time job. She had significant debt and no health insurance. She lived with roommates in Little Village, and she reflected in her interview:

My first few years here I was, like, really wanting . . . a full-time job that offered a salary and benefits and stuff. . . . I thought I needed to live a *good life* and then . . . I got a different job that I didn't really expect and . . . it was a job . . . where you could [have] a random Tuesday off . . . an open sort of flexible schedule that, like, allowed me to . . . see a different future for my life that I hadn't thought of before. So I had more time to do things that I liked, like writing and stuff.[47]

Then the pandemic hit, and both she and her roommate lost their jobs. She ended up having to move multiple times to find rents she could afford on unemployment. One of her roommates managed to keep a job waiting tables and sometimes covered Samira's costs, and Samira's siblings helped her survive.

I conducted two interviews with Samira, and in both, she was very vague about applying for social assistance. She told me she had to struggle to get unemployment, and then she got cut off when the system was transferred into a new platform, and it took her weeks to get her unemployment back. But she refused to call regularly. When I asked if she signed up for Medicaid, she said something noncommittal: "Well I tried to one time, but then honestly, I can't remember what happened. I don't know. I stopped signing up? Never finished. I don't know."[48] During her second interview, when I asked about applying for food stamps or rental assistance, she said, "Life just moves too fast for me . . . I think about it and I'm like, oh, I need to do these things. And then I have something else happen and then, that's more pressing."[49] Then she explained that her wisdom teeth are impacted and causing her pain, but she has not gotten coverage to see a dentist.

In both interviews, if I pushed Samira to reflect on her dire economic conditions or her lack of motivation to apply for social assistance, she would start to cry and become despondent. In some ways, I thought she believed her life would be different from her mother's, so applying for social assistance seemed like a step backward, tarnishing her belief in upward mobility. At other points, I thought that facing her struggles was simply too hard—she tried to put them out of her mind as much as she could. For example, when asked about George Floyd, she started crying and told me that it was a "very traumatic moment during the pandemic," one that she tries to avoid thinking about on a daily basis. When she does remember, it's simply too painful. "My brain just sort of pushes past it [*crying*]. I'm sorry. . . . It's weird 'cause if I'm just passively thinking about the past couple years, it's like . . . I don't know, it doesn't affect me in the same way. But if I really try and *remember* . . . it kind of sucks."[50]

In the fall of 2021, Samira was able to secure a very part-time job teaching violin to children five hours a week. She said that finding work had been difficult, but she also does not want to work in a job just to survive—she wants to wait and find meaningful work:

> I wouldn't want to be put in a position . . . to just work a job simply to survive and pay for my rent. I want to work a job that, uh, makes me feel like I have worth and . . . gives me time to live my life as well. . . . I feel like people . . . must have felt that way before [the pandemic], but [the pandemic showed] . . . how impermanent jobs and life is . . . [and it] made people realize that they shouldn't have to work a job that's so grueling, just to skirt by.[51]

While Samira struggled with the everyday, she was also challenging ideologies of the good life and trying to imagine something different for people of her generation. She did not want to face her conditions of existence in certain ways, but she was also attempting to challenge the necessity of working just to survive the mundanity of slow emergencies. She wanted to find work that was meaningful to her and would give her autonomy to live the way she wants.

Samira was not the only younger person I interviewed who felt they did not want to work simply to survive. Kelly, a young Black woman who lives in Albany Park, also told me that before the pandemic, she was working several jobs to make rent. When she went on unemployment and things slowed down, she started baking and painting and selling her products online. She said she realized she wanted something different for her future:

> Pre-COVID . . . Honestly, I was, like, in this really crazy mindset—well not crazy, but I was in this mindset of, like, I need to do better. . . . I was working two jobs before COVID hit. . . . I worked this shitty job at this company [that was] willing to replace me in a heartbeat, you know, rather

than pay me a livable wage, so that I don't have to work two jobs. . . . We're being underpaid, and we're being overworked. And, you know, treated like shit. . . . Before COVID . . . I should have left but didn't just because, like, fuck! I needed some money and . . . the job search wasn't too great.[52]

Kelly was fired when the pandemic began, and several months later, her previous employer contacted her to see if she would work for them from home, but "they had the audacity to offer me a lower wage. . . . COVID definitely helped me realize that . . . money can be made doing something that I actually *care* about."[53] Kelly and Samira both defied their unfair labor conditions. During the pandemic, many young people began to demand better wages and more meaningful work. Yet, being able to choose one's work was not an option available to others.

Miguel has lived undocumented in the US since 1977. He moved to Chicago to be close to his uncle's family. He lives in Albany Park. Miguel works for a company that provides cleaning services to offices and schools. To make ends meet, he lives with two roommates he does not like and barely sees. Miguel cannot access social assistance, and he has witnessed and been the target of rising crime in Albany Park. He is judgmental of people who resort to crime instead of working hard, and he has contradictory views on social assistance. "So the other people are very exasperated and they want money. Then some people get money also from the government. I think in the beginning of the pandemic, of course, [it] was [a] very serious, very extreme situation. But not now," in March 2022.[54] Miguel critiqued people who committed crime out of desperation. He told me:

> During the pandemic, more people who I know personally, and I experienced with them, we were suffering because we didn't have jobs, our money was running out of our checking accounts, we didn't have money to pay. We didn't go to commit any crimes. It's not why we came to the United States. . . . Because in the end, I am the victim. I am the victim. And I can't tell you how many times I felt extremely unsafe on the train. I use the train every day because I don't have a car. I use the bus every day and I felt extremely scary moments.[55]

Miguel has not experienced the upward mobility he expected in the US, even though he still dreams it. He wants to continue to work hard and make his life better, but he barely survives from paycheck to paycheck, working long and hard hours. He said:

> We stretch the dollars. We stretch the dollars. I don't have TV, first of all. I don't have cable. You have to give up a lot of things. I give up a lot of

things. I give up my car because I don't have money. . . . You only have one [pair of] shoes. I mean, you limit how often you go out. So we make some sacrifices. Very tough sacrifices. Yes . . . Yeah, it's very tough.[56]

He explained that after the shelter-at-home order was lifted, he returned to work as soon as he could. He believed that people whose work was deemed "essential" should have been compensated for the risks they took. He said, "We felt that were ignored. We felt that, really, they don't appreciate our work."[57] Nonetheless, the imminent emergencies that caused him to emigrate to begin with were far worse. He was thankful he came to the US, and he fought to stay. Miguel accepted food donations during the pandemic, but he emphasized that he does not want to rely on government assistance:

> I don't want to stay like this. A lot of people who I talk to who are also immigrants, we don't want to stay this [way], depending upon the government. We want to get and work . . . on our own and build ourselves, you know, have our own home. And just to be dependent on the government . . . I see the evidence, that [it] is not always helpful, because *it's kind of a way to keep you poor forever*. . . . We are not coming here to have things given to us. We don't want . . . things here given to us for free. We came here to work and work hard. But sadly even if you work hard, you don't earn anything. You keep working hard and hard and hard—*we still end up poor*. Better of course than where you came from, but it's still poor.[58]

Miguel's language is loaded. He is suggesting that Black Americans engage in crime when they are desperate and they rely on welfare, which makes them generationally poor—unlike immigrants who come to work. This anti-Black racism is often expressed by Latinx immigrants by insisting that racial groups embody different work ethics. But he is also criticizing the ways in which welfare regulates poor people and keeps them impoverished. Miguel is conflicted. He does not want his community to be poor forever, and though he wants to work, his constant struggle is not changing his circumstances. He does not want to accept social welfare, but he does support educational grants and free health care. Miguel envisions the autonomy afforded by well-paying work—this fantasy is not so different from Samira's and Kelly's.

I found that people living in emergency conditions are not attached to unrealistic fantasies that keep them from recognizing their conditions of existence. They are hyperaware of the racist systems that keep them from thriving, but they also resist being devalued and degraded. They imagine work conditions that are meaningful and appreciated, and they strive to actualize certain kinds of autonomy. In some ways, the pandemic blurred the line between the crisis ordinariness of slow emergencies already in the making and the eventful crises instigated by pandemic precarity—the present and some eventual future blur into each other, and there is no longer a nonemergency to return to.[59] This can cause people to rethink and disrupt what is considered normal, to instigate a politicization of emergency conditions. It can also strengthen the politics of care.

The Politics of Care

Social reproduction—the often unvalued and unseen reproduction of life forces under capitalist exploitation—has always sustained communities marginalized and subjugated by racial capitalism. In his analysis of the queering of family life produced by the contradictions of slavery and Jim Crow, Roderick Ferguson argues that surplus populations that exceed the demands and restrictions of capital are often critical of existing systems.[60] Cultural and structural formations that disrupt normative regulation and racial boundaries, that continue to sustain life in the wake of devaluation and letting die policies, hold radical potential. When and where the state recedes, people take up the political work of fostering life that challenges racial biocapitalist relations.

While there are multiple examples I could give about the life-giving work people provided one another during the pandemic, here I will present one example and return to this theme in the last chapter of the book. Marlin and one staff member, Shanice, run a small mutual aid organization in Austin. It offers a recovery program, violence prevention, and mutual aid. When the COVID-19 pandemic began and Marlin made a deal with a local laboratory to provide testing services, he converted a small storefront into a testing site. He employed the people in his recovery program as testing volunteers, and they earn a small amount of money for every test they complete. This is a way to support people in his community. In addition, Marlin and Shanice collect donations and hand out food, and they help people navigate applications for food stamps, unemployment, and other relief programs run through the city. Shanice explained, "There are some resources out there, but people don't know how to get them. Our organization tries to fill that gap in. . . . Small community organizations fill in the gap between the government and bigger nonprofits."[61]

I visited the storefront and church where Marlin and Shanice hold meetings with volunteers and host support groups for people in recovery. Most of the volunteers are also in recovery—they feel they were given compassion and support when they were most in need, and they want to do the same for others. I held a focus group discussion with volunteers in July 2022.[62] When I asked the volunteers why it was important to them to provide testing and mutual aid to people in Austin during the pandemic, they responded in similar ways:

> I grew up without. I've always saw the need to help the next person, you know, we were raised to share whatever it was that we had, even if it wasn't much. You know, the next person may not have what you have and if you give them a little bit of what you have, that person has as well . . . And that's what being in this community is all about.

> There are no resources anywhere. People don't have anywhere else to go. We help them. People don't have support to go to places, so we go to their homes when they don't have kin to help them.

This organization also goes well beyond its mission statement. Its workers do not simply do testing and recovery—they provide food, they help connect people to existing city resources, they hold funerals for community members, and they go out into the community to provide violence prevention services. Members of the focus group explained:

> This organization has been helping people for years. They feed the homeless. They fight the pandemic that is destroying our community like hellfire. They make house calls and come to you. They also do drug recovery, so if someone comes to do a COVID test and a volunteer sees drug addiction, they try to help with that. This organization does a lot, but there is a lot still to be done.

> This organization is hands-on. We go to you if you can't come to us. We always open. People can call after hours and someone is on call. We work an eight-hour shift, but someone is on call. We could do more. I'm really struggling. But if people took their minds off "what am I gonna get if I do this," and think more about how they can help others and how that will help the community as a whole, then we'd be better off. I had a bad background, but this organization accepted me and they empowered me. People ask, "Are you all just doing COVID testing?" No, we're not. We will help you with what you need.

Community members are critical of existing welfare infrastructure because it is porous and difficult to access. Austin residents do not always know what services are available to them or how to apply, and during the focus group, volunteers told me that they help connect people to services:

The city could do more, but we never find out about the resources that are being made available. Politicians don't communicate with everyday people. We have to find out about these resources and then spread the word to the community.

Among politicians, there is a lack of care for people in poor communities. We have to beg to get free money. They tell us to help ourselves, but then they put up barriers to getting everything. The system is a long haul. There is so much red tape. People don't know where to go. We do the research and let them know how to do it.

Shanice also explained that with city agencies and larger nonprofit organizations, there is a lot of red tape and bureaucracy required to access services. Not only does Marlin's organization help people navigate bureaucratic barriers, but it also offers services without the need for identification or proof of need. "We work around the red tape," Shanice told me. "You don't need to fill out forms for me to feed you, I'm just going to feed you."[63] Shanice and Marlin, though, also recognize the downside of this—they did not get money from the city to provide services in Austin. That money went to a larger organization, which nonetheless relies on these smaller mutual aid organizations to connect people to care. As Marlin explained, "When they get that money, they don't even reach down to the little organizations, right . . . but we're down here, ground level fighting this war, while they're actually reaping the benefits."[64]

But there are some benefits, as well, to remaining smaller—being able to fill in the gaps and avoid bureaucracy. The community trusts this work and the people who provide it. While many Austin residents do not trust government officials or agencies, they do trust these volunteers who work for free to help the community survive. These volunteers understand the struggle and the hustle, so they are best positioned to help, as one of the volunteers underscored during the focus group discussion:

We need more organizations like this one. We need to grow bigger. We grew up here in the struggle. We know how to cope. We learn to cope and help others. No one knows better than someone who went through the same thing. . . . People who haven't lived in Austin, don't know what it's like. This is why this organization is so important.

Marlin explained that he started the organization because "if we don't take care of where we grew up at, who will?"[65] Shanice explained that they do not see themselves fighting the system—they see themselves teaching people how to survive. She said:

> You know, no one is above help. I don't care where you come from, you
> know, what your financial status is, everybody's going to need some help
> at some point and time in their life. . . . It's not, you know, to beat the sys-
> tem. No, we're not teaching them that. We're teaching them to survive
> in a life . . . that was dealt us.[66]

And in the end, through this radical politics of care, members of this organization are surviving the letting die policies of a state that devalues Black and
Brown life—that leaves people to fend for themselves with broken systems
and underresourced institutions. Marlin's organization is teaching people
to value their commitments and the care they give to one another to perse-
vere another day amid their slow emergencies.

*   *   *

The causes of slow emergencies are difficult to identify because they stem
from a conjuncture of historical racist policies, interactions, and ideologies.
Slow emergencies are easy for politicians to ignore when designing welfare or
emergency programs. This chapter has shed light on the processes by which
racism is masked when it is embedded in infrastructures and bodies, and
the effects this concealment has on racially marginalized subjects. Although
structural racism was given momentary recognition after the racial
uprisings that erupted in the summer of 2020, it soon faded back into
the background, where it could be easily ignored by state actors and those
who benefit from white supremacy. But those who experience the effects
of racism in everyday interactions with state agents and medical establishments or in institutionalized settings (e.g., recovery homes, prisons, hospitals) come to embody its effects in the form of distrust, chronic conditions,
and mental health challenges. These same effects put people at risk of hospitalization and death from COVID-19. Although state actors claimed they
sought to redress racial inequalities in coronavirus outcomes or vaccine access, they ignored the very conditions of slow emergency that caused these
inequalities in the first place. Social assistance was expanded in unprecedented ways during the pandemic, but its patchwork and paternalistic form
concealed how welfare provision instantiates and exacerbates institutional
racism. Barely providing minimal aid in means-tested and paternalistic systems includes (documented) racially marginalized subjects within the body
politic, but through exclusionary and contingent means—means that rely
on the uptake of regulatory and disciplinary norms. Undocumented people
are included in the US imaginary, as the economy is reliant on their labor,
but they were excluded from the extension of pandemic aid. The extension
of aid (and not just social abandonment) constitutes a primary mechanism

of racist state neglect in the contemporary US. And yet, the people in this study resisted—not just through political organizing or visible social movements but also by reimagining their relationship to work and welfare and by taking care of one another in the face of racial devaluation. In so doing, they resisted their emergency conditions and forged new political formations in the shadow of racial biocapitalism.

5: SACRIFICING "ESSENTIAL" WORKERS

It was partially a *racial thing*... I've seen people gettin' treated as though they were *sacrificial lambs*.... It's like essential workers were getting categorized as essential, but it was a hollow label.... A lot of essential workers were underpaid or not paid.... You got some people puttin' their life on the line ... [but] they haven't been treated like *essential* workers.

MARLIN, Black resident of Austin interviewed on April 21, 2021

People in jobs deemed "essential" by the State of Illinois, which required them to work during the shelter-at-home order, included people working in agriculture and food production, meatpacking and production, transportation, clinics and hospitals, government agencies, and delivery and shipping industries. Although higher-income "essential workers," such as government officials and physicians, were celebrated and compensated for their heroism, lower-income workers were largely invisibilized and sacrificed to safeguard the biosafety of the norm. In Chicago, low-wage frontline laborers were predominantly Black and Latinx, making their sacrifice a "racial thing." Marlin's quote that opens this chapter points out the paradox that lower-income, racially marginalized workers faced during the pandemic: the term *essential* implies value, but being underpaid and unprotected reveals a subtle racial devaluation of their sacrifice. Racialized "essential" workers are valued as a class because they enable the enhancement of capital but are devalued as individual humans putting their lives at risk. Racism creates a system of differential human value that capitalists exploit to accumulate profit and safeguard the norm. This logic has been embedded within the racial biocapitalist system in the United States for centuries, but it was named and publicized during the COVID-19 pandemic—momentarily exposing the ways in which racism is a structuring logic of capitalism.[1]

Rodrigo, a Mexican American resident of Little Village, spoke extensively in his interview about the various paradoxes that lower-income and undocumented Latinx workers experienced, especially in the early months of the pandemic:

> We're essential . . . but they don't treat us essential . . . 'Cause we are the guys. We are the ones that feed you, clean and pick the fruit, and work the soil, and make the factories run, and make the restaurants run. . . . We immigrant communities make this nation run. Because of us, this nation runs, so they care that we do stuff for *them*, but when it's time for us to go home [and be protected], we're forgotten because all they want is our service, but not [to] service us.[2]

In addition to being exploited for their labor in undesirable but crucial industries, Rodrigo points out that many workers may have chosen not to work during the pandemic and lose the income, but for so many lower-income Latinx families, the "choice" was between exposure to a deadly virus or watching their families starve. As he explained, "either we work or we don't eat because we don't have the luxury that other communities have."[3] And this situation was deemed acceptable by the government and middle-class Americans because "essential," lower-income frontline workers were treated as replenishable and disposable. I asked Rodrigo, "How high are the COVID-19 rates in Little Village?" He responded:

> Really high because we couldn't stay home. We had to go and work. We had to be your home caretaker. We had to be your person making your food . . . so we couldn't stay home. As much as we wanted to stay home, we couldn't afford it, or we didn't have the choice. The label of "essential" is hypocritical. Because when you're essential, you're appreciated. . . . You're one of a kind, but they don't treat us like we're essential. They treat us like, "Oh, well, one more Mexican. We've got more coming anyways." . . . Like we're disposable. Right, so I think that was just wrong and inhumane on the part of the city, on the part of the mayor, on the part of the aldermen and the state and the county.[4]

Here, Rodrigo suggests that the term *essential* implies distinctiveness, but in practice, frontline workers were deemed fungible. Further, workers were given no protections or hazard pay. "The country did not take care of us. The state did not take care of us," Rodrigo said. He explained that other states gave undocumented residents temporary housing when they needed to quarantine and provided cash assistance so they could pay their rent or keep from infecting others at work, but "the city [of Chicago] has learned to ignore the undocumented community."[5] He scoffed again at being labeled "essential": "essential means that you care, that you matter . . . so then we were not essential at all."[6]

Rodrigo points out the paradoxes of being deemed essential, *critical*, crucial to the nation, but expendable, replaceable, and invisible at the same time. This was a distinct form of exclusionary inclusion used by state actors during the pandemic: the declaration of emergency enacted an overt sacrifice of "essential workers," who were asked to risk their lives for the sake of the nation and the economy's health. Although this form of exclusion was publicized during the pandemic, sacrificial labor logics enabled by differential racial valuation epitomize a constitutive though often hidden feature of US racial biocapitalism. As mechanisms of exclusionary inclusion, slow emergencies and sacrifice supplement each other. Conditions that create slow emergencies, such as neighborhood disinvestment, overpolicing, paternalistic workfare, and citizenship limitations on welfare make lower-income, racially marginalized people compliant workers, readily exploitable in low-wage jobs with few benefits or protections.[7] Racism assigns differential value to certain populations, who are then exploitable as disposable surplus labor. As a *class*, frontline lower-income workers were valued as "essential" because their labor enabled the ongoing pursuit of capital and the protection of the norm. As *people*, however, they were rendered disposable and fungible.

In what follows, I provide background on racial capitalism and the differentiation of value. I then present statistics that illustrate the economic vulnerability of frontline workers. Next, I explain the policies that were implemented in Illinois around "essential work" and how they exposed certain communities to disproportionate risk. Finally, I describe how the people I interviewed experienced the various paradoxes of "essential work" during the pandemic.

RACIAL CAPITALISM AND
DIFFERENTIAL VALUATION

> Capital is dead labor, that vampire-like, only lives by sucking living labor and lives the more, the more labor it sucks. The time during which the laborer works, is the time during which the capitalist consumes the labor-power he has purchased of him.
>
> KARL MARX, *Capital*

In this quote, Marx argues that capitalists rely on the living labor power of workers, who own no property other than their labor and must sell their labor power to the capitalist as a commodity.[8] Capital can only accrue through this "vampire-like" arrangement in which the capitalist lives off of and profits from the living labor of the worker. Because, as Cedric Robinson argued, racism permeates the social structures of capitalism, this exploitative bloodsucking is stratified by race and nationalism.[9] Racial projects assign differential value to human groups, which capitalists then exploit in their competitive pursuit of profit.[10] Jodi Melamed explains this process of accumulation and devaluation:

> Capital can only be capital when it is accumulating, and it can only accumulate by producing and moving through relations of severe inequality among human groups.... These antinomies of accumulation require loss, disposability, and the unequal differentiation of human value, and racism enshrines the inequalities that capitalism requires.[11]

Certain racial groups are valued because of their disposability and replaceability as laborers, and this differential valuation has deep historical roots in the origins of capitalist development.

Settler colonial dispossession, chattel slavery, indentured servitude, debt peonage, sharecropping, and successive waves of manipulating social policies to ensure cheap labor through immigration or war have all operated to supply US capitalists with readily exploitable and fungible pools of racialized laborers.[12] Neoliberalism operates in a cyclical way, where the imposition of austerity and structural adjustment on countries in the Global South creates entrenched inequality and economic vulnerability, which then spurs migration to the Global North where immigrant workers can then be hyperexploited and criminalized.[13] Immigrant workers are both valued for their labor and criminalized as perpetual "aliens," often subject to deportation when their labor value is no longer useful.[14] This is one mechanism through which capitalist and racial logics operate to create a class of devalued racialized laborers who are forever exploitable and replenishable. Another mechanism is the retrenchment of social assistance and the creation of necropolises that contain American-born surplus populations, who must adhere to the stringent, paternalistic logics of workfare in order to barely scrape by.[15] The struggles Phyllis and Dolores described in chapter 4 perfectly illustrate this logic of exclusionary inclusion. Relying on immigrant labor within racially segmented labor markets and rolling back or offering fractured social assistance to lower-income Americans of color are two neoliberal means of creating forever exploitable and racialized reserve armies, who must then accept poor wages and minimal work protections to survive. Discourses that paint Latinx immigrants as perpetual "illegal aliens" and stigmatize Black Americans as "welfare queens" or "lazy and demanding" workers create compliance with deplorable and risky working conditions. These sacrificial logics of exclusionary inclusion were already in place when the coronavirus began to circulate. The pandemic simply exposed and exacerbated these conditions, rendering lower-income workers at risk of immediate premature death owing to the conditions of racial biocapitalism. During the pandemic, industries and governments relied on the labor of "essential workers" without providing hazard pay, personal protective equipment (PPE), quarantine conditions, or other safety measures.

This chapter explains how Latinx and Black workers were exploited and sacrificed during the pandemic, but it also highlights the disproportionate vulnerability that undocumented workers experienced. Olayo-Méndez and colleagues found that 69 percent of immigrants and 74 percent of undocumented immigrants worked in "essential," critical infrastructure jobs in the US during the pandemic.[16] Agriculture and meatpacking are two industries in which undocumented laborers were hyperexploited during the pandemic. Although President Donald Trump imposed strict immigration control during the early months of the pandemic, farm industrialists protested, arguing that a supply of immigrant laborers were essential to food production and national security. Therefore, an exception was allowed so that mostly Mexican and Central American male migrants could access H-2A visas to work on farms during the pandemic.[17] Immigrant farm workers were given transportation, housing, and low wages for their labor, but this created conditions of total dependence on employers, and farm workers were subject to wage theft, substandard housing, illegal fees, and retaliation against whistleblowing. Further, migrants on H-2A visas were given no pathway to citizenship and were subject to deportation once their labor was no longer valued. Further, coronavirus outbreaks were common among farm workers, who were not given access to health care or proper quarantine accommodations and were not prioritized for vaccination.[18] This is a particularly egregious example of rendering an entire population disposable and sacrificial for the sake of American health and prosperity.

Similarly, meatpacking plants were declared "critical infrastructure," and under the Defense Production Act, this designation allowed meatpacking industries to restrict workers' applications for time off. Ian Carrillo and Annabel Ipsen suggest that long before the pandemic started, undocumented workers faced "precarity convergence" because the informalization of working conditions, racial segmentation of the market, and inaccessibility of social welfare overdetermined their precarity.[19] When certain industries were designated "critical" and their workers deemed "essential," already precarious working conditions turned deadly. Workers were given no sick leave, no PPE, and no unemployment benefits. The government deemed both agriculture and meatpacking industries critical to national security, but the workers who made these industries run during lockdown were left vulnerable to not only exploitation but also a deadly pathogen. The state actively participated in the sacrifice of workers within these industries.[20]

Making exceptions to allow agriculture and meatpacking industries to operate (and prosper) during the pandemic exposed undocumented workers to coronavirus infection and death. Yet, many other lower-wage frontline workers were rendered disposable through mechanisms of racial devaluation and capitalist exploitation. Neoliberal restructuring and the flexibilization of labor, the gutting of care infrastructures (and restrictions on access based on citizenship), and COVID-19 economic and health precarity converged into an overdetermined conjuncture of risks placed on lower-income frontline workers who were sacrificed to safeguard the economic norm. As such, a racialized and devalued surplus labor pool served as what Marx labeled a "lever for capitalist accumulation."[21]

Those who are consigned to slow emergencies and those who are sacrificed through exploitative labor conditions (and these groups often overlap) occupy ambivalent positions in American society. They are exceptional because their exclusion defies American democratic ideals and they are essential to the workings of racial biocapitalism, and yet neither group is given full recognition and entitlements. The boundaries of their exclusion are plagued by crisis tendencies, which leads to a constant negotiation and rearticulation of the norm. People ensconced in slow emergencies are slowly let die through the retraction of economic and social supports, yet remain constantly entangled with the state, whereas people who are sacrificed through low-wage labor are essential to capitalist accumulation but are completely extinguished in the process—their social reproduction is withheld or threatened to the point of exhaustion, until others take their place in a system of renewable exploitation. People may suffer from slow emergencies and sacrificial labor logics at the same time or move from one to the other category during their lives.

And yet both groups are ostensibly "free" to choose otherwise. Free in the sense Marx describes: "They are free from, unencumbered by, any means of production of their own" and are therefore free to sell their labor power on the market.[22] Both excluded groups occupy structurally vulnerable positions that require them to labor for the benefit of the nation, but their exploitation and abandonment are premised on their freedom. The flexibilization of labor that accompanied neoliberal reform externalized risk from the corporation to the shoulders of the worker. Low-wage, contingent laborers can choose *not* to work without protection, in dangerous conditions, and if they assume the risk and get sick or hurt, the responsibility is their burden to bear. Similarly, state assistance is made contractual and is contingent on the performance of behavioral norms (around "responsibilized" reproduction or minimum-wage work) and when structural conditions make these requirements impossible to achieve, the fault lies with the recipient and not the system.[23] In both cases, then, exclusion is premised on individual "choice." Without freedom, one cannot be held responsible for one's sacrifice or abandonment.

In the next section, I provide some statistics on the economic vulnerability of lower-income workers that forced them to work in an "essential" labor force during the pandemic. I also review the Illinois policy on "essential work" and explore some of its paradoxes. In the latter part of the chapter, I provide data from my interviews on how people experienced these conditions during the pandemic.

ECONOMIC VULNERABILITY
AND FRONTLINE LABOR

Alejandro Olayo-Méndez and colleagues argue that Latinx workers faced two kinds of exclusionary processes during the pandemic: (1) those who had to continue to work were exposed to illness because government and industries failed to protect them, *and* (2) those who worked in service industries were fired without means of subsistence because of limitations on federal benefits for the undocumented.[24] And yet, this double bind affected all lower-income, racially marginalized frontline workers because economic vulnerability is racially stratified. Black and Latinx workers were not only more likely to experience unemployment during the pandemic, but they were less financially stable before the pandemic and therefore had a harder time responding to the economic volatility the pandemic introduced. In contrast, white workers experienced the lowest rates of unemployment during the pandemic and were in better financial positions to weather job losses because of their greater liquid assets and accumulated wealth. Undocumented Americans were barred from accessing any social assistance during the pandemic, but the unemployment rates in Black communities lasted much longer than in Latinx communities as the pandemic dragged on. Nationally, the Black unemployment rate reached its peak of 16.7 percent in April and May 2020, and the Latinx unemployment rate reached its highest point of 18.9 percent in April 2020. As figures 5.1 and 5.2 illustrate, Black residents of Illinois as a whole and Chicago in particular continued to face high unemployment in 2021, even as other racial groups rebounded.[25]

Many people I interviewed lost work and were struggling to survive by cobbling together meager federal aid with help from family and friends. But for many undocumented Chicagoans, they simply watched helplessly as their debt accrued. Lorenzo, whom I introduced in chapter 4, is a fifty-three-year-old undocumented Mexican man who worked as a waiter in

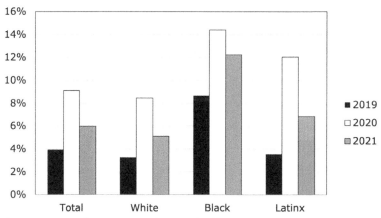

Figure 5.1 Unemployment Rates by Race in Illinois, 2019–21
Source: Basic Monthly Current Population Survey.

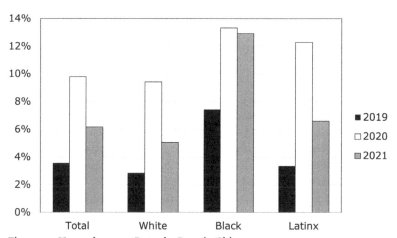

Figure 5.2 Unemployment Rates by Race in Chicago, 2019–21
Source: Basic Monthly Current Population Survey.

Little Village. He lost his job at the start of the pandemic and could not find another job. Because he's undocumented, he could not access unemployment. His savings of $2,000 lasted only two months, and he was four months behind on rent when I first interviewed him. He explained, "I was paying everything but the rent. The unemployment made me miss four months of rent. And by the time I paid it, I owed a lot of money. I paid one month. [The landlord] said, 'You already owe four months.'"[26] This accrual of debt was profoundly destabilizing for many lower-income Chicagoans.

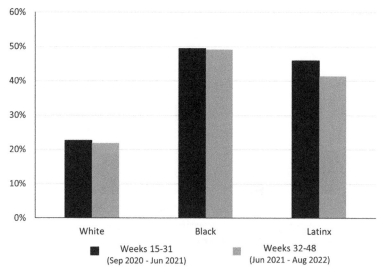

Figure 5.3 Families Who Struggled to Pay for Food, Rent, and Childcare, by Race, 2020–22

Source: US Census Household Pulse Survey Data Public Use File.

As figure 5.3 indicates, Black and Latinx families were struggling to simply make ends meet during the pandemic.[27] In the Household Pulse Survey, respondents in the greater Chicago area were asked, "In the last 7 days, how difficult has it been for your household to pay for usual household expenses, including but not limited to food, rent or mortgage, car payments, medical expenses, student loans, and so on?"[28]

Fifty percent of Black families and 46 percent of Latinx families indicated that they struggled to meet the basic needs of their families during the pandemic. Families of color were also more impacted by the closure of schools and childcare centers during the pandemic, which affected their ability to keep steady employment. Figure 5.4 illustrates how stresses from school and childcare center closures disproportionately affected families of color during the pandemic.[29] For this question, respondents in the Household Pulse Survey were asked, "Which if any of the following occurred in the last 4 weeks as a result of childcare being closed or unavailable?"[30]

These figures reporting on data from the Household Pulse Survey illustrate that Black and Latinx Chicagoans suffered from much higher rates of economic vulnerability during the pandemic. Family members who were unable to work (because industries closed or they needed to stay home with children) had to rely on those who managed to keep their frontline, "essential" jobs. Economic vulnerability within the family led directly to people

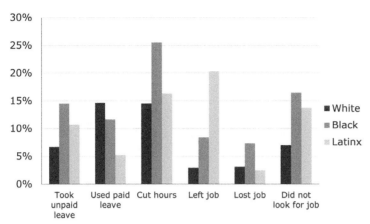

Figure 5.4 Disruptions in Childcare Affecting Work/Employment, by Race, 2021–22

Source: US Census Household Pulse Survey Data Public Use File.

"choosing" to expose themselves to the coronavirus in risky work conditions. Economic vulnerability and exposure through "essential" labor were intimately linked in low-income households.

Black and Latinx workers were more likely than white workers to work in frontline jobs. Nationally, Black and Latinx workers made up 17.0 percent and 16.3 percent of the frontline workforce, respectively, in 2020.[31] In Chicago, 35.7 percent of frontline workers were Black, while 25.5 percent of frontline workers were Latinx.[32]

Figure 5.5 illustrates that Black and Latinx Chicagoans were overrepresented in the frontline labor force.[33] Historically, the concentration of Latinx and Black Chicagoans in the lowest-paying jobs in Chicago was caused by neoliberal restructuring and labor market segmentation. In 2016, half of Latinx workers and one-third of Black workers did not earn a living wage, which means they spent at least 30 percent of their earnings on housing and could not afford food or other basic necessities.[34] Just before the pandemic, Martha Ross, Nicole Bateman, and Alec Friedhoff estimated that in the Chicago metropolitan area, 42 percent of workers were low wage, with a wage median of $10.67 per hour. Eighteen percent were Black, and 33 percent were Latinx.[35] According to data collected in the first three months of the pandemic, frontline laborers working in labor and customer service (including production/manufacturing, cleaning and maintenance, construction, and food preparation) were largely Latinx and male, lived in predominantly Latinx neighborhoods on the West Side of Chicago, had low median incomes, lacked health insurance, and were most vulnerable to both economic and health risks. This description applied to 30 percent of workers

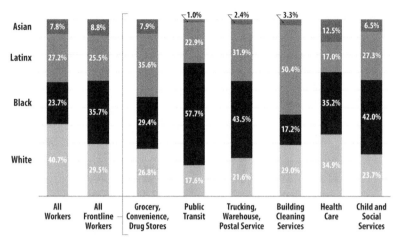

Figure 5.5   Racial Demographics of Frontline Workers in Chicago
Source: Decoteau et al., *Deadly Disparities*, 102.

in Chicago.[36] Black women were highly concentrated in lower-income home health care, and Black men were highly concentrated in security and protective services.[37] Frontline industries that require English-language skills, college degrees, or US citizenship, as well as those with a history of strong union representation, were filled with predominantly Black workers in Chicago.[38] These industries include nursing, postal services, transportation, education, and child and social services. Therefore, Black and Latinx residents were overly represented in "essential" jobs in Chicago.

ILLINOIS POLICY ON "ESSENTIAL" WORK

The Illinois Executive Order that outlined the directive for Illinois residents to shelter at home was signed by Governor JB Pritzker and went into effect on March 21, 2020. It also indicated which industries were considered "essential" and were therefore exempt from sheltering in place. These industries included government, critical infrastructure (food production, construction and utility maintenance, sewage/garbage, internet and telecommunications, distribution, mail services, and transportation), and health care. "Essential" businesses were also identified, including grocery, pharmacy, laundry, hardware, construction and critical trades (electricity, plumbing), charitable and social services, media, gas stations, financial institutions, education and childcare, residential services, hotels and motels, and funeral services.[39] Despite being deemed "essential," most of these industries failed to protect their workforce. They did not implement safety precautions such as social distancing or provision of PPE, or they did so in a piecemeal fashion over a long stretch of time. And they did not offer sick leave or hazard pay, and so workers showed up to work sick, creating a risk of contagion that was condoned by corporations and city officials alike.

A Federally Qualified Health Center (FQHC) physician I interviewed told me that the city looked the other way as many industries remained open and failed to protect their workers during the shelter-at-home order. In this way, employers exploited workers' precarity. He explained:

> Many of our patients get sick in their place of employment ... for example, this person calls me:
>
> [*imitating patient*] Hey, I don't feel well. I have this, this and that.
> [*provider*] That sounds like COVID.
> [*imitating patient*] Yeah, but my employer, I have to go to work. I need a note to go to work because my employer is asking me for this thing.
> [*provider*] First, you're sick. Second this sounds like COVID. And third, we are in a stay-at-home mandate now. How come your employer is asking you to go to work? What industry do you work for?
>
> If this guy was sick, then the person next to him was sick, and the next person was sick as well. . . . Workers are forced to jeopardize public health and not seek care in order to remain employed ... [because] they are ... financially dependent on these industries. They don't have savings. . . . Our populations are vulnerable because they work for employers that don't protect their employees. . . . Employers really took advantage of people's desperation, and the city did nothing to help.[40]

As this health care provider explains, the risks associated with working during the pandemic were externalized by industries by placing the onus on the worker to get a doctor's note, attesting to the worker's safety.

City officials were aware of the risks of "essential work." In chapter 3, I discussed how Chicago Department of Public Health epidemiologists marveled at the new "occupational risk" category they were witnessing in the data—a new vulnerability that arose in a population that was buttressed from existing definitions of vulnerability by their employment. In April 2020, the communities with the highest positivity rates were neighborhoods that were predominantly Latinx (Little Village, Pilsen, and Belmont Cragin), and the city invited community groups from these neighborhoods to join the Racial Equity Rapid Response Team. But the city did *not* institute citywide policies on worker protection, offer sick and hazard pay, or even provide PPE to businesses deemed "essential." The city did provide additional resources to FQHCs and safety net hospitals for these kinds of services, so only those in higher-paid positions were protected. Lower-wage workers were knowingly sacrificed and exposed to a deadly virus.

Gabriela, reflecting on the city's lack of protection of Latinx workers from her community of Little Village, said:

> [The city's response] could've been so different. I think it's a question of priorities, again, like ... what are you thinking of first. [The city] could've had a policy that focused on the safety of those, quote, essential work-ers or they could've really taken into account the realities of working-class people, who are often people of color. . . . Then the messaging . . . wouldn't have been so [focused on] "stay at home." Some people don't have that option. You could've focused on ... allowing more people to, I guess, stay off work, but more importantly, making sure that workplaces are safe where people continue to work.[41]

Gabriela went on to explain that instead, the city focused on prioritizing the most privileged people and left the workers to fend for themselves.

As occurred in most states, Governor Pritzker instated a progressive re-opening plan in Illinois. Phase 1 was characterized by the rapid spread of the virus and strict sheltering-in-place and social distancing restrictions. The shelter-at-home order was in effect from March 21 through May 28, 2020. Phase 2 of reopening occurred in early May, when retail stores could open for curbside pickup and delivery but the shelter-at-home order was still in place. Phase 3 began on May 28, when manufacturing, offices, retail estab-lishments, and salons could reopen. Phase 4 started on June 26, 2020, at which point restaurants and bars could reopen at 25 percent of their seating capacity, gyms could reopen at reduced rates and with mandatory distanc-ing, childcare centers reopened, and travel could resume. Although other businesses slowly reopened over time, full reopening did not occur until June 11, 2021, when vaccination was widely available to the public.[42]

Chicago Mayor Lori Lightfoot largely followed the governor's reopening stages, though she did express concern that infection could spread more easily in Chicago, with its high population density and public transporta-tion. However, she also pressured Pritzker to let bars and restaurants reopen earlier than June 26, but he did not allow this.[43] Residents I interviewed commented on Lightfoot's prioritization of bars and restaurants over other critical infrastructure in the city, often presuming Lightfoot felt pressure from these industries to prioritize their profits. For example, Gabriela said:

> I think there's a misalignment of priorities. . . . I still don't understand in the country as a whole and in Chicago specifically how we could

be comfortable opening bars and events before we had figured out schools. . . . The most at-hand things seem to be giving more leeway to bars and restaurants. . . . The mayor has a lot more pressure, I guess, from those industry sectors directly in Chicago.[44]

Many residents were acutely aware that the city government was prioritizing businesses and Chicago's economic vitality over providing care to the most vulnerable. Ana, a Mexican American woman from Little Village, expressed this view:

It seems like as mayor . . . [Lori Lightfoot is] probably trying to protect Chicago as, like, the hub of the Midwest . . . and she's trying to keep tourism going. And probably create revenue for the city. . . . I think she probably is trying to keep businesses open or something. I don't know. I just feel like she's not protecting vulnerable people.[45]

In fact, four progressive alderpeople wrote a statement criticizing Lightfoot's economic recovery task force because it was stacked with industry and corporate elites, including Republicans. They claimed she was prioritizing industry profits over the protection of workers.[46]

The federal government also prioritized industry profits over workers' lives. The federal government did not require that employers protect their workers during the pandemic. The Occupational Safety and Health Administration received thousands of complaints about employers not enforcing safety standards, but there were minimal sanctions or citations given.[47] Further, certain corporations (Amazon, Lowe's, Costco, Kroger, Walmart) gave their "essential" workers temporary pay increases, but these increases expired in the summer of 2020 when workers were still facing ongoing risks in their places of work.[48] The lack of hazard pay, enforceable safety standards, or provision of PPE to "essential workers" made it exceedingly clear that lower-income frontline workers' lives were devalued. This revelation was not lost on the people I interviewed, who were acutely aware that white, middle-class lives were protected, while low-income racially marginalized lives were not.

THE PARADOXES OF "ESSENTIAL" WORK

Protecting White Life

As I have explained, differential devaluation of human life is an essential feature of racial biocapitalism and is used to amass profits within industry by sacrificing racially marginalized surplus laborers. During the pandemic, white, middle-class Americans were able to work from home during the pandemic *because* Black and Latinx workers continued to labor in agriculture, meatpacking, shipping, delivery, and food industries. Across the country, middle-class workers were able to work from home and maintain the security of full employment while also limiting their exposure to the coronavirus, and several surveys revealed that remote workers were most likely to be white and have higher median incomes.[49] The people I interviewed were hyperaware of this dynamic. Kim, a Filipina American woman from Albany Park, told me:

> [White people] are probably more likely to have jobs that let them work at home, and so they're not going out—they're probably less likely to be essential workers. They can afford childcare . . . so that they can continue to do their work uninterrupted. When you have your job, you still have health care, so you can continue to take care of yourself in that way. . . . Black and Brown people, rightfully so, have reasons to distrust the government when it comes to things like health. In the past there has been lots of ways, too, that the government has harmed us. I think there's less distrust with white people because they know that—they can live knowing that their government's gonna protect them.[50]

As Kim so vividly points out, the spatial privileging of white life, sequestered in the home with childcare and health care intact, reinforces the valuation of white life. Kelly, a young Black woman from Albany Park, echoes the view that middle-class Americans had safety nets to fall back on if they lost work:

> I think a lot of it has to do with finances. I think that a lot of Black and Brown people who are affected, and myself included, with this pandemic are now out of work and relying on government assistance to help but I find, like, [in] a lot of the more affluent areas in Chicago, the people are able to stay home. . . . They're able to work from home . . . they're able to . . . have groceries delivered . . . [so] they don't necessarily need to leave the house. And then . . . also health insurance comes in with work and stuff like that. . . . This person who has money is gonna probably come out way better and have a better chance of not contracting it [than] someone who doesn't have that type of, like, net.[51]

As Kim and Kelly make clear, the protection of the white, middle-class norm was enabled not only by government legislation and mitigation policies but also by residential racial segregation and the wealth gap. The valuation of whiteness is institutionalized through current and historical policies and infrastructure and is often invisibilized through "colorblind" racist policies.

But during the pandemic, this differential valuation was made very evident, especially in cities such as Chicago.

Further, despite the city's efforts to enact "racial equity" measures, white, middle-class spaces were prioritized for resource allocation, especially in the early months of the pandemic. The prioritization of white space was automatic and did not require exceptional mitigation strategies to enact because white supremacy is taken for granted within the US. For example, Sholanda explained that testing sites were abundant in white neighborhoods, whereas Black residents of her Austin neighborhood struggled to access testing throughout the pandemic. She said, "In reality, where did the first testing resources [get] started? . . . Areas where people [live] whose income is six figures or better. . . . They started in suburban areas . . . with people who had money."[52] When vaccines were first rolled out to health care workers and the elderly from December 2020 through April 2021, a *Chicago Tribune* exposé revealed that most people being vaccinated lived in zip codes with the highest wealth in the city: "An analysis of more than 1 million first doses given in Chicago found nearly 60% of shots went to suburbanites and residents of neighborhoods deemed to have the lowest risk of COVID-19."[53] The fact that white, middle-class Americans could shelter at home, rely on their accumulated wealth to protect them from precarity, and easily access testing and vaccines was axiomatic because the valuation of white life is so naturalized in the US infrastructural and policy landscape. The sacrifice of lower-income, racially marginalized laborers to protect the white normative population is also hegemonic—it has characterized racial biocapitalism since its inception. Labeling frontline workers "essential" during the pandemic momentarily unveiled this historic practice of differential devaluation, and workers themselves had to live with that paradox.

The Polarized "Essential" Workforce

Many respondents commented on how higher-income workers deemed "essential" during the pandemic, such as physicians and government officials, were not only widely heralded but given PPE and hazard pay. In fact, funding from both the Coronavirus Aid, Relief, and Economic Security Act in 2020 and the American Rescue Plan Act in 2021 provided additional money for the medical profession, including expanding telehealth technology, PPE, and staff hazard pay. Of course, this funding was crucial to the effort to support the medical workforce during a health crisis. And yet, lower-income laborers whose work was deemed "essential" were often invisible and worked without a boost in pay or work protections. Several workers in these positions commented on this paradox in their interviews.

Sara, a young woman whose family is Pakistani, explained that her mother works in a hospital emergency department as a social worker, and she was not given the kind of specialized treatment doctors received:

> ["Essential worker" is] kind of an empty title. Because if you're describing doctors and nurses, I would say that those are people who know their value, because they're paid their value, like they knew that already. My mom . . . is a caseworker. She [is] not a doctor or nurse, she's also paid a normal salary . . . it's not like they paid her more at all. It's not like they paid her hazard pay. Really, anything like that. So it's, like, what does it really do that she got called an essential worker? Also, a lot of my friends are . . . waiters and hosts [in restaurants]. I would say that they were out there every day. They didn't get to do remote work or work from home. But they weren't really, really considered essential workers, like saving people's lives. And they especially don't see that reflected in their pay. So I don't really know who that title is meant for.[54]

Sara explains that salaries are a means of unpacking differential value. She says that if a person is considered truly "essential," then she should be paid for her sacrifice and be "valued" through work protection. Sara explained in her second interview that her mother could have done a lot of her work with clients via telehealth, but her mother was not given the opportunity to work from home because she was not properly valued as a caseworker.[55] Sara provided yet another example of how lower-income workers were undervalued when she explained that they were not prioritized for vaccination:

> I think the label "essential workers" is kind of like PR [public relations]. . . . Lots of people got to be essential in the beginning, like . . . doctors, nurses, but also streets and sanitation, or service workers. . . . But then when vaccines started to get rolled out, Tier One [those who were designated first in line for vaccines] wasn't for . . . all people who used to be [considered] *essential* workers. It took a long time to get a lot of people who were, like, supposedly essential vaccinated . . . [so] when you hold up a title like that, like essential workers, to . . . harsh light, it doesn't hold up.[56]

Again, Sara points out that the term *essential* implies value—it implies being given pay and protection for your labor and being prioritized for vaccination. And yet, only certain "essential" workers were treated with value and respect, and others were ignored and abused. Other respondents expressed similar disdain for the implicit stratification of value hidden within the label "essential."

Cheryl, a Black woman from Austin, worked as an in-home caregiver for the elderly, and she reflected on how her work was "essential," but she was not offered hazard pay or additional compensation for putting herself at risk during the pandemic:

> The people that work within the hospital, they are called essential workers, right? They get hazardous pay. . . . If you're in the health care profession working with seniors and whatnot, you don't. That's not fair. . . . It's a lot of people of color that is doing all the work. Amazon. Post office. Uber. Lyft. They tryin' to keep they head above water. Trying to make sure their family are okay, but they are not [categorized as] essential workers. No, they are essential workers, but they don't get the hazard pay. That's not fair. That's not fair at all.[57]

Gabriela called the label *essential* a euphemism—a cover-up for differential devaluation:

> It feels a little bit like a euphemism—trying to elevate these professions that otherwise are actually very low in prestige. It feels like it's at odds with the reality of how these people are treated, and what these professions are. How much they are paid, also. I think it can feel really cruel for people who are working in these industries to be called "essential," on one hand . . . and then being paid the way they are, on the other.[58]

Miguel, whom I introduced in chapter 4, works the night shift for a company that provides cleaning services to offices and schools. He explained that the sacrifice he made, working in risky conditions, was unseen and taken for granted:

> We felt that we were ignored. We felt that, really, they don't appreciate our work. I felt that. Not all people were working from home, some workers were in the offices, and we would take care of them. We were cleaning for them. And we were not appreciated. . . . I was working almost a month or so after the lockdown. And I see on the buses, a lot of Hispanics and African Americans who were also essential workers and we went to work in the restaurants, or cleaning . . . no, of course we were not recognized. I see faces here in my neighborhoods, maybe in other places of course you will see other faces. People who work in the field also, they were not recognized.[59]

Miguel could see the faces of people in his neighborhood who did frontline work so others could stay home, but they were invisible to the privileged. Their work and sacrifice was assumed but not appreciated.

Having No "Choice"

Luis, an undocumented man from Albany Park whom I introduced in chapter 4, explained that he had no choice but to continue to work if he and his family wanted to eat and pay the rent:

> It wasn't possible to [shelter at home] because . . . the company where my wife was, the company closed down. And then obviously you have less money for food or whatever, so there was no way to stay home. There was no way. We had to risk working. . . . My wife was nervous, right? She says she wasn't, but I could observe her and she was nervous, she was scared about the pandemic, a lot of people, even me too. . . . There was no other option.[60]

For lower-income workers, who were not given protections to continue working, there was a subtle placing of blame on their shoulders for assuming the risk of exposure. Yet, most found themselves in situations where structural precarity made their "choice" for them. Many primary breadwinners felt their family needed them to work, even if it also meant they might bring the virus home with them.

Sickness also brought about vital work interruptions, so risk and vulnerability were overdetermined, as Tomás, a man from Little Village, described:

> It's even more stress and, you know, they have to be extra careful not to pick up COVID when they step outside of their house or when they go to work. But also being even more aware of the fact that if they do end up picking up COVID, right, not only is their health in jeopardy but also their employment and their source of income, not only for themselves, really for their family and whatever other household members live with them.[61]

Because the undocumented did not qualify for federal pandemic relief aid, they had even fewer choices about whether to continue to work. Tomás continued:

> The fact [is] that a good amount of community members are also undocumented. So when we talk about providing them assistance, many of the times they don't qualify for that assistance, you know, they definitely didn't qualify and receive a government aid check. Which was nothing, to be quite honest. But at the same time, they didn't even receive that.[62]

Tomás explained the paradox of choice perfectly:

> There are people who are working . . . you know, getting paid *cash*, and if they don't go to work, there is no insurance for them, there is no financial

security. So yes, they're going to leave their home and they're going to expose themselves and potentially others. Because they *need* to have a source of income to then pay for everything else. You know, and I think not having that safety system established for communities or for individuals, . . . you know, it's one of those unfortunate realities that we have here in the States.[63]

Without a social safety net, many undocumented people and other precarious community groups did not have a choice *but* to expose themselves at work to support their families. In the next section, I provide specific experiences of being undocumented and labeled an "essential" worker.

Experiencing Dual Risks of Undocumented Status and COVID-19 Exposure

Maria is an undocumented single mother who has lived in Little Village for about fifteen years. She lost her job at a manufacturing plant at the start of the pandemic and began working for temp agencies, like the ones I described in the historical section of the introduction to this book. This work was flexible, but not reliable—often requiring her to work at night—but she could not find childcare for her two elementary school-aged children. And work through a temp agency offered her no benefits or work protections. No matter how hard she worked, she was not making as much as she had been at the plant. She contracted COVID-19 in September 2020 but continued to work daily because she could not pay her rent or buy food for her children without daily wages. Maria explained that the pandemic made it even harder for her to find more permanent, stable work. Given that basic essentials became so expensive, she really struggled to make ends meet. Maria lived in a basement two-room apartment with no windows and paid $900 a month in rent. She wished she could afford a better living environment, but she could not. She described her situation:

> [When] the cold weather comes, the work decreases, so now I am afraid that it will decrease more because . . . there may be sickness. Well, sick people get laid off, because it has happened to me that the companies and these people with the flu or headaches, they send them home. So that's what I'm afraid of, I'm afraid of getting sick with just the flu and losing my job. . . . Every time I take a break from a job, I start thinking about what I'm going to do, if I can't make this month's rent. But then, as I said, I take another job, but it's still three days, two days, a week, and the longest I've lasted is a month. . . . Even though I have my siblings, they have their family, so they have to work for their family, so I don't

feel that I have their full support, economically. So I have to keep looking day and night, I have to look for work.[64]

The stress of trying to remain healthy, looking for work regularly, and
taking care of her children was overwhelming. Maria felt stuck and unable
to do anything other than continue to work for survival.

Rodrigo said that temp agencies took advantage of people during the
pandemic, which contributed to people's suffering because the pay was
minimal and there were no safety precautions:

> So a lot of restaurants closed, a lot of restaurants let people go.... So we
> were pushed to those day labor temp agencies, they were *flooded* with
> people, the temp agencies, and they were raping them right there. You
> had to pay your transportation, you were not getting paid the minimum
> wage, you were told, come back today, but not tomorrow. So a lot of peo-
> ple ... didn't know how to pay their rent, they didn't know how to pay
> their bills.[65]

The pandemic drove wages even lower, while prices increased, and undocumented workers felt they had no choice but to work in increasingly precarious positions. Temp agencies capitalized on people's desperation, and
workers were treated as disposable labor pools, while simultaneously being
exposed to new health risks.

Before the pandemic, Luis and his wife both had steady employment in
metal factories in the suburbs of Chicago and their son was in college full-
time, but when Luis's wife's factory closed at the start of the pandemic and
then he was also let go, they slowly started to slip into emergency conditions. Luis found new work at another metal factory, but he got paid seven
dollars less per hour and did not work full-time. He told me:

> I went to work for another company, but they wouldn't give us a job that's
> full-time, you know? We worked three days, sometimes four days, and
> well, we resigned ourselves to that kind of situation and we had to face
> problems paying the rent. I borrowed money to pay the rent, everything
> fell apart ... sometimes there are serious economic problems, family
> problems, problems with the owner of the house we rent ... I am telling
> him to wait a little bit but then ... they get upset. So I end up borrowing
> to be able to cover at least the rent and food.[66]

This situation left Luis really anxious and worried. He said quietly, "I'm
sorry to say it, it's not because I'm lazy, but sometimes I run out of money.
Totally. Right now my car has a quarter tank of gas and that's not enough to

get to work."[67] And he explained that he was often up late at night worrying about how his family would survive. "The stress, the worries about the lack of work or the lack of money always affects you in some way that sometimes it becomes more difficult to sleep at night."[68] If he had been given some form of social security—housing assistance, stimulus checks, unemployment, food stamps—he would not be overcome with precarity and fear.

Not only could undocumented Americans not access social assistance, despite the fact that they were engaged in "essential" labor that put them at risk of infection, at the onset of the pandemic, social assistance was weaponized as a tool of immigration enforcement. On February 24, 2020, as the coronavirus began to circulate in the US and abroad, President Trump's Public Charge Rule went into effect, penalizing immigrants who use public assistance from achieving permanent resident status.[69] Although this policy was later retracted by the Biden administration in March 2021, many immigrants stopped seeking medical care for fear of being exposed to immigration enforcement while using Medicaid.[70] The Public Charge Rule contributed to fear, confusion, and distrust of medical institutions at the precise moment when COVID-19 began to devastate Latinx communities. According to the US Census Bureau, in 2021, 17.7 percent of Latinx Americans were uninsured.[71] The risks posed by working in unsafe environments were compounded by the fear of exposure to US Immigration and Customs Enforcement while seeking health care.

Luis said that his anxiety about becoming infected never diminished. Each time a new variant emerged, his worries accumulated. In his second interview in late 2021, he told me:

> I think we all feel fearful, everyone, everyone. At work we still talk about the same thing; even at work, we still maintain the social distance, in the cafeteria there is only one person per table. . . . But everyone talks about the variants, everyone talks that it is [be]coming stronger. Everyone is talking about how many people are dying that they knew or that the infection numbers that were going up because many people were not being responsible with the vaccinations, with taking care of themselves. . . . I think we all have that fear of getting sick.[72]

Family Ties

There was a great deal of media attention placed on "multigenerational households" as sites of broader infection, especially among those who continued to work in front-facing jobs during the pandemic. Social scientists cautioned against blaming families for the spread of disease, when familial networks were also important lifelines of support, care, and financial commitment.[73] And yet, it was certainly true that the precarity that caused many lower-income workers to continue to labor during the pandemic reverberated back to their families and communities, which overdetermined already existing structural vulnerabilities.[74] Further, many families who lost work moved in with their kin, leading to conditions of "doubling up," which posed constraints on the ability to quarantine when a family member got sick. These conditions of "doubling up" were often invisible to policymakers, and rental assistance programs were inept at helping those who left precarious rental situations to live with family.[75]

Camila, a Mexican American woman from Little Village, told me a heartwrenching story of family infection early in the pandemic. Camila worked at the information desk of a large hospital on the city's West Side, and she described how frightening it was when the first COVID-19 patients came into the hospital. Masks were optional, but her boss told her she should protect herself. Camila had just had a baby five months before the pandemic began, and she was terrified she would infect her daughter. Because it was so unclear how the coronavirus was transmitted in the beginning, she described coming home from work and changing out of her work clothes on the porch, putting them into a plastic bag, and then showering immediately. "I was paranoid about everything . . . just to even think of me bringing it back home . . . I thought of quitting," but she didn't because her family needed her salary.[76]

And then it happened. She brought the coronavirus home.

She called off from work one day because her day care center was closed, and while running errands, her muscles began to ache. The next day, she lost her voice and called into work. Her boss told her to get a coronavirus test. By then, she felt like she had a bad case of the flu: "My back was hurting, I was having, like, runny nose, nausea, chills, I had a fever."[77] The next morning, she got a call from a nurse at the clinic, who informed her she had contracted the coronavirus. She recalled her reaction:

> That's when my heart dropped. I remember I started crying . . . I was holding my daughter. And I was breastfeeding her and I was, like, oh my goodness. So when I was breastfeeding her, like, I just completely stopped. And I asked the nurse, "What am I gonna do? I have a five-month-old and I'm breastfeeding her, should I stop? What do I *do*? What is the protocol? I mean, we only have one bathroom." It was a [house with] one bathroom, one living room, one bedroom. Just a small kitchen. I mean, we're in this house. What am I gonna do?[78]

She ended up weaning her daughter right then and had her mother-in-law come pick up her baby: "I stopped breastfeeding at that moment.

Yeah, I had to give her a bottle. It was horrible [*crying*]."⁷⁹ She also had a two-year-old son, who stayed with her, as did her husband. And she lived with her parents and her brother. She wore a mask and gloves and told her son not to touch or hug her, and she cleaned constantly. But in the end, the whole family got sick. Her father had to be hospitalized because at some point, he was unresponsive. Her husband could not get off the couch. Even walking to the bathroom winded him. The family suffered lingering symptoms for weeks and weeks—loss of taste, shortness of breath, and memory loss. Her father still suffers from intermittent dizzy spells.

And then her baby daughter ended up infecting her parents-in-law and their entire extended family. Then the extended family ostracized Camila because they blamed her for spreading the infection. For six months, Camila's immediate family did not see their extended family, and eventually, Camila and her immediate family moved into another household.

When Camila brought the coronavirus home from the hospital where she worked, at a time when no one understood how the coronavirus was transmitted, it splintered her family. This story illustrates the many ways in which COVID-19 could destabilize even strong networks of care and support. Luis also faced increasing strain in his family as he was forced to borrow more and more money from his son. He believed this caused tension between his son and daughter-in-law, and Luis's other son had to drop out of college to help support the family. Although familial networks often buttress against the isolation and precarity that stems from racial devaluation in the US, there were certain ways in which the mounting vulnerability from COVID-19—from illness, from interrupted work, from meager or nonexistent social assistance—strained family ties.

When Camila went back to work, she was terrified: "I wore two masks. I did not get close to anyone . . . it was frightening to get back to work. Especially just to know that I was the one that brought it home. I felt so guilty. It was so much guilt just to know, you know, it was me . . . who brought it back." Camila told me that she got livid at work when people without masks came up to the information desk where she works: "Why are people not listening? Why are people not getting vaccinated? I mean, don't they have family members to go home to . . . [and] then they don't think that we have family at home? . . . I mean, we're already two years into this—just wear the mask!"⁸⁰ So dealing with recalcitrant members of the public highlighted the risks she was taking every day to continue doing her work to help others. This risk, and the toll it took on her family, made the stakes of "essential work" so much clearer for Camila.

Workplace Risks

Lola Loustaunau and colleagues argue that being labeled "essential" led to very precarious workplace conditions.[81] There were many definitions of "essential" in circulation, so some workers at the beginning of the pandemic were uncertain whether they would retain their jobs or for how long. People who were initially let go were sometimes uncertain when they could return to work. Further, Loustaunau and colleagues argue that management was often slow to implement COVID-19 protocols (e.g., social distancing, required masking), and corporations and states were not forcing compliance. Then, once mask and vaccine mandates were in place, it was often the responsibility of lower-paid employees to impose these policies, which could become burdensome and dangerous. The interviews I conducted confirmed these findings.

Shantal, a Black woman from Austin and a former nurse, commented on the constant anxiety and exhaustion that accompanied "essential" work as she reflected on the work done by her former colleagues:

> I feel bad that, uh, it wasn't enough relief, where they didn't have to work the seven days a week, because when you're burnt out, that puts you at risk for catching these things. When your immune system is worn out. You're . . . sleepy, you're tired . . . you're overworked. Your family is at home, you're taking a risk of taking something back home to your family because you *got* to come to work to *provide* for your family. . . . The burnout is a lot.[82]

Candice, a Black woman from Austin, worked at a court-mandated treatment facility. She told me that in March 2020, there were sixteen patients she was overseeing, and the next day, there were only two because the others had been sent to quarantine facilities. This moment is when the gravity of the pandemic hit her, she said. She spoke about how management and the corporate leaders stayed home during the pandemic, whereas she was required to keep working:

> All the high management like financial, the CEO, HR [human resources], the director, all them was working from home. . . . I felt like everybody should have been [at work]. Everybody should have been there. We was there, everybody should have been there. You know, if we're an essential worker program . . . why did you get to stay home out of harm's way? And we didn't? [If] you felt like it was that bad that *you* couldn't come to work, then why you just didn't shut the facility down? Yeah, so. But . . . I know how it's, you know, played. Especially in the Black community, the

poor community, and the community I stay in. You know, it is what it is. It always been like that even before the pandemic, so I wasn't surprised.[83]

Candice also did not believe that she was properly compensated for the risks she was taking. She told me there was a pool of additional money workers could get if they never missed a day of work: "They took some of the money they got for businesses during the pandemic and they was issuing it out to us essential workers but we couldn't miss a day. So every two weeks when you got paid, you got an extra $350 but you *couldn't* miss a day. So if you missed a day, you didn't get the $350."[84] Such a policy incentivized working while sick.

Sholanda worked for FedEx, and she talked extensively about how lax the company was in meeting COVID-19 protocols to protect their staff:

> To me, FedEx was slow to react to it. Some stores you go in now, you see those little plastic Plexiglass screens up so people don't be right up on you. FedEx never done that. They still haven't done that. To me, they're not doing enough to protect their people. I just feel FedEx can do so much more. . . . We had to start *whining* about it. We had to start complaining, that hey, where is the protection? I mean . . . we were going out with our own money, buying hand sanitizer, buying things to protect our-selves. . . . We wasn't even made to make people wear masks. . . . And only time they did that was when [a coworker] got COVID, that's when FedEx decided to do something.[85]

When that employee's illness occurred, FedEx made everyone stay home for two weeks. However, the company asked employees to take their sick leave. Sholanda informed her coworkers that the company could not make them use their sick leave for a mandated leave of absence. She told me she looked up the policy on the corporation's website, printed it out, and handed it out to her coworkers on all the shifts, informing them of their rights.

Dolores, who worked as a member of the cleaning staff for a hotel, said that she was not given proper PPE:

> I consider myself a frontline worker 'cause I work with the public . . . I work with the public 'cause people come from all over to our hotel. You know what I mean? So, and then we don't wear PPE, we just wear masks and gloves. That's not the proper PPE to wear in that kind of environ-ment. Because you get people coming from all over and everybody don't wear masks, you know what I'm saying, like they should.[86]

When Dolores contracted COVID-19, she was required to stop working for ten days, but without pay, and she did not feel that was fair given the risks she was taking.

Isa, a Filipina American woman from Albany Park, explained that she knew people who were not complying with the policy at her workplace whereby people had to remain home without pay if they tested positive for COVID-19:

> If they do get sick, then they're like, "Okay, you gotta go through all these hoops before you can come back and work." Sometimes they're sick. I've heard a lot of people say, "I can't call off." I'm like, "Why not? You're sick." Isn't this the whole point of the guidelines? . . . I get it. If you miss a day of work, [according] to CDC's guidelines, it's ten days. So, guess what? You're gonna miss ten days of work, and that's an income you've lost. It definitely disproportionately puts down more risk.[87]

Many respondents discussed these policies for mandated sick leave but remaining at home for 10 days with no pay, was a serious constraint on peoples' economic survival. Such policies pit economic and health risks against one another.

Sara, who earlier described her mother's caseworker position at the hospital, also worked as a barista in a coffee shop, and she discussed how hard it was to implement the vaccine mandate that was in place from January 3 through February 28, 2022, during the Omicron surge. Chicago had a citywide vaccine mandate. To work out in a gym, eat in a restaurant, or attend events where food and drink were served, Chicago residents had to show a proof-of-vaccination card.[88] But it was up to workers to police customers on the mandate. Sara told me:

> We started checking for vaccination cards . . . but what happened is . . . there was just enough outrage and lack of support for the move that we were told to stop checking for vaccination cards, even though we had a sign on the door that said like, "Oh yeah, we're gonna check." They said, "Stop asking people." And I really didn't like that, that made me, like, really uncomfortable. It like felt like very explicitly condoning . . . people [coming in] unmasked, unvaccinated. Especially when so many people had gotten sick *while* at work. And so that was rather uncomfortable. To feel like they did not care at all.[89]

Even though she felt uncomfortable confronting recalcitrant customers about the policy, Sara felt it was safer, as a work condition, than not doing so.

In this section, I explained a few of the workplace uncertainties and hassles that emerged for frontline workers during the pandemic, at their places of work. They were exhausted and overworked. Their bosses were slow or failed to implement COVID-19 safety protocols and were vague or unfair about hazard pay or sick leave, and they often left it up to workers to implement vaccine and mask mandates or failed to comply with them. Therefore, not only were frontline workers being sacrificed, but their work conditions were also precarious and anxiety-producing.

*   *   *

The neoliberal flexibilization of labor *and* the retraction or fractured nature of social safety nets left Black and Latinx workers without any choice but to sacrifice their health to earn a living during the COVID-19 pandemic. During the pandemic, "essential" laborers were seen as a necessary yet disposable supply of cheap labor. Policymakers treated the sacrifice of low-income, racially marginalized workers as a necessary price to pay to safeguard the economy and the middle class. The exclusion of Latinx and Black workers from protection by the state was predetermined by historical forces but also newly rearticulated during the pandemic. As Pulido explains, "The devaluation of Black (and other nonwhite) bodies has been a central feature of racial capitalism for centuries and creates a landscape of differential value which can be harnessed in diverse ways to facilitate the accumulation of . . . power and profit."[90] During the pandemic, differential valuation allowed state actors and corporations to safeguard the middle class and the economy until "normal" exploitative conditions could resume. The sacrifice of low-wage workers operates in conjunction with slow death. Those ensconced in slow emergencies are slowly let die through lack of resources, and "essential" workers are immediately sacrificed through labor exhaustion. But the paradoxical nature of their exclusion and the ultimate outcome are similar. I end with a story that highlights the mechanisms of disavowal and paradoxical devaluation of those deemed "essential" and disposable.

Linda, a Black woman from Austin, proudly declared in her interview that she "works for COVID." She was employed as a manager of one of the unregulated pop-up testing centers that emerged all over US cities in the winter months of 2021–22, as the Omicron variant was quickly spreading. Linda explained, "I work for COVID now . . . I take COVID tests. I run the whole team. Yeah. Me. That means I can hire someone, up under a W-9 contract. I can, uh, put them to work. . . . Train them, and all that. And test them and turn my tests in."[91] Although she seemed proud when she first explained it to me, she then expressed anger at how little she was being paid for the risk she was taking:

> You think because they . . . allowing us to do free COVID tests that that's paying us? Man, some of that money that they paying the doctor, do you know how much the doctor make for one specimen? . . . He make $2,000

and some dollars, ma'am, look it up. That's the money that they could have gave to somebody out here. I just told you they don't pay me but $20 for a test. . . . I'm on the front line just like the doctor. Where my money? You understand what I'm saying? . . . They playing games with people lives.[92]

She went on to explain that to her, this situation was similar to paying certain people to stay home while others needed to keep working in frontline jobs. Linda said, "If they would have been paying me to stay home, I would've did it, too [*chuckles*]. Unfortunately, I didn't have that." She also told me that the stimulus checks did not stretch far enough, and people's needs far exceeded what they were able to receive. Linda told me she thought that the high prices caused by inflation in 2022 were taxing people for having received stimulus checks the year before: "You see how much chicken cost? You see how much a dozen eggs cost? Do you see how much milk cost? They taxing us for this shit." She said that pandemic policies clearly illustrated the wide-scale devaluation of Black and Brown lives, and she ended the interview by explaining to me that the government was prepared to just let people die. To her, the ending of pandemic aid was a clear message that the government was ready to move on and leave all the vulnerable people to die: "Man, these people know what they doing. They killing us off. . . . Just open up the cemetery. Shit. And act like it's God's work and not ours."[93] Such is the outcome of differential racial devaluation during a pandemic.

6: TRUST AND DISTRUST IN PANDEMIC TIMES

Yeah, I'm not gonna take no vaccine 'cause I don't know what's in it.
I don't know what's goin' on. . . . I think that . . . they wanna eliminate
Blacks. They wanna use us as guinea pigs. . . . The politicians, the
presidents, all these CEOs, the billionaires . . . the high society people,
they know what's goin' on. They puttin' this out here. They know what's
goin' on. We not dumb. We just don't have no rights 'cause we don't
have money.

JADA, Black resident of Little Village,
interviewed on December 16, 2020

It has become sociologically commonplace to suggest that racially marginalized populations express broad sentiments of distrust in the state and in the medical establishment.[1] Prior to the onset of the COVID-19 pandemic, however, there was little scholarship linking vaccine hesitancy among nonwhite groups to distrust stemming from medical neglect and harm.[2] During the pandemic, however, a great deal of public commentary and academic scholarship blamed "misinformation," conspiracy theories, *and* medical distrust for the lower rates of vaccine uptake among especially Black but also Latinx Americans.[3] Jada's quote that introduces this chapter expresses sentiments I heard repeatedly in interviews with Black Chicagoans. Many Latinx Chicagoans I interviewed also expressed doubts about vaccine safety. Based on my interviews, vaccine distrust is linked to experiencing racial devaluation within the US racial biocapitalist system. And yet, popular media portrayals and academic scholarship often conflate feelings of distrust with health behavior.[4] Many people I interviewed did not believe that the state or the medical establishment cared about protecting Black and Brown lives, but they nonetheless got vaccinated. This chapter explores the paradoxes of trust and vaccine hesitancy in the era of COVID-19, among those who feel racially devalued within the United States.

Black, Latinx, and Indigenous communities consistently had lower vaccination rates than white Americans throughout the pandemic.[5] Consider figure 6.1, which depicts rates of vaccination by date in Chicago among designated racial groups.[6] This figure only captures completion of the initial vaccine sequence, which became available to all Americans aged eighteen or older in April 2021. In May 2021, children aged twelve or older could receive the vaccine, and around late October or early November 2021, children ages five through eleven could receive the initial vaccine sequence. Figure 6.1 indicates how many people who identify as Black, white, Latinx, or Asian received the initial vaccine sequence—the values are not weighted by population percentage. Because white, Black, and Latinx Chicagoans each make up approximately one-third of the population, figure 6.1 clearly indicates racial disparities in vaccine uptake.

As of March 2023, Black communities in Chicago had the lowest vaccination rates: 64.3 percent of Black Chicagoans had received one dose of a vaccine (compared with 81.0 percent of Latinx and 78.0 percent of white Chicagoans), and 57.1 percent of Black Chicagoans had completed one vaccine series (compared with 72.0 percent of Latinx and 70.0 percent of white Chicagoans).[7] When vaccine boosters became available in the fall of 2021

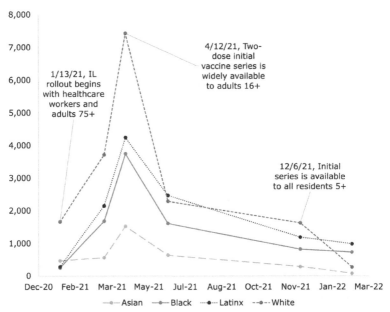

Figure 6.1 Average Daily Vaccination Series Completed by Racial Group in Chicago, January 2021–February 2022

Source: City of Chicago, "COVID Dashboard."

and again in 2022, racial disparities in vaccination rates were even more pronounced. White Chicagoans were much more likely to receive boosters than either Latinx or Black Chicagoans.[8] And yet, the reasons for failing to vaccinate may have shifted over time. A recent study found that although racially marginalized groups may have originally distrusted the safety of new vaccines, once the vaccines proved effective, distrust was no longer an obstacle to vaccination.[9] As the pandemic progressed, racially marginalized people increasingly struggled to *access* vaccines. Therefore, while vaccine uptake rates remained consistently low, distrust may have only been an explanatory factory early in the pandemic.[10] Access barriers may become even more pronounced moving forward since the cost of COVID-19 vaccines is no longer covered by the federal government. People must pay for them with private or public health insurance or out of pocket if uninsured.[11]

The academic literature on vaccine beliefs and behaviors during the COVID-19 pandemic paints distrusting communities with broad cultural brushstrokes.[12] There is an overrepresentation of scholarship focusing on the role of social media "misinformation" and generalized medical distrust.[13] These articles conflate feelings of distrust with health behaviors, such as vaccine uptake, and yet the relationship between belief and action is complex and often context specific. In interviews with me, Black and Latinx Chicagoans discussed an array of factors and interactions that caused them to distrust both state and medical actors and institutions, and while this distrust often led to questions and concerns about vaccines, it did not always lead to vaccine avoidance, which was quite varied. Further, there is a subtle insinuation in the scholarship on and social media coverage of vaccine hesitancy that people who buy into "misinformation" or "conspiracy beliefs" are irrational. Yet, such a presumption discounts the very real concerns the people I interviewed shared about whether or not they could trust the state or the medical establishment to protect their lives.

The distrust expressed in interviews was often warranted, given people's experiences with differential racial valuation and their multiple, negative, racialized interactions with state authorities (e.g., police, parole officers, social welfare agents) and medical professionals (whom they often feel are overly surveillant of Black and Brown patients). Respondents also explained that the constancy with which public health advice changed during the pandemic made them distrust public health experts. Many people in this study are HIV positive, have a history of drug or alcohol addiction, or are survivors of domestic violence—these conditions are heavily medicalized, and people often feel surveilled, disciplined, and pathologized by both state and medical actors involved in their therapeutic governance.[14] Such feelings can cause system avoidance and suspicion. Backlash from the Public Charge Rule, which I explained in chapter 5, also led some immigrant groups to distrust medical institutions and staff. Finally, many Black and Latinx Chicagoans felt that their broader social vulnerability was ignored, and city and public health officials only cared whether they got tested and vaccinated. These experiences of harm and devaluation could lead to an accumulation of distrust that is difficult to counteract.

And yet, a community group I was introduced to through this research countered vaccine hesitancy with an epistemic approach that encouraged structural critique and recognized racial devaluation but nonetheless taught people to trust vaccination as a politics of survival. One-third of the respondents I interviewed in Austin were recovering from substance use addiction. I offered fifty dollars per interview, and I found that many people in Austin were sharing the interview flyer with contacts from their recovery group. Fifty dollars can go a long way in economically insecure times, and so people shared information about participation in this study to help one another survive. By accident, I tapped into the close-knit recovery and mutual aid group run by Marlin and Shanice, which I discussed in chapter 4. Many members of the group had been in recovery for over a decade. While I did not intentionally recruit participants who were members of this recovery group, the emergence of this network in the sample allowed me to see how belonging to a trusted social group can provide an outlet for processing distrust and uncertainty.

People who deal with substance use in their daily lives are very familiar with the slow grind of addiction and how its consequences extend across kin networks. But they are also accustomed to urgent crises of overdosing. People in recovery programs, then, are primed for navigating the slow and immediate emergencies of state disinvestment and devaluation. Recovery groups are also very exclusive and intimate because survival is dependent on honesty and life-giving support. Although certain recovery programs are court mandated or sponsored by state or medical institutions, the recovery group I accessed in Austin functioned more as a long-term mutual aid recovery group. It was not linked to state or medical services or oversight. This recovery group was well poised to offer an alternative politics of care amid the necropolitics of state pandemic policies. Marlin's organization provides recovery support to its members, as well as resources for people who are HIV positive, violence prevention, and a food pantry, and the organization developed a testing site to respond to the needs of the community during the COVID-19 pandemic. Many members of the group are in long-term recovery, are HIV positive, and have dealt with gun violence in their families. In many ways, this organization fulfilled the welfare role that the state has abandoned, and it allowed its members to survive the slow and fast emergencies of COVID-19. It also provided an important epistemic lens for acknowledging distrust but nonetheless encouraging vaccination.

I begin by explaining the varied forms of distrust that Black and Brown Chicagoans expressed in interviews with me. In doing so, I illustrate that distrust is warranted, linked to experiences of being racially devalued and neglected, and often accumulates over time. I then review some of the vaccine beliefs I heard in interviews, alongside a critical account of vaccine policies in the city. Finally, at the end of the chapter, I provide evidence of the ways that Marlin's recovery group countered fear, isolation, and distrust, while also offering broad structural support that the state failed to provide. Distrusting the state and medical establishment does not always lead to vaccine avoidance. Distrust is relational and context specific, and a politics of care can affirm a structural account of inequality while also offering an alternate narrative about vaccination as a means of counteracting racial devaluation.

CONDITIONS OF ACCUMULATING DISTRUST

Distrust tends to accumulate over time when it is compounded by multiple experiences of racial harm. And it often begins with a generalized sense of anomie linked to knowledge that state and medical agents devalue Black and Brown lives. Citing historical instances of medical abuse (e.g., the Tuskegee experiment, mentioned in chapter 2) or espousing suspicion that the government purposefully introduced crack or HIV into Black communities as a form of population control is a rational way people make sense of the US racial state and its ongoing violence and abuse of Black and Brown populations.[15] When state agents continuously illustrate racist intent through punitive and disciplinary policies and racial violence, people distrust the state to protect their lives. And this sense of devaluation was heightened during the COVID-19 pandemic, especially as news began to surface of the disproportionate racial toll the pandemic was taking. It was exceedingly common for people to mention population control in interviews with me. Consider these statements made by Bernice and Alicia, two Black women from the Austin neighborhood:

> I think they just dropped [COVID-19] . . . on us . . . to try to take down some of the population. I think it got outta control and they can't secure it. . . . Donald Trump did that. . . . Think about it. It's not enough jobs for people. It's not enough of nothin', really, for us, period. . . . He dropped it there. . . . I don't know how he did it, but he did it.[16]

> I believe that [COVID-19] was targeted for poverty, and Black Americans and Hispanic and Latino. . . . I believe that the government had to come up with this pandemic, because [Trump] was trying to, he was trying to stay and be reelected.[17]

In these framings, COVID-19 was constructed by government agents to control the size of the population because there are limited resources or to exterminate racially marginalized groups because they might vote against the incumbent president Trump. Naming COVID-19 and the vaccines as mechanisms of racist population control was a common refrain in interviews, especially among Black respondents. Acknowledging a history of racialized abuse, these sentiments reflect deep distrust of the state, steeped in racial devaluation. People also expressed distrust of scientific and medical experts.

Because expert advice kept changing, people felt incapable of making sense of wildly shifting policies. Shantal, a Black woman from Austin who was a nurse before she retired, told me:

> I was on a call with some young Black, *educated* men . . . when they started talking about how they wasn't gonna take the vaccine, and they was talking about the Tuskegee Airmen, and (*pause*) I was *so* sick to my stomach, I didn't know what to do! . . . Because [the pandemic] happened so fast, and [the coronavirus] was unknown. . . . But then, too, . . . the people giving out information, there was such a discrepancy, sometimes in the information that was given. So if you're already a nonbeliever, and this person is saying one thing, who's an expert, and this one is saying something else . . . I think a lot of that added to the fear.[18]

Phyllis, another Black woman from Austin, explained that she tried to follow expert advice, but it kept changing, leading to ontological insecurity:

> I try to watch the news and keep up on any information every day. But even from the same person . . . they may say different information. . . . Like right now is the masks a mandate, or isn't a mandate? And you might hear in one breath where it's a mandate here, but it's not a mandate here. . . . So you don't know what the heck you're dealing with! It's a lot of confusion. It is! It's a lot of unanswered stuff. . . . But in this case, no one knows what to do. Even the people who are *studying*—the doctors and all that, that's supposed to have all the answers . . . they don't know.[19]

As Phyllis affirms, the constantly shifting advice from scientific leaders asking for public trust contributed to suspicions about expert competence.

Dolores, also a Black resident of Austin, reflected on both the contradictions in expert knowledge and the uncertainty of the bodily toll of exposure to unknown viruses and vaccines over time.

Because I wasn't expecting these other variants . . . You know, it's another variant now. And they always say, "Well, we got control." Ya'll had the Omicron under control [*laughs*]. . . . Y'all had all the other stuff contained and look what happened. Now they talking about [requiring boosters] six months from [now, then] next year. . . . So we gone keep taking shots? Then what's the side effect of all this stuff in our bodies over the years? . . . What's the point of getting the shot if I'm gone get sick anyway? . . . Because you know in the beginning they was saying take this shot and you gone be good. And that shit was a lie. People still dying from it that been vaccinated. It's just that the death rate is not as high with vaccinated people.[20]

Here, Dolores expresses exasperation that whereas initially the vaccines were celebrated for stopping transmission, in the summer of 2021, when the Delta variant emerged, experts realized the vaccines did not completely protect against infection—only reduced the likelihood of hospitalization. She indicates that this shift in rationale made people wary of vaccination.

In fact, when policies were explicitly changed for obvious economic rationales, people's trust in public health experts declined because it illustrated the political as opposed to scientific motivation of public health advice. Dolores, for example, discussed shifts in quarantine policies. She reminded me that originally public health experts advised people to stay home for ten days but then switched the recommendation to five days "because of the economy." I quoted her in chapter 1 expressing her exasperation, "They grasping at straws, right? . . . How do you protect yourself? Right? When you steady getting wrong data. If y'all don't know, y'all don't *know!*" Shifting expert advice caused people to distrust public health officials *and* led many to avoid boosters, even if they had originally been vaccinated. Because of a history of violent interactions with both the police and medical authorities, Dolores explained, people are primed to be suspicious: "Like with the syphilis when they were deliberately giving Black people syphilis and having them to suffer through that. So, um, you don't know that you can trust this." Despite all this suspicion, Dolores got vaccinated because "I don't want to be a statistic . . . I didn't want to end up one of the dead people."[21] This illustrates that people can have a lot of distrust in the government and medical expertise, and still get vaccinated.

Other respondents spoke about a lifetime of experiences with racist state agents. Robert Vargas argues that when people have a series of negative experiences with authority figures, including hospital staff, social workers, and welfare agents, then they are less likely to register for Medicaid, even when it's available.[22] Many of the people I interviewed discussed racist

interactions with police, hospital emergency department staff, and staff at
court-mandated recovery programs, which also sometimes resulted in distrusting views of state or medical institutions. Recall Reginald, a Black resident of Austin whom I introduced in chapter 4, who discussed his negative
experiences with hospital staff who treated him "like shit" because he was
unhoused, and who also believed he was "railroaded" by the police and
the judicial system because he was poor and could not afford a decent lawyer.[23] People who have experienced a lifetime of racialized mistreatment
from agents who are charged with protecting them often end up distrusting
the system as a whole.

Other people I interviewed felt disgruntled because it seemed that state
agents did not care about meeting robust community needs for economic,
food, housing, childcare, and health support, and they only cared whether
people got vaccinated. Because the pandemic intensified already existing
social vulnerability, many people were *more* concerned with resolving their
health, financial, and housing precarity than with getting vaccinated. Some
research suggests that broader social vulnerability is linked to vaccine hesitancy. In one study, people who were having difficulties paying rent were
seven times more likely to avoid vaccination because vaccination was not
a priority.[24] A Kaiser Family Foundation study from September 2021 found
that nonelderly adults without health insurance had the lowest rates of vaccine uptake of any group.[25] Since free vaccines were accessible to those
without insurance at this time, this statistic must capture other measures
of social vulnerability.

And yet, city officials were keen to get people of color vaccinated. Equitable vaccine metrics were one way Mayor Lori Lightfoot proved her success
in mitigating the disproportionate impact of COVID-19 on communities of
color in Chicago. In 2021, the mayor asked community-based organizations
(CBOs) working in communities that were prioritized for vaccine outreach
through the COVID Community Vulnerability Index (CCVI) to vaccinate at
least 50 percent of their constituents. One community organizer who works
as and trains health ambassadors who go door-to-door in a predominantly
Black neighborhood in Chicago explained this problem:

> So sometimes community doesn't even want to talk about it, right? Be-
> cause the message overwhelmingly is "get the vaccine." Get the vaccine,
> and that's it. . . . And so . . . are people really addressing their concerns?
> And if they're not, and if the only thing they're saying is "get the vac-
> cine," yes, people are tired of it.[26]

The Chicagoans I interviewed understood that health stems not simply
from medical prevention and treatment but also from safe homes and

neighborhoods, good food and clean water, affordable housing, and financial security. So when government agents expressed a sole interest in getting people vaccinated, often this narrow focus resulted in pushback.

Some interviewees turned their distrust toward their own communities, often invoking racially pathologizing narratives of one another. Given widespread uncertainty and isolation, these people parroted postwelfare logics prominent in the news and within agencies promoting workfare and self-responsibility. Monique, a Black resident of Austin, told me she was scared to go out in her neighborhood because youth might steal her groceries out from under her:

> You coming home with the groceries, people robbed me. I'm on the West Side of Chicago. And that's what they do. They look for the weakest link. I'm not the weakest link. I'm gonna fight back. But still, that's what they go for. You know, they rob you for your groceries and anything they can get 'cause for them to sell to get them some money. Because of the virus, [there] ain't no jobs.[27]

Others blamed members of their community for taking advantage of the social welfare made available during COVID-19, as if everyone had to compete for scarce resources. Adela, a Mexican American woman from Little Village, argued that people in her community were taking advantage of the available social assistance. According to Adela, her tenant received rental assistance but made enough money to pay her rent. Adela went on to make racialized claims about welfare dependency:

> I assure you that if they didn't give [government assistance/welfare], even if it is selling tamales or whatever, people would get ahead. I mean, we are in a country where nobody is starving, there are pantries, there are places where you can get food. That is what I have been doing. I say they should take away all the assistance ... [because] as long as the government is giving money to people, they're not going back to work. The government is giving money. . . . I assure you that it is not good, now they are already rich, with all that the government has given them. But that's why they don't want to work, because with everything the government gave them, they don't need to go out to work because they were making more than working.[28]

Several residents told me that people in their neighborhood were taking advantage of small business loans, which made the government close the system for everyone. Phyllis contended:

> The reason why rental assistance and food assistance are not offered or continued is because people don't do what they're supposed to do with

it. One example is, I think it was money offered to some businesses. And the only thing you had to do is say that you had one and then apply for this money. And they would give you so much amount of money to help you stay afloat. A lot of people were using that money that never had a business. And then when they got the money, they didn't use the money to help their situation, they still weren't paying bills, they weren't trying to keep a roof over their head, or none of that. They were going to Vegas. They were splurging on things that they wouldn't normally even buy, and things like that. So that makes it hard for the next person that really does need it that would do the right things with it.[29]

Therefore, widespread distrust often filtered into community relations and caused people to distrust one another, blaming each other for taking advantage of a system that was barely helping those who most needed it.

In this section, I have provided a whole host of ways in which people expressed distrust during the pandemic, illustrating how distrust can pile up and extend out, based on an accumulation of experiences with state and medical authorities. Often when distrusting experiences do accumulate, people feel isolated and may express greater resentment of public health advice. Despite the myriad reasons people felt distrusting in the midst of the pandemic, this distrust did not always lead to a failure to vaccinate.

VACCINE BELIEFS AND COMPLICATIONS

In my interviews with racially marginalized Chicagoans, vaccine concerns were widespread. These beliefs were consistent with those circulating on social media during the pandemic, and with findings from other research.[30] The most common misconception expressed was a concern that the vaccine *causes* coronavirus infection. The rationale was that the US government has a history of medically abusing Black Americans by purposefully giving them syphilis, which is how the Tuskegee experiment is widely understood among residents I interviewed (as Dolores explained in a quote in the previous section). This rationale was not unrelated to the second widespread sentiment, that COVID-19 was created by the government (on purpose or by accident) with xenophobic or necropolitical intent, as several of the quotes I discussed earlier indicated. Deion, a Black man from Austin, expressed a belief that the vaccine was meant as a population control measure:

Once the population gets too big or they feel like the United States is too crowded . . . [then] they got to get rid of people, so I feel like if I get the vaccine then . . . it's gonna be a lot of people that die from it.[31]

A third concern was that vaccinations cause extended illnesses, which can disrupt already attenuated work schedules, making survival more difficult. Maria, an undocumented single mother from Little Village whom I introduced in chapter 5, feared getting vaccinated because she could not afford to miss work from the side effects: "Well, the truth is, people that have had [the vaccine], some say that it . . . hurts the way they breathe or that it alters their heart and they have a headache . . . [so] I'm afraid of a reaction afterwards."[32] She told me that she worries about getting COVID-19 because she has no one to care for her children, but she also worries that the vaccine will make her sick. She is not sure which is worse:

> I'm afraid of getting sick or something bad happening to me and leaving my children. I mean . . . I try to take care of myself, to wash my hands, to be covered whenever I go out, whatever it is. But I also don't want to get vaccinated for the same reason. So it's like half and half: I'm afraid of getting sick, that something will happen to me, but I also don't want to get vaccinated for the same reason.[33]

Despite fearing vaccination, Maria does follow other public health advice such as masking, washing her hands, and social distancing. This illustrates that distrust is not monolithic and often leads to variable expressions of hesitancy.

Fourth, people from both Black and undocumented communities told me that vaccines were installing invisible tracking devices under the skin. A health ambassador from Austin told me that her organization required organizers to write down people's names and addresses when vaccinating them, which made residents suspicious about being surveilled:

> They don't want to give us any information. We have to take their ID and ask if they have insurance. But people, and rightfully so, are worried about where this information is going and why they have to give it. People think we're giving away their information . . . [so] I understand why they're scared.[34]

Communities who are highly surveilled by both the criminal justice and medical systems are often skeptical of any service that requires documentation of their personal information. Anthony Urea found this skepticism to be true among Black, queer youth being encouraged to adopt preexposure prophylaxis for HIV.[35] In the case of COVID-19, needing to show an ID sometimes made people wary of vaccination.

As I already mentioned, some people who originally got vaccinated became skeptical of boosters once it became clear they do not prevent infection from new variants, even if they do protect against hospitalization and death. The possibility that people may need repeated boosters as new variants emerge caused some interviewees to waver in their support of vaccination. As Rodrigo put it:

> If the first vaccination didn't work, and the second vaccination didn't work . . . what makes me feel secure that the third would? . . . I've been vaccinated two times and that's it. I'm good, I test myself and I've been negative. . . . If you're telling me that (*sighs*) what I have in my body is not going to cover me from this variant, then I do not know if I want to trust what you are telling me right now. Like, I have then a little doubt.[36]

In this way, what starts as vaccine trust turns into circumspection as more and stronger variants emerge. Yet, Rodrigo still gets tested, and he believes that he is protected against the worst outcomes from COVID-19 because he received the full initial vaccine series.

Finally, there were concerns about certain adverse effects of vaccines being hidden from the public. People often discussed these matters in oblique ways with me, but community organizers reported that men feared testicular swelling and impotence and women were concerned about disruptions to menstruation and infertility. And in fact, because city and state officials were hesitant to provide forthright information on adverse vaccine reactions (before population data could be gathered), silence about side effects fueled people's concerns. Members of a community organization in a predominantly Black neighborhood suggested to city officials that they publish information on physical vaccine reactions, so people were properly informed. The organizer told me:

> The men having pain in their groin, you know, testicular swelling. There are all types of reactions that are heard of that I feel like should be more publicly talked about, so that people can be informed, they don't have to be caught by surprise once they get vaccinated. Because then that gives them the idea that they've been tricked, or they've been lied to about what could possibly happen after being vaccinated. . . . We recently had a virtual meeting with those who facilitate Chicago Public Health Dashboard to give them feedback, and we definitely let them know that one of the resources that we felt like should be recorded are the reactions . . . just to give the community a sense of normalcy among what symptoms are happening more frequently. Because if it's just me by myself, and I'm having these adverse reactions, if I don't see that there are communities of people that are working through these same reactions with me,

I'm going to feel very isolated, paranoid, and that's going to impact the way I'm healing.[37]

Another worker at the same CBO suggested that publicizing adverse reactions would combat misinformation. There has been no scientific evidence indicating that testicular swelling is a confirmed adverse reaction to vaccination, which likely explains city officials' reluctance to discuss this matter with residents.[38]

Another community organizer in a predominantly Latinx neighborhood explained that a lack of open conversation about the impact of the vaccine on menstruation was also a barrier to vaccine uptake.

> One of the things that we have noticed very recently, a lot of our staff members are predominantly female. So they have had very, very, very, very large complaints that their bodies have not been the same after the vaccines. . . . I think that maybe very recently, [a woman's] period has become something that women are more comfortable talking about. But within a minority community, that's really not something that we talk about. . . . We have had two meetings, and . . . [staff] will check and say, . . . "Hey, I've been feeling this. Am I the only one?" And I think that that's the component that's scary, because people are going through these things, but they're not talking about it, or they're not asking anybody because they don't know who to ask. . . . We have heard women tell other women, like, "Don't get it because it messed up my period," or "Don't get it because what if it causes infertility?" . . . And as a woman, I can't in good conscience say, "Oh, get it, nothing's gonna happen."[39]

In both of these examples, community workers want to build trust by openly discussing adverse vaccine reactions with residents. When side effects remain undiscussed, distrust percolates, calling the knowledge and trustworthiness of the very organizations charged with countering fear into question. While there is no scientific evidence testicular swelling occurs after vaccination, reports of disruptions to menstruation after receiving the COVID-19 vaccine are exceedingly common.[40]

As I explained earlier, CBOs were also involved in going door-to-door to improve vaccination rates in neighborhoods prioritized by CCVI data. Some residents were distrustful of these visits, and CBO organizers were sometimes regarded as simply another state agent out to control or surveil the community. One CBO worker in a Black community explained:

> It's really just the history that . . . people of this community . . . have had with . . . public officials, government offices. . . . People are very hesitant to move toward things that are kind of just pushed on [them]. Like, we

keep hearing the phrase "herd immunity." And ... especially during vaccine rollout ... a lot of people will refer back to Tuskegee, and other experimental things that have kind of plagued the relationship between ...
Black and Brown communities and, you know, government.... So there's
that hesitancy.... We are the COVID response team ... and even if
we're coming to, you know, someone's doorstep ... with grant information, ... the first thing that they see is uniforms coming from a ...
government agenda, so to speak.... Residents are thinking, you know,
we're the census, or that we're FEMA [the Federal Emergency Management Agency], or, something of that nature coming to kind of police how
people are taking care of themselves in the community.[41]

Because Black and Brown Chicagoans have learned about and experienced
extensive racist state violence and surveillance, vaccine ambassadors were
often interpreted as being state agents who could not be trusted.

A history of negative interactions with the medical establishment had a
similar effect on people's willingness to get vaccinated, as one community
leader in Austin related:

A big obstacle for a lot of people in in these neighborhoods ... is the
lack of trust in doctors.... With Black and Brown communities, right-
fully so, because they've had their ... fair share of negative experiences
in hospitals. And that's from getting a health care check, all the way to,
you know, maternal-child health, and having a mother who is in pain
or in need of a certain level of attention, you know, not having their
voice heard.[42]

Therefore, ongoing racist treatment within medical settings can also fuel
vaccine hesitancy. And certain medical policies introduced during the pandemic contributed to already existing fears. Rodrigo said that when Latinx
patients were hospitalized and died from an illness that was not COVID-
related but their death certificate indicated they died from COVID-19, people began to believe the myth that COVID-19 was a hoax:

They probably died of another illness, but they got categorized COVID,
and it was not even COVID.... That's what made our community say, "Is
this bullshit?" ... 'Cause my kid had a kidney failure, and he got categorized as COVID-19. That's why they were believing the bullshit Trump
was saying.... Yeah, and then they started telling their family member,
"This is all like a joke. It's a hoax. It's not something serious." That made
our community confused, and it was chaotic.[43]

This issue may have arisen because death certificate policies shifted during the pandemic. In an effort to capture as many COVID-19 deaths as possible, the practice of naming only the ultimate cause of death on the certificate was changed to including COVID-19 even when it was only present and not the cause of death.[44] This policy change may have unintentionally fueled distrust.

Given the data presented in this chapter on the various sources and reasons for distrust, it may be surprising how frequently Black and Latinx Americans *did* get vaccinated and remain vigilant in following public health advice. I found that among people who experience accumulated distrust across their lifetimes, those who were involved in a close-knit community group in which they could openly and honestly discuss their fears were more likely to vaccinate in the midst of widespread uncertainty.

RECOVERY AND TRUST

> African Americans . . . say "They tryna kill me [with the vaccine]." I say they've been did that when they give you drugs, alcohol, and guns . . . they don't have to give you a vaccine to kill you. . . . You know they had a few people who get vaccinated . . . [and] passed away. But . . . 2 or 3 people versus 700,000 people. I mean, that's . . . not good math for evidence for me, right? That . . . 3 people died . . . through vaccination, but 700,000 died from COVID. I'll take my chances with the vaccine.
>
> MARLIN, Black resident of Austin, interviewed on December 13, 2021

I found that people who had been in a trusted recovery group for an extended period of their life and forged a lasting solidarity with community members came to express structural critiques of the racist biocapitalist systems that ensnared them in slow emergencies, but they nonetheless saw vaccines as a lifeline that would allow them to survive yet another racialized threat aimed at their communities. As Marlin explains in this quote, state violence against Black and Brown lives is constant, so he sees no reason to distrust the vaccine specifically.[45] For him, the benefits of the vaccine outweigh the risks, and the vaccine offers a means of surviving racial devaluation and necropolitics. Beyond encouraging vaccine uptake, the recovery group in Austin, led by Marlin and Shanice, was well rehearsed in responding to both slow and urgent emergencies in Austin. And they were practiced in countering the state's neglect of their community through mutual aid.

People who suffer from substance use are familiar with state abandonment. Although people are often court mandated to enter institutional sites of recovery, once those programs end, people must forge trusted networks of support to continue to survive addiction. And the state offers very little by way of support. Further, there are few biomedical resources to help with addiction, especially as a chronic, lifelong condition. Therefore, people in long-term recovery are accustomed to state and biomedical neglect, and to the broader public's misunderstanding of their experiences with addiction. This is what makes long-standing, community-based recovery groups so important: people learn to trust each other, when institutional and familial assistance falters or fails. I spent time with Marlin and Shanice in the storefronts they converted into a church and recovery space and a testing site, and I conducted a focus group with members of the group. People told me over and over again that Marlin literally saved their lives, and so they felt obliged to give back to others who desperately needed support and had nowhere else to turn. As Shanice affirmed, "We do it because someone did it for us. . . . [Marlin] saved my life, so I got to give back."[46]

In addition to recovery and COVID-19 testing, Marlin's group engages in violence prevention in the neighborhood, responds to overdoses by providing naloxone, offers food donated from the Greater Chicago Food Depository, and provides a network of support to people living with HIV.[47] Group members also help one another apply for federal or state assistance programs, such as unemployment insurance, rental assistance, or Supplemental Nutrition Assistance Program benefits. In the early part of the pandemic, Marlin's group held outdoor grieving sessions, so that people who had lost family members but could not properly mourn them in funerals could process their loss in a productive and supportive environment. Marlin told me about these informal grief sessions:

> They talk, they're talking about, you know, losing a loved one, trying to come back from losing a loved one, right? Trying to put their life back together, right? And just talk about ways to grieve. Some people, one person may give a problem, the next person will give a solution, right? It's like that because we don't have any professional mental health people coming out so we got to service ourselves the best way we can.[48]

Members of this group also raise money within the community for people who overdose because families are often unwilling to pay for funeral services. Therefore, this mutual aid group provides a means of accessing services that the city fails to provide and that families may withhold. Shanice told me that during the pandemic, many people felt they could not trust one another, but this was not the case for the members of the recovery group: "A lot of people trust us because we're here. We sit in the community, and we have open door policies. Most of the times when we say that we're gonna do something, we do it. . . . And that means a lot to the community, especially for our community. . . . Trust right now is everything for us."[49]

Members of this Austin recovery group learned to openly discuss their fears surrounding vaccination. Destiny stated:

> We do better when we know better. People just need a little help to get there. And the government needs to help more. People think, "Why take the shot if I'm still gonna get COVID?" and I tell them, "Because your chances are better. We don't know how COVID will get you. For some people they get it and die, and others [are] asymptomatic, but you don't know. So get the shot, and get the knowledge."[50]

Jamilah told me that just watching the numbers of Black deaths mount, day after day, year after year, had a profound effect on her: "Watching the news every day, then listening to the numbers, seeing the different spikes and just knowing that it was here, and that this . . . wasn't something that was gonna go away anytime soon . . . That affected my personal decision [to get vaccinated.]"[51] Countering an obvious politics of death was often reason enough to get vaccinated, and Jamilah shared her thoughts with others who were skeptical of vaccination.

Like Marlin, many people in the group felt as though vaccines counteracted the broader devaluation of Black and Brown lives so obviously on display during the pandemic. Tanisha contended that if professionals were getting vaccinated, then her whole network should follow suit:

> Everybody. All of us agreed to take the vaccine. . . . My whole group that I operate with, we just waiting for them to okay us to come and take our vaccine. We ready. . . . When I started seeing all the big peoples like the lawyers, the doctors, or nurses in the hospital . . . they done took the vaccine . . . so I feel like they were safe, I'm safe.[52]

Sharing knowledge about the vaccine became a means of combating the necropolitics associated with devaluing Black and Brown lives. This mutual aid group serves as an epistemic community that orients not only people's health beliefs but also their approach to survival.[53] Marlin explained to me how the testing site became a means of educating people about COVID-19 more generally, which brought the community together in new ways:

> At first, people didn't have much information. Right. And it's [a] funny thing about . . . poor urban communities, right. The only information they probably obtained is through Facebook. Whatever somebody say on Facebook, that's what it is. So what was happening was [Shanice and I] was paying attention to CNN, we was downloading PubMed materials, right . . . and we would pass it out. And anytime we had the opportunity

to explain it to people, to the best of our ability, we would do so. Right. . . .
We probably test anywhere from . . . uh, five hundred to a thousand people a month, we test that many people now. Yeah, because people are
more . . . receptive, and they're more informed now about COVID. Right.
And I'll tell you one thing COVID has done. Sad as it may seem and it's
hard to kind of see, but COVID brought people together even at a time
when they tell us we shouldn't be together; COVID has brought a lot of
people together.[54]

Fear of the unknown is familiar to people living in long-term recovery, and
comfort with uncertainty is something that not only brought this community together but also made its members better able to manage the many
ambiguities of COVID-19. Further, Marline and Shanice shared the expertise they gained from reading the research about COVID-19. During the
focus group I conducted, Jamilah pointed out that "we have a sense of the
structure of public health, and so we alert people to the fact that COVID is
real and ongoing, and how to deal with it."[55] And the group took a strong
line on vaccination and its benefits. According to Marlin, "people that's
vaccinated, gone be vaccinated and the ones that's not, they don't stand a
chance. . . . We're gonna get some more dead people because they not gone
adhere to . . . what society have to embrace . . . they just don't want to buy
into what's happening. How it got here? I don't know. I just know it's here
and they've found a solution, how to keep us alive, and so I have to go with
that."[56]

Sharing information about the coronavirus and vaccination was not the
only lesson this mutual aid group imparted. This epistemic community was
also committed to teaching people how to survive structural inequality. As
Shanice put it, "we're teaching people to survive the life that was dealt to
them."[57] In the focus group, Tanisha elaborated, "In this organization, I got
brothers and sisters who care about others, and they help to the best of their
ability to help. When they brought us on, they taught us. I'm motivated because I want to do something for my community."[58] And part of what they
learn in the recovery group is to endure both slow and urgent emergencies.
When I was first interviewing Marlin in the spring of 2021, a member of
the recovery group dropped by to pick up a collection box for a friend who
"passed away from fentanyl. He decided to let his addiction creep back in
and get the best of him, and it killed him." The two men discussed how crucial the recovery work they do together is. "Recovery. That's the throughline
through all of us. It is a lifeline," Marlin said.[59] There are many slow emergencies that plague the residents of Austin. Residents cannot find work,
or they work for meager wages, and they hustle to pull together welfare

to supplement their rising household costs. They struggle with chronic ill-nesses (e.g., HIV), substance use, street violence, and trauma. They are overpoliced and underserved. And when COVID-19 hit, all this precarity was heightened and ignored by city officials. And yet, this mutual aid or-ganization is well poised to respond to these existing and new slow emer-gencies, as well as urgent crises such as death from overdose, gunshots, or COVID-19. When I arrived in the area for the focus group discussion in July 2022, Marlin explained that he had just stopped two shootings in the area that week and had "Narcaned" someone who overdosed on fentanyl that day.[60] As we walked together down the sidewalk on Cicero Avenue, he stopped to shake people's hands, introducing me to ten people in one half block. They were all people he knew, who used the services his small store-front provided when they could. The volunteers who work for his organi-zation help one another survive a series of endemic emergencies that are invisible or inconceivable to people living in other parts of the city. People who participate in this group fill in where the state lacks, and they provide an epistemic orientation that acknowledges racial devaluation and mounts structural critique but also responds with a politics of care.

Racially marginalized lower-income Chicagoans feel as though the gov-ernment abandoned them during the pandemic. Their communities have been the hardest hit and the least protected, and throughout this book, I have illustrated how they see their suffering being discounted and ignored by government and public health officials. While the literature on distrust often paints Black and Brown communities as homogeneous and widely distrustful, such a portrayal fails to illustrate the complex, layered, and relational means by which people manage distrust and make health decisions. Distrust can accumulate as one interacts with racist institutions and agents, but it can also be countered or at least better situated within a structural analysis of valuation, through strong community solidarity. People in Marlin's recovery group realize that not getting vaccinated sim-ply exacerbates state neglect, contributing to pandemic precarity and vulnerability. As Marlin emphasized, "These our people, this our life. These our lives at stake."[61]

CODA: LEST WE FORGET

"The time is out of joint."

HAMLET, in William Shakespeare,
Hamlet, act 1, scene 5

We are a forgetful society. Throughout the pandemic, I heard people claim again and again how shocked they were to live through a pandemic of this size and impact. I don't know how many times I heard, "I never would have thought . . . this could occur in the US . . . in this day and age." Such shock and dismay reveal profound *epidemic orientalism*—the presumption that pandemics of this nature only occur in non-Western countries.[1] But as a scholar of HIV/AIDS, I had to remind people that we are *still* living with a pandemic of this size and impact, in the United States, in this day and age. HIV may not infect as many people as it once did, but 1.2 million Americans currently live with HIV, and so many more live in constant threat of contracting it. The ongoing and devastating toll HIV has had on Black Americans has been largely ignored by the popular media.[2] In 2008, I wrote an article about how amnesic and ignorant American culture had become about HIV—that antiretrovirals were accepted as analgesic and prophylaxis, and as such, those infected were rendered spectral and out of joint.[3] But in fact, the public health experts who built the COVID-19 response were all HIV experts. HIV infrastructure and knowledge were crucial to the COVID-19 response. A robust social safety net has been key to reducing the impact of HIV on marginalized communities, but this knowledge did not translate into the COVID-19 response. Rather, state and public health experts adopted epidemiological modeling and technocratic quick fixes—touting an ideology that recognizes the social determinants of health while simultaneously ignoring the lessons they learned from years of working on HIV.[4] And once again, four years after COVID-19 began to ravage our population, we are already forgetting. Well, some are. Others may never have that privilege.

On May 11, 2023, the federal government ended the official COVID-19 public health emergency.[5] The expiration of emergency measures halted the remaining pandemic social assistance in place—COVID-19 tests and vaccines were no longer federally funded, and Medicaid expansion concluded.[6] Masks were no longer mandated in schools, restaurants, or health care settings.[7] The Centers for Disease Control and Prevention stopped tracking positivity rates. In early May 2023, 76,000 people were still contracting and 250 people were still dying from COVID-19 on a weekly basis in the US.[8] As of January 2024, more than 1.1 million people have died of COVID-19 in the US alone—more than the number killed in World Wars I and II combined.[9] Nearly one in five people who contracted COVID-19 experiences symptoms of "long COVID."[10] Many people are struggling to survive the legacies of enduring poverty, inflation, sickness, and loss. The termination of pandemic aid, alongside rising inflation, caused surges in housing and food insecurity.[11] Yet, the nation has moved on, ready to live with COVID-19 as an endemic illness. How quick we are to consign the most vulnerable among us to the "viral underclass."[12]

Kelly, a Black woman from Albany Park, discussed how she felt when pandemic unemployment insurance expired in the fall of 2021. She emphasized that the state sent a clear message that it devalues vulnerable Americans when it treated the pandemic as a *temporary* crisis:

> We're disposable . . . in our time of *need*. . . . We're supposed to be the country of . . . freedom that cares about its people. And we have a clear-cut moment where we need to care about our people. And it's, like, "Okay, we did that already. You know, we gave y'all a year of [unemployment]. But now it's time to get back to work. We got to make money." It shows us that this country only gives . . . a shit about money. Money and numbers . . . and things like compassion and grace and shit just goes straight out the window.[13]

While white, middle-class families who weathered the COVID-19 storm could anticipate a hopeful future with fewer restrictions and more freedom when the pandemic was declared "over," many vulnerable communities had no such expectations. For marginalized populations who faced tremendous loss of life and financial, housing, educational, and food precarity, bouncing back is still uncertain.

COVID-19 could have been a moment of reckoning. William Sewell reminds us that in "times of structural dislocation, ordinary routines of social life are open to doubt, the sanctions of existing power relations are uncertain or suspended, and new possibilities are thinkable."[14] The pandemic could have been a portal, as Arundhati Roy proclaimed, a historic about-face that would reverse market fundamentalism and state racism and secure a robust social safety net for all.[15] The billions of dollars of federal relief that poured into cities throughout the nation could have been used to build infrastructure that served the most vulnerable people: community clinics, public housing, schools, food banks, and community gardens. Such a move would acknowledge that fifty years of neoliberal economics have decimated racially marginalized communities, who were then left to die from COVID-19. In fact, in a *New York Times* editorial, Matthew Desmond explained that the child tax credits, unemployment insurance, increases in food stamps, and rental assistance programs sponsored by billions of dollars of federal investment during the pandemic lowered child poverty and instances of eviction to levels unseen in decades.[16] Yet such measures did not go far enough to counteract the insecurity and compounded structural disadvantage the poor suffer as a result of years of neoliberal restructuring. Improvements in poverty measures during the pandemic, Zachary Parolin explains, do not counteract or eliminate "the disadvantages associated with cumulative poverty exposure."[17] Further, aid was still doled out through means-tested, paternalistic, and highly bureaucratic systems. Desmond explained that America is "addicted to poverty" because the middle class and the wealthy benefit from it.[18] Pandemic aid constituted a small and fleeting shift in the country's antipoor agenda. Now even that has passed. And the rates of poverty and housing and food insecurity are climbing at breathtaking speeds.[19]

Although COVID-19 posed possibilities for more radical structural transformation, the opportunity was undermined by a series of political rollbacks, constituting a return to the neoliberal normal. For example, President Joe Biden was unable to pass budgets that would sustain social safety nets and COVID-19 supports, the US Supreme Court decision in *Dobbs v. Jackson's Women's Health Organization* criminalized abortion and reduced reproductive health care access in multiple conservative states throughout the country, and the termination of Medicaid expansion left many residents of conservative states without health insurance. The convergence of these backlashes to COVID-19 transformations, has led us toward a recommitment to even more fragmented and patchwork social assistance and health care for the nation's most vulnerable people.

During the pandemic, however, there were moments when a larger economic and racial reckoning did seem possible. Kelly told me:

> There's no way in hell . . . all of the different pressure points that I feel like COVID set off for different groups of people . . . in terms of race and ethnicity and . . . social class and . . . right versus left. All this different shit that it set off and has been awakened in people. There's . . . literally

no way we'd be able to go back to whatever it was before that. . . . The world was, like, kinda shitty [*laughs*]. It still is. But I mean, . . . I feel like a lot of stuff that was just kind of *bubbling under the surface*. Like, even though it took a lot of . . . death, a lot of famine, a lot of negative shit for it to happen . . . a lot of the stuff needed to get to the damn surface, so that we could at least *witness* it and see it and try to move forward from it.[20]

There were and continue to be moments when the public collectively recognizes and grapples with the racism and market fundamentalism that has always bubbled beneath the surface. But these moments are fleeting, drowned out by novel news cycles and crises, and delinked from the underlying causes of our failure to contend with COVID-19. The emergency of COVID-19 and the way it exacerbated already existing slow emergencies and sacrificial logics has just slightly reoriented business as usual. Rather than "Apocalypse Now," as Susan Sontag puts it, it's "Apocalypse From Now On"—an ongoing catastrophe happening in such slow motion that those who are not ensnared by it fail to see it.[21] Like 9/11 or HIV/AIDS, COVID-19 has fundamentally reshaped society. Annie, a Korean American woman from Albany Park, told me, "The groups that were most affected, definitely have this living memory of the way that they were treated and the way that they were disregarded and left to die."[22] People's bodies are marked by these living emergencies and ongoing devaluations.

COVID-19 arose because of radical shifts in environmental, economic, and scientific practices over the past fifty years, but this fact is being ignored by the global political authorities who could use those lessons to mitigate the inevitable destruction the next pandemic will unleash.[23] The infrastructural lacks and racial violence that COVID-19 both intensified and exposed are also being ignored, and in fact worsened by the termination of emergency conditions. These failures will both haunt us and shape our futures.

On February 28, 2023, Mayor Lori Lightfoot lost her bid for reelection—the first time an incumbent mayor has been denied reelection in Chicago since 1989.[24] Immediately, other Democratic mayors and state officials took notice—would Chicago be a lesson to the nation? A real reckoning with the legacies of COVID-19? Many commentators simply blamed Lightfoot's harsh negotiating style, but most focused on her inability to successfully contend with crime in the city.[25] Only a few blamed her pandemic policies and practices of racial injustice.[26] The runoff election between white candidate Paul Vallas, former CEO of the Chicago Public Schools, and Black candidate Brandon Johnson, a little-known former schoolteacher and union organizer, was painted as symptomatic of the tensions Lightfoot's loss unveiled: a hard-on-crime candidate who promised to fund the expansion of policing versus a critic of the police who campaigned on investment in schooling and mental health. Johnson was elected Chicago's fifty-seventh mayor on April 4, 2023. Clearly, this election constituted a reprisal in Chicago—voters were tired of neoliberal business as usual and wanted to see whether a progressive mayor could do more to heal the city's deep racial and socioeconomic divides. Only time will tell whether the new administration can rectify the decades of racist infrastructural disinvestment, devaluation, and labor market segmentation that has led to both concentrated slow emergencies and sacrificial labor logics.

Lightfoot named racism a crisis, invested in epistemic infrastructure to track racial disparities, and gave voice and resources to community organizations to guide the COVID-19 response in racially marginalized neighborhoods, but she ignored the root causes of racism, social vulnerability, and poor health; presumed scarcity; and used canonical neoliberal tactics that served to sustain and exacerbate ongoing slow emergencies and sacrifice racially marginalized workers to protect the economy. I have argued that COVID-19 should be analyzed as a convergence of emergencies—a declaration of emergency by the state that facilitated the enactment of a temporary set of mitigation strategies that obfuscated links to slow emergencies and the sacrifice of lower-income frontline workers.

States governed COVID-19 through emergency by enacting temporally bounded policies that presumed scarcity and delinked the effects of racism from its structural causes. Once the privileged could regain a semblance of normalcy, the emergency was declared over. As Charles Mills explains, the epistemology of ignorance structured into white supremacy allows white Americans to construct a reality for themselves, knowingly misinterpreting the world, in order to sustain their privilege.[27] In the case of liberal leaders during the pandemic, this epistemology of ignorance was rearticulated as race-conscious business as usual. Rather than completely ignore state racism, state actors such as Lightfoot, acknowledged racism's toll and invested in epistemic infrastructure to track its effects, but this nonetheless served to obscure the ongoing means by which racism operates and functions. Liberal state actors offered a distorted, "officially sanctioned" reality, backed up with epidemiological data, that nonetheless diverted attention and political will away from the fundamental causes of racism.[28] Because slow emergencies happen at a protracted pace, their root causes are detached from their effects, facilitating willful political ignorance. Using data to track racial disparities further disembeds race from its structural context.

I have argued that contemporary racial biocapitalism operates through exceptional governance in multiple ways. First, it does not simply abandon but extends aid to exceptional, racialized subjects—those whom the data deems most vulnerable during an acknowledged political crisis. In other words, a liberal, Black mayor could not abandon her Black residents when their deaths were mounting without suffering political fallout, so she extended aid, but she presumed scarcity and economized her public health approach. Second, though, I have argued that Black and Latinx Americans are not just excluded—they are the target of exclusionary inclusion.[29] In various ways, they are needed to uphold the norm of white supremacy and racial biocapitalism but prohibited from reaping its benefits, except in exceptional moments. Latinx and Black low-wage workers were absolutely essential to the COVID-19 state emergency—without them, the privileged would have suffered, and the economy would have tanked. People trapped in slow emergencies were also turned into political clout—transformed into metrics that could prove "woke credentials" and secure political and symbolic capital.[30] The suffering of Black and Latinx Chicagoans during the pandemic was capitalized upon by political actors. Meanwhile lower-income, racially marginalized communities were made to wait for assistance because resolving their vulnerability was deemed an intractable problem—one that any one political administration could not possibly address. In this way, the slow emergencies the racially marginalized suffer are turned into ontological truths. Policies and discourses surrounding frontline work were similarly paradoxical. Frontline workers were recognized by the public, but their sacrifice was disavowed.

Black and Brown Chicagoans (and Americans) were socially vulnerable targets of state racism and neglect long before the COVID-19 pandemic, but their social precarity was also exacerbated by pandemic conditions and policies. They have lost neighbors and family members; their bodies have undergone compounded weathering and new viral assaults; they have accumulated debt and economic precarity; their housing, health care, and mental health care are unstable; and they are riddled with ontological insecurity. These are the enduring legacies of COVID-19 among the racially marginalized, and unless we continue to reckon with the structural causes of inequality and racism, their exceptional dispossession will, once again, be forgotten and ignored.

ACKNOWLEDGMENTS

I want to begin by acknowledging the debt I owe to the 110 residents of Chicago who spoke to me on the phone about some of their most intimate experiences of the pandemic. Their fear, uncertainty, and trauma were palpable, and I am so grateful that people shared their thoughts, practices, and critiques with me. As a result, I was able to glimpse something other research on COVID-19 may miss—how vulnerable people navigated and survived despite being forgotten and sacrificed, how they experienced racial devaluation, and how they challenged existing policies and structures. I hope their experiences and analyses are what readers of this book most remember, and that their accounts will help shape readers' considerations of the pandemic.

I also want to thank the experts who dedicated a very precious sixty to ninety minutes with me, amid their countless duties and efforts. While I am critical of the city's approach to the pandemic, the doctors, epidemiologists, organizers, and policy experts I spoke with cared deeply about helping the people of Chicago survive the pandemic. And they worked tirelessly and with tremendous dedication. They also taught me a great deal about the inner workings of Chicago politics.

There were so many people who worked on this project and contributed to its success. First and foremost: Cal Garrett. Cal served as the project manager for the entire duration of our research, and I literally could not have pulled off a project of this magnitude without them. Cal's organizational skills, compassion, dedicated hard work, and astute analytic viewpoint constantly impressed me, and I relied upon their expertise and skills on a daily basis. Cal and I also wrote multiple articles together, and I really appreciate their sociological imagination. Cal's sense of humor and willingness to engage in long conversations about dinosaurs with my son also made the work more enjoyable.

Amanda Lewis and Iván Arenas were also key contributors to this project's success. Their critical insights, knowledge of Chicago's communities, willingness to support the project financially and administratively, and intellectual mentorship were vital. Both Amanda and Iván are exemplary scholar-activists, and I learned so much from following their guidance and advice. Despite their incredibly busy lives, they were both always available to troubleshoot and provide support.

In the first year of the pandemic, Cal Garrett, Fructoso Basaldua, Cindy Brito, and Bianca Perez helped to conduct interviews with one hundred Chicago residents. We met weekly, and these conversations and our constant reworking of our recruitment tools and interview guides enabled the collection of rich, poignant interview data. They were also coauthors of the Institute for Research on Race and Public Policy (IRRPP) State of Racial Justice Report, *Deadly Disparities in the Days of COVID-19: How Public Policy Fails Black and Latinx Chicagoans*. Their dedicated hard work and contributions to this project are legion. Chris Poulos also worked on the Household Pulse Data that I report on throughout the book—his critical sociological analysis and statistical skill are most appreciated. AJ Golio is a coauthor on a paper about housing that emerged from this research. His excitement about the findings in our IRRPP report led to a collaboration that has been very rewarding.

There were multiple other graduate and undergraduate students who worked on this project in various ways. Yesenia Vargas, Irma Ramirez, Dakari Finister, and Ni'Shele Jackson helped with Institutional Review Board clearance, grant applications, and transcription. Tirza Ochrach-Konradi stepped up at the last minute to help with formatting the book. A host of undergraduate students helped transcribe and summarize interviews, including Julissa Guerrero Cruz, Leen Tajeddin, Ariel Maldonado, Henry Hodge, Alexis Ruiz, Dino Numanovic, Kristi Leach, Dahlya El-Adawe, and Emily Chavez.

I received funding from multiple institutes and centers at the University of Illinois at Chicago, including the IRRPP, the Institute for Policy and Civic Engagement, the Center for Clinical and Translational Research, and the Chancellor's Creative Activity Funds. Amy Sporer and Louise Martinez spent hours helping me craft funding applications.

I am extremely grateful to people who read drafts of the book. Nik Theodore and Alice Street both read early chapters and offered critical advice. I held a book workshop in May 2023. Paige Sweet, Michael Rodríguez Muñiz, Anthony Ryan Hatch, and Steven Thrasher read an entire draft of the manuscript and offered extremely supportive and critical advice on how to improve the book. My analysis is indebted to their brilliant insight. I must also thank the anonymous reviewers for the University of Chicago Press, who provided crucial critiques that have greatly improved the analysis. Andy Clarno has read the book multiple times, and I could not have completed it without his encouragement and acumen.

Elizabeth Branch Dyson at the University of Chicago Press met with me after I had conducted the research but was still honing my analysis for the book. Her early excitement for the project and generous support and feedback have been incredibly important to my success. I really appreciate Mollie McFee, Stephen Twilley, and Olivia Aguilar for ushering the book through the University of Chicago Press production and promotion process. And I thank Lori Meek Schuldt, who copyedited the book, and Derek Gottlieb, who put together the index, for their amazing attention to detail. Although this labor is often invisible to readers, producing a book is definitely a team effort.

I have presented components of this book in multiple venues both near and far, and I greatly appreciate people's feedback and advice in each instance.

COVID-19 was obviously incredibly isolating, and there were months on end when I could not see my extended family (beyond their faces on a screen). But they supported me from afar when they had to and up close when we could be. Huge thanks to Nancy, Jim, Liza, Alex, Mirabelle, Jenna, Kevin, Kenzie, Grant, Charlie, Drew, and Lucy for the love and enjoyable diversions you've offered.

I have dedicated this book to my parents, Pam and Jack. The isolation, disorientation, and fear during the first year of the pandemic were very difficult for them, and then they suffered from a series of health challenges. These past few years have reshaped their lives in irrevocable ways, and it has shown me how much I depend on their constant and unwavering support and love. My parents have always been my biggest champions, and their pride in me is a bulwark.

My biggest thanks, as always, are owed to Andy and Felix, who put up with my sleepy grumpiness and singular determination with giggles and hugs. Felix's entire early childhood was structured by COVID-19 policies and our efforts to stay safe. He got so used to wearing a mask, he often forgot to take it off at home. So many of his early childhood milestones took place amid lockdown, closures, and mandates. Yet his critical and empathetic gaze toward the world, which never ceases to amaze me, stems at least in part from asking questions about and learning from pandemic politics. Andy's brilliant analytic talent, compassionate activism, and knowledge of Chicago shaped this project in innumerable ways—it is often difficult to detect where his brain ends and mine begins. To you both, thanks for the tickle parties, game nights, and dinosaur romps that got us through the dark times. I would never want to do this without you.

APPENDIX A: TIMELINE OF IMPORTANT COVID-19 DATES

US AND GLOBAL	2020	ILLINOIS AND CHICAGO
January		
US confirms its first case of COVID-19	21–31	
US declares COVID-19 a public health emergency		
February		
First US death from COVID-19	6	
March		
US surpasses 1,000 COVID-19 deaths	11–13	Governor JB Pritzker closes Illinois schools
President Donald Trump declares national emergency		
Trump signs Family First Coronavirus Response Act (FFCRA) that provides $3.5 billion in emergency allocations, halts Medicaid unenrollment during the declared public health emergency, and includes a 120-day moratorium on evictions	18–21	First shelter-in-place order in Chicago Pritzker issues stay-at-home order for Illinois
US leads with most COVID-19 cases of any country in the world	26–27	
Trump signs $2 trillion stimulus package including $1,200 checks to individuals		

(continued)

US AND GLOBAL	2020	ILLINOIS AND CHICAGO
April		
US Centers for Disease Control and Prevention (CDC) recommends that people wear face masks	3–7	Mayor Lori Lightfoot initiates Racial Equity Rapid Response Team (RERRT) in Auburn Gresham, South Shore, and Austin neighborhoods
HHS announces $186 million in additional funding to state and local jurisdictions for the COVID-19 response		Chicago Department of Public Health releases data showing that, despite being about 30% of the population, Black people account for 68% of the COVID-19-related deaths in Chicago
Trump issues first guidelines for reopening in the United States	16–17	Schools in Illinois are closed for the rest of the school year
Trump signs Paycheck Protection Program and Health Care Enhancement Act into law	23–30	Pritzker issues Executive Order 2020–30 to extend his previous moratorium on evictions
		Illinois issues mask mandate
May		
Trump declares "Operation Warp Speed" for development of medical measures to counter COVID-19	6–15	Lightfoot extends RERRT initiative to Belmont Cragin, Little Village, and Pilsen neighborhoods
Unemployment rate in the US reaches 14.7%—the highest since the Great Depression		
	20–24	Chicago allots $2 million for emergency rental assistance
		Pritzker signs bill allocating $300 million for housing assistance; $324 million dispersed by December 30, 2020
George Floyd murdered by Minneapolis police; nationwide protests follow	25–28	Protests spread throughout Chicago
Recorded death toll from COVID-19 in the US surpasses 100,000		

(*continued*)

US AND GLOBAL	2020	ILLINOIS AND CHICAGO
June		
Moderna and Pfizer vaccines enter Stage 3 clinical trials	3–27	Restore Illinois Plan to reopen the state begins
		Businesses in Chicago reopen
August		
Trump signs executive order on rental assistance	5–8	Chicago Public Schools decide on remote learning for fall 2020
September		
CDC issues federal moratorium on evictions	4–16	
US Department of Health and Human Services produces plan to administer vaccines		
December		
Emergency Use Authorization issued for Pfizer vaccine, then Moderna vaccine	11–18	Illinois health workers become eligible for vaccination
Coronavirus Response and Relief Supplemental Appropriations Act of 2021 signed by Trump in one of his final COVID-related actions before leaving office after having lost the 2020 presidential election in November	27–29	
Internal Revenue Service and Treasury Department begin to deliver a second round of direct payments to individuals		

US AND GLOBAL	2021	ILLINOIS AND CHICAGO
January		
President Joe Biden signs an executive order requiring masking and physical distancing in federal buildings, on federal lands, and by government contractors	20–21	
Biden releases National Strategy for the COVID-19 Response		

(continued)

US AND GLOBAL	2021	ILLINOIS AND CHICAGO
January		
CDC issues federal mandate to wear masks on airplanes and public transportation; refusal to wear a mask becomes violation of federal law	25–30	Frontline essential workers and residents aged 65 or older become eligible for vaccination in Illinois
February		
US surpasses 500,000 COVID-19 deaths	1–25	Protect Chicago Plus is launched: Chicago's vaccine distribution plan to vulnerable communities
An estimated 2.5 million women and 1.8 million men have left the workforce since the start of the pandemic in the US		Residents with high-risk conditions become eligible for vaccination in Illinois
March		
Biden signs American Rescue Plan of 2021, which provides additional relief to address the continued impact of COVID-19, including an increased child tax credit for 2021	1–11	Phased reopening of Chicago Public Schools begins amid tensions with Chicago Teachers Union
Biden administration announces $10 billion investment to expand access to COVID-19 vaccines and address vaccine hesitancy	22–29	Government workers and higher education staff become eligible for vaccination in Illinois
		Restaurant staff, construction workers, and religious leaders become eligible for vaccination in Illinois
April		
CDC updates mask mandates so that fully vaccinated people no longer need to wear masks outdoors	12–27	Any Illinois resident aged 16 or older can be vaccinated
		Lightfoot announces $9.6 million for Healthy Chicago Equity Zones to advance health equity in Chicago
May		
CDC updates COVID-19 guidance on masking: fully vaccinated people can stop wearing masks in most places	13–17	Pritzker signs Emergency Housing Act into law, sealing eviction records for those who were economically impacted by COVID-19

(continued)

US AND GLOBAL	2021	ILLINOIS AND CHICAGO
May		
Children ages 12–16 eligible for vaccination		Mask mandate for vaccinated Illinoisians is lifted (following CDC guidelines)
Only 56% of women in US are now working for a salary, the lowest rate since 1986		
	24	A 2021 round of housing assistance begins, with $80 million to be dispersed by Chicago
June		
COVID-19 Delta variant becomes the dominant variant in the US and begins a third surge in infections	1	
July		
Because of Delta variant increase, CDC updates its guidance and recommends that people in substantial or high COVID-19 transmission areas wear a mask indoors	27–30	Pritzker adopts CDC guidance on masking for Illinois, recommending masks
CDC moratorium on evictions expires		
August		
Biden administration creates new 60-day moratorium on evictions, but it is struck down by US Supreme Court	3–21	Pritzker makes masks mandatory in schools regardless of vaccination status
CDC recommends first vaccine "boosters" for people with compromised immune systems		Delta variant pushes COVID-19 average daily cases in Chicago over 500
September		
COVID-19 cases, fueled by Delta variant, peak at 172,500 average daily cases in the US	13	
Pandemic unemployment benefits expire		
October		
	3	Illinois eviction moratorium expires

(*continued*)

US AND GLOBAL	2021	ILLINOIS AND CHICAGO
October		
	27	Chicago City Council passes Lightfoot's $16.7 billion budget proposal for 2022, including $1.9 billion in COVID-19 relief funds, with $31.5 million earmarked for direct cash assistance
November		
CDC's Advisory Committee on Immunization Practices recommends the Pfizer-BioNTech pediatric COVID-19 vaccine for all children ages 5–11	2–26	
CDC urges everyone aged 18 or older who received an initial vaccine series to receive a booster		
WHO designates the COVID-19 Omicron variant as a "variant of concern" because of its increased transmissibility		
December		
CDC shortens recommended isolation period for people with COVID-19 from 10 days to 5 days, followed by 5 days of masking	27	
US AND GLOBAL	2022	ILLINOIS AND CHICAGO
January		
Reported COVID-19 cases reach a new peak in US at over 800,000 cases per day, fueled by Omicron variant	1–15	Reported cases in Chicago peak at nearly 7,000 cases per day
March		
Biden declares COVID-19 "endemic" in his State of the Union address	1–26	
CDC estimates that about 55% of all current COVID-19 cases in the US are caused by Omicron BA.2 variant		

(*continued*)

US AND GLOBAL	2021	ILLINOIS AND CHICAGO
September		
Updated booster vaccinations for new variants are released for people aged 18 or older	1–18	
Biden announces that "the pandemic is over" in interview on TV news program *60 Minutes*		

US AND GLOBAL	2023	ILLINOIS AND CHICAGO
February		
	28	Lightfoot loses mayoral reelection
March		
Emergency Supplemental Nutrition Assistance Program benefits expire	1	
April		
	4	Brandon Johnson becomes Chicago's 57th mayor
May		
World Health Organization declares an end to the COVID-19 global health emergency	5	
US National Emergency and Public Health Emergency expire, ending free COVID-19 tests, treatments, and vaccines, and ending continuous Medicaid enrollment; CDC stops tracking positivity rates	11	

APPENDIX B: METHODS

When the pandemic first began, I was on a fellowship, finishing up edits on my second book. Amanda Lewis, director of the Institute for Research on Race and Public Policy (IRRPP) at the University of Illinois at Chicago, put out a call, asking to meet with scholars interested in studying the disproportionate toll that COVID-19 was taking on racially marginalized communities in Chicago. I attended the meeting alongside six other faculty, and I was hailed to lead what was imagined to be a multidisciplinary, multi-institutional initiative—mostly because of my expertise in studying how pandemics impact marginalized populations. The work began immediately and was intense and fast-paced. We needed to conceive of the project, apply for funding and Institutional Review Board clearance, hire graduate students, and begin interviews, in order to capture how Black and Brown Chicagoans were experiencing the decimation of their communities in real time. Soon all the other faculty dropped away—focusing on projects of their own—and I became the sole faculty investigator, managing a team of four graduate students.

This was unlike any other project I have taken on. First, the project is not global in scope but situated in Chicago, and I was keen to get to know my hometown as a researcher. Second, the project was initially conceived and sponsored as research necessary to produce an IRRPP State of Racial Justice Report—a series of policy reports that are written in accessible language to provide data on racial inequality in Chicago, used by policymakers and community organizers. We published our report, *Deadly Disparities in the Days of COVID-19: How Public Policy Fails Black and Latinx Chicagoans*, in December 2021, and I took part in a series of public launches, community-engaged discussions, and op-ed reports. This was my first foray into policy writing and reporting, and I learned a great deal in the process.

I am an ethnographer at heart, and this project required conducting interviews on the phone with people I would never meet in person. And I had to rely on interviews that graduate student assistants conducted. I did interview some people in this study twice, and I spent some time with community organizers in the neighborhoods we report on. But I am used to spending years getting to know the respondents in my projects. Because of the social distancing restrictions of the pandemic and the speed with which we engaged in this research, to capture people's real-time experiences and reflections, long-term ethnography was not an option. But this was a new and often alienating research experience for me.

In the first year (August 2020 through May 2021), I worked closely with four graduate students to engage in recruitment and interviewing: Cal Garrett, Fructoso Basaldua, Cindy Brito, and Bianca Perez. We met weekly, and we communicated very openly and regularly about recruitment, obstacles we were facing in sampling the populations we needed, and in revising the interview protocol time and again. At the outset, we expected to recruit hundreds of interviewees to sit for ninety-minute interviews on phone or video call platforms.[1] These expectations were challenged by the social conditions created by COVID-19.

We chose three neighborhoods in Chicago to sample based on their population demographics and whether they were targeted for additional resources by the city. We interviewed residents from Austin, Little Village, and Albany Park. Austin is a predominantly Black, lower-income neighborhood on the West Side of the city, and 44 percent of the interviewees lived in Austin. Austin is both geographically and in terms of population one of the largest neighborhoods in Chicago. Little Village is a predominantly Latinx, working-class community on the Southwest Side of the city, and a significant proportion of residents are foreign-born and undocumented. Nineteen percent of the interviewees lived in Little Village. Albany Park is a more economically and racially diverse neighborhood on the Northwest Side where residents include affluent homeowners, undocumented migrants, and front-facing, low-income workers. Thirty-one percent of the interviewees lived in Albany Park. Austin and Little Village were targeted with health equity initiatives by the City of Chicago, and Albany Park was not. All three neighborhoods had high rates of COVID-19 infections and death, compared with the city average.

Figure A.1 indicates the percentage of interviewees from each neighborhood. The category of "Other neighborhood" indicates interviewees from the neighborhood of West Ridge, which we had originally included in our sample. Initially, we wanted to include Indigenous and Asian populations in our sample. West Ridge is a northeastern neighborhood with a large Asian population, but we were only able to recruit white subjects from West Ridge despite multiple attempts to reach the various Asian communities in the area. Therefore, West Ridge was dropped from our sample. Albany Park is also home to large Asian and Indigenous populations and hosts community organizations dedicated to providing services to Indigenous, Korean, Filipino, and Arab communities. So we were able to include some Asian interviewees in our sample.

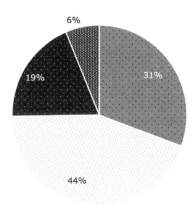

Albany Park   Austin   Little Village   Other neighborhood

Figure A.1 Interviewees by Neighborhood

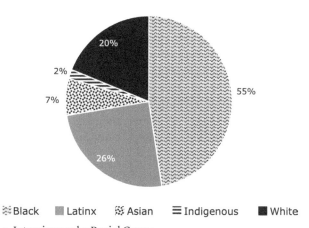

Black   Latinx   Asian   ≡ Indigenous   White

Figure A.2 Interviewees by Racial Group

In the end, however, I focused on vulnerabilities specific to Latinx and Black Chicagoans. Comparing Latinx, Black, and white Chicagoans' experiences is important because Chicago is made up of almost equal proportions of each group and because the city only targeted initiatives toward Black and Latinx communities. Of the 110 residents interviewed, 55 percent were Black, 26 percent Latinx, 7 percent Asian, 2 percent Indigenous, and 20 percent white. Respondents could designate more than one race or ethnicity when indicating their racial identity, which is why these percentages exceed 100 in the aggregate. Figure A.2 illustrates the racial makeup of my sample. Sixty-eight percent of the interviewees identified as women and 32 percent as men.

To be eligible for an interview, Chicago residents had to live in Albany Park, Austin, or Little Village and be either a designated "essential worker" or have lost work or employment during the pandemic. Based on the Illinois Executive Order that Governor Pritzker signed in March 2020, "essential workers" included people working in government, grocery, agriculture, pharmacy, mail, laundry, hardware, construction and critical trades (electricity/plumbing), charitable and social services, media, transportation, gas stations, financial institutions, education and childcare, residential services, health care, hotels and motels, and funeral services.[2] Most of the interviewees who identified as "essential workers" worked in jobs that were lower-income, but we did interview some higher-skilled professionals as well. As figure A.3 indicates, 11 percent of our interviewees identified as "essential workers" in the health care industry (though some were lower-income workers in medical facilities), and 33 percent identified as non–health care "essential workers." Fifty-one percent of the interviewees were not working, 3 percent were self-employed, and 2 percent worked from home.

We used typical methods of recruitment for qualitative interviews, adapted to meet COVID-19 restrictions, including distribution of flyers in public places, sending out electronic flyers on email LISTSERVs, and using our own social networks to contact potential interviewees. Our flyers had to be especially informational and clear, with contact information and a QR code linked to a study website, because many people were minimizing their time in public spaces. All written materials, including flyers and the study website, were bilingual, in English and Spanish. We also posted

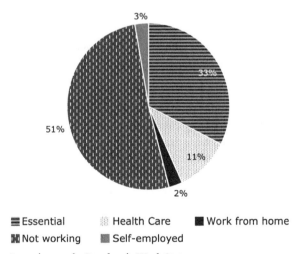

Figure A.3 Interviewees by Pandemic Work Status

project information via social media, and we asked local clinics, community centers, churches, and food banks to distribute flyers.

We offered fifty dollars per interview to residents because we believed it was ethical to do so, given people's financial and time constraints. It also helped with recruitment, as many people were in need of the additional funds, and people often shared our study with friends and family members who needed supplemental income. Some potential interviewees were undocumented and had concerns about sharing information over the phone. We addressed some of these concerns by changing the wording of our materials to emphasize that interviewees need not share any sensitive information. But at first we struggled to interview undocumented Chicagoans, until Cindy Brito, one of the research assistants, who is fluent in Spanish, did some focused recruitment with Latinx undocumented communities in Albany Park and Little Village.

Potential interviewees who contacted the study were asked to enroll via text message, phone call, or email by responding to a series of fourteen questions in English or Spanish. Basic demographic information that interviewees were comfortable sharing was collected at this time, including work, education, age, gender, race or ethnicity, household size, housing type, number of children, and language spoken. Eligibility was determined based on whether they were a health care worker, other essential worker, did not work, or had experienced some loss of work or employment precarity because of COVID-19. The enrollment questionnaire was also used to match interviewees to researchers based on availability and language. Race matching was not possible due to our small interviewer team and scheduling constraints. Consent and information documents were provided electronically to enrollees via email or a link to our study website where these documents were posted. In total, the study reached 162 confirmed contacts and enrolled 118 interviewees.

Scheduling and completing resident interviews proved to be one of the components of research that was most impacted by COVID-19. Interviewees often had unpredictable schedules or difficulty finding times to talk when they would be in a comfortable and quiet space suited to a long conversation. This is something that we simply had to adapt to. In all cases, we called or texted interviewees multiple times to confirm good times to talk and often rescheduled at least once. We told interviewees of the expected length of the interview and asked if they had the time and space to dedicate to it. Some of us completed interviews in multiple parts over several days, and others adapted the interview protocol to complete essential questions during a forty-five-minute break in an interviewee's day—sometimes while the interviewee was driving or otherwise in transit. The interview protocol also transformed substantially over the course of the study, as we adapted it to ask residents to reflect on current pandemic conditions, local or federal events, or policy shifts. Our efforts to be flexible were not always success-ful: 17 interviewees ultimately were unenrolled because we were unable to complete an interview with them, and 1 interviewee withdrew early in the study because of anxiety about sharing personal information over the phone. One hundred completed interviews were conducted between August 2020 and May 2021.

In the fall of 2021 and spring of 2022, I personally reinterviewed 25 peo-ple we had interviewed in the previous year. Cindy Brito reinterviewed five of the original undocumented interviewees in Spanish. I recruited 10 addi-tional participants from Little Village and Austin. I wanted to conduct these interviews myself, and I wanted to capture people's experiences with the Delta and Omicron variants, the termination of pandemic social assistance, and the shifting of federal policy away from emergency measures.

Conducting interviews with residents over the phone was not ideal, but in certain cases, the relative anonymity this provided respondents proved useful. Many people opened up and spoke to me for hours about their ex-periences, sharing intimate details of their lives and allowing themselves to be very vulnerable. The difficulty was that I often could not gauge their reception of me or the questions, and there were times when respondents suddenly began crying, and I had been unaware they were getting emo-tional. Being able to ascertain bodily cues is a primary feature of good ethno-graphic interviewing, and the pandemic robbed me of this opportunity. And yet, many people told me how cathartic they found the interviews. Opening up and reflecting on how the pandemic affected their families and bodies and lives in the midst of such isolation, grief, and fear was difficult, emotional, but in some cases also therapeutic. Others found themselves getting angry all over again at city or state officials, community organizers, and health care staff. As the interview quotes reveal, people were extra-ordinarily thoughtful about pandemic policies and their effects on vulner-able communities.

From January 2021 through May 2022, I also personally interviewed 65 experts (most often with research assistant Cal Garrett), including govern-ment officials (at the state and city level), Chicago Department of Public Health staff and epidemiologists, epidemiologists involved in the Racial Equity Rapid Response Team, hospital staff, administrators and clinicians, housing advocates and lawyers, alderpeople, mental health care workers, and community organizers. Many of these experts were generous with their time and genuinely glad that we had an interest in the details of their work. To understand their personal expertise, we generated individual-ized interview guides for each expert based on the organization where they work, their professional responsibilities, and some of our specific research interests. We did not gather demographic details of expert interviewees (e.g., race, gender identification), but interviewees reflected the demographic profile of Chicago.

All the graduate research assistants and I engaged in multiple phases of coding, especially to generate the policy report. I then engaged in more purposive flexible coding over the course of two years, to determine core themes and patterns in the data. I also engaged in systematic archival research of the COVID-19 coverage in the *Chicago Tribune*, *Chicago Sun-Times*, and *New York Times*, and I collected and coded policy documents that were pertinent to the analysis. I have tried to represent the conditions in Albany Park, Little Village, and Austin accurately and to provide a snapshot into Chicago's COVID-19 mitigation efforts. If I have failed in this task, I bear the fault.

NOTES

Sources are cited in short form in the notes. For full source citations, see the list of references.

INTRODUCTION

1. Flynn, "'Those Numbers Take Your Breath Away.'" In appendix A, I provide a timeline of major national and Chicago-focused events during the COVID-19 pandemic.

2. Office of the Mayor, "Racism a Public Health Crisis."

3. These five laws were the Families First Coronavirus Response Act (FFCRA) enacted March 18, 2020; the Coronavirus Aid, Relief, and Economic Security (CARES) Act enacted March 27, 2020; the Continuing Appropriations Act 2021 and Other Extensions Act, enacted October 1, 2020; the Consolidated Appropriations Act 2021, enacted December 27, 2020, and the American Rescue Plan Act of 2021 (ARPA) enacted March 11, 2021 (Bitler, Hoynes, and Schanzenbach, "Suffering," 41).

4. The full list of benefits include unemployment insurance (UI), and Pandemic Unemployment Assistance (PUA), which extended eligibility to those who are self-employed or in the gig-economy; Supplemental Nutrition Assistance Programs (SNAP); Special Supplemental Nutrition Program for Women, Infants and Children (WIC); the Child Tax Credit; stimulus payments (called Economic Impact Payments, or EIPs); Earned Income Tax Credits; school lunches and summer lunch programs; housing vouchers and rental assistance; and Medicaid expansion (Miller and Parlapiano, "European-Style Welfare State"). Medicaid is a federal-state initiative for people with lower incomes, whereas Medicare is a federal insurance program for Americans who are aged sixty-five or older. Some older adults may qualify for both Medicare and Medicaid.

5. Parolin argues that when poverty is measured through a once-per-year indicator of household economic status (as these figures are), we fail to grasp the long-term risks and consequences associated with ever having experienced poverty. The effects of living in poverty linger, Parolin argues, and produce uneven risks such as poor health conditions, lower educational attainment, and lack of long-term economic opportunity (Parolin, *Poverty in the Pandemic*, 16). For the statistics on child poverty and health care uninsurance, see Bitler, Hoynes, and Schanzenbach, "Suffering"; Miller and Parlapiano, "European-Style Welfare State."

6. I use the terms *Black* and *Latinx* to refer to broad racial groups who make up two-thirds of the population of the city of Chicago. (I prefer the gender-neutral term *Latinx*

over *Latino* or *Latina*.) I recognize that some people are both Black and Latinx, but none of the respondents in this study identified as such. When describing respondents, I name their specific racial/ethnic identity (e.g., Mexican American).

7. Interview with Shantal, a Black woman from the Austin neighborhood, September 17, 2020. All names of residents provided in this book are pseudonyms. Experts are referred to by job title. In providing quotes from my original interviews, I maintain some of my interviewees' speech patterns, tone, and style, but I have lightly edited them for clarity and readability. I indicate when an interview was conducted in Spanish and later translated.

8. Data-driven policymaking has become a core tool of neoliberal governance. It relies on the quantification of social problems and utilizes quantitative assessments to determine policy success. It is meant to be efficient and to allow for public accountability (Garrett and Decoteau, "Data Citizenship"). I critique the quantification of emergency governance in chapter 3.

9. The interviews were conducted by me as well as a team of graduate students, as I explain in appendix B, which provides details on my methods and analysis. To avoid volleying between the first person singular and first person plural, I consistently write in the first person singular when I discuss the interviews, but I want to acknowledge my debt to the graduate students who conducted many of the interviews I draw on in my analysis: Cal Garrett, Cindy Brito, Fructoso Basaldua, and Bianca Perez.

10. I use the gender-neutral terms *alderperson* and *alderpeople*, but the official governmental title is *alderman* (or plural *aldermen*). Each of these officials is elected by one of fifty wards in Chicago to serve on the City Council, the legislative body of the city. When quoting from interviews, I maintain the original language used by the respondent. The background section later in this chapter provides details on the three sampled neighborhoods: Albany Park, Austin, and Little Village.

11. Interview with community organizer, Latinx neighborhood, October 15, 2021.

12. Bitler, Hoynes, and Schanzenbach, "Suffering"; Moffit and Ziliak, "US Safety Net"; Aaron, "Social Safety Net."

13. Undocumented Americans were excluded from all three stimulus payments, and mixed-status families were excluded from receiving the first two stimulus payments (Ruiz-Grossman, "Undocumented Immigrants"). Olayo-Mendez and colleagues explain: "To be eligible for unemployment insurance and the stimulus check cash assistance program funded by the CARES Act, immigrants had to demonstrate that they had filed taxes in 2018 or 2019 with a valid social security number or receive Social Security benefits and are not required to file taxes. This includes resident aliens, green card holders, DACA recipients and workers with H1B and H2A visas. Individuals filing taxes using an Individual Taxpayer Identification Number (ITIN) rather than a social security number do not qualify for stimulus checks, nor do households filing a joint return if either spouse lacks a social security number" (Olayo-Méndez et al., "Essential, Disposable, and Excluded," 619–20. Undocumented people living in Illinois were also excluded from unemployment benefits (Zamudio, "Undocumented Workers").

14. Nixon, *Slow Violence*. Theorists of "slow death" include Berlant, "Slow Death"; Berlant, *Cruel Optimism*; Anderson, "Emergency Futures."

15. Sewell, *Logics of History*, 102, 9.

16. Ruth Wilson Gilmore defines *racism* as "the state-sanctioned or extralegal production and exploitation of group-differentiated vulnerability to premature death" (Gilmore, *Golden Gulag*, 28).

17. Foucault, *Power/Knowledge*, 195–96.

18. Wagner-Pacifici, "Restlessness of Events"; Wagner-Pacifici, *What Is an Event?*

19. The term *longue durée* is from Fernand Braudel, who explains that historical change occurs in imperceptible ways because it takes place over such an extended period (Braudel, "Histoire et sciences sociales").

20. Kotsko, "What Happened to Agamben?"

21. This is an argument also made by Weheliye, *Habeas Viscus*. Goldberg, *Racial State*, theorizes the racial state.

22. In *Society Must Be Defended*, Foucault argues that racism is a basic mechanism of biopower and normalization, and that it operates in all modern states (62, 254, 256). Ann Stoler explains, "Racism does not merely arise in moments of crisis, in sporadic cleansings. It is internal to the bio-political state, woven into the weft of the social body, threaded through its fabric" (Stoler, *Education of Desire*, 68–69).

23. Agamben, *Homo Sacer*. See also Decoteau, "Exclusionary Inclusion."

24. Foucault, *History of Sexuality*.

25. For scholarship on racial capitalism, see Carmichael and Hamilton, *Black Power*; Robinson, *Black Marxism*; DuBois, *Black Reconstruction*; Gilmore, *Golden Gulag*; Clarno, *Neoliberal Apartheid*. Wienbaum, *Afterlife of Reproductive Slavery*, uses the term *biocapitalism* to refer to the role that human reproduction plays in sustaining racial capitalism. I am using the term differently. On apparatuses of security, see Piven and Cloward, *Regulating the Poor*; Eubanks, *Automating Inequality*; Willse, *Value of Homelessness*; Wacquant, *Punishing the Poor*.

26. Foucault, *Society Must Be Defended*.

27. Willse, *Value of Homelessness*.

28. On marginalized groups being required to perform their identity or history in a way that forces them to violently translate their realities to achieve recognition, see Decoteau, *Ancestors and Antiretrovirals*; Giordano, *Migrants in Translation*.

29. Anderson et al., "Slow Emergencies."

30. Anderson, "Emergency Futures."

31. Anderson et al., "Slow Emergencies."

32. Anderson, "Emergency Futures," 473.

33. This view is similar to Wacquant's causal account of social abandonment (Wacquant, *Urban Outcasts*). I focus not simply on abandonment but on the paradoxical extension of aid amid conditions of disadvantage.

34. Nguyen, "Government-By-Exception."

35. See also Murphy, *Economization of Life*.

36. Nguyen, "Government-By-Exception," 209.

37. Agamben, *Homo Sacer*.

38. Wagner-Pacifici, *What Is an Event?*

39. Bonilla, "Coloniality of Disaster," 2.

40. Bitler, Hoynes, and Schanzenbach, "Suffering."

41. Faberman and Krawchenko, *Impact of Chronic Underfunding*.

42. Interview with community-based organization (CBO) activist, December 17, 2021.

43. Moffitt and Ziliak, "US Safety Net."

44. Corallo and Moreno, "Medicaid and CHIP Enrollment."

45. Bitler, Hoynes, and Schanzenbach, "Suffering."

46. Bitler, Hoynes, and Schanzenbach, "Suffering."

47. Moffitt and Ziliak, "US Safety Net," 5.

48. Bitler, Hoynes, and Schanzenbach, "Suffering," 53.

49. Interview with Candice, a Black woman from Austin, February 22, 2022.

50. Thebault, Tran, and Williams, "Killing Black Americans." Emphasis added.

51. Milloy, "Cure for Racial Disparities." Emphasis added.

52. Nowicki, "Virus Plateau." Emphasis added.

53. Pence quoted in Attwood and Almeida, "Food-Worker Deaths." Many of these quotes were also cited in a *New Yorker* article by Keeanga-Yamahtta Taylor, who also argues that the multiple crises facing Black Americans were largely ignored in the initial political response to the pandemic (Taylor, "Black Plague").

54. Interview with Racial Equity Rapid Response Team (RERRT) epidemiologist, April 22, 2021.

55. Nash, *Birthing Black Mothers*; Johnson, "Triumph of Black Lives Matter."

56. On colorblind racism, see Omi and Winant, *Racial Formation*; Bonilla-Silva, *Racism without Racists*.

57. Taylor (*#BlackLivesMatter*) argues that institutionalized racism (Carmichael and Hamilton, *Black Power*) was facilitated by colorblind policies such as welfare retraction. I am arguing that race-conscious, data-driven strategies claim racial equity while buttressing the continuation of colorblind policies that disguise white supremacist goals.

58. Omi and Winant, *Racial Formation*.

59. Interview with Chicago Department of Public Health (CDPH) official, March 19, 2021.

60. Interview with RERRT epidemiologist, April 22, 2021.

61. Interview with CDPH official, November 2, 2021.

62. Interview with Sophia, a Mexican American woman from Little Village, November 23, 2021.

63. Hatch, *Blood Sugar*; Wailoo, "Spectacles of Difference"; Noble, "Teaching Trayvon"; Davis and Ernst, "Racial Spectacles."

64. Noble, "Teaching Trayvon"; Davis and Ernst, "Racial Spectacles."

65. Wailoo, "Spectacles of Difference," 621.

66. Krupar and Ehlers, "Biofutures."

67. Krupar and Ehlers, "Biofutures."

68. Krupar and Ehlers, "Biofutures," 224.

69. Flynn, "'Those Numbers.'"

70. Ewing, "Memes."

71. Drake and Cayton, *Black Metropolis*; Wacquant, *Urban Outcasts*; Wilson, *Truly Disadvantaged*; Krause, *Model Cases*.

72. Henricks et al., *Three Cities*.

73. Because of my choice of neighborhood sites, I concentrate my attention on the West and Northwest Sides of the city. There are a number of studies focused on the historical disinvestment in Chicago's South Side, including Drake and Cayton, *Black Metropolis*; Wilson, *When Work Disappears*; Venkatesh, *American Project*; and N. Moore, *South Side*.

74. Hirsch, *Second Ghetto*.

75. Lugalia-Hollon and Cooper, *War on Neighborhoods*.

76. Hirsch, *Second Ghetto*; Wacquant, *Urban Outcasts*.

77. Fernández, *Brown in the Windy City*, 24–25.

78. Betancur, Cordova, and Torres, "Incorporation of Latinos," 110. Because I recruited by neighborhood and Little Village is home to mostly Mexican Americans, I did not interview many Puerto Rican Chicagoans, so I mostly focus on the history of Mexican migration and Mexican Americans' living and working conditions.

79. Amezcua, *Making Mexican Chicago*.

80. Amezcua, *Making Mexican Chicago*, 4.

81. Lugalia-Hollon and Cooper, *War on Neighborhoods*; Fernández, *Brown in the Windy City*.

82. Fernández and Amezcua both offer detailed histories of Mexican settlement in these regions of Chicago: Fernández, *Brown in the Windy City*; Amezcua, *Making Mexican Chicago*. Hirsch, Wilson, and Lugalia-Hollon and Cooper offer histories of Black settlement in Garfield Park, North Lawndale, and Austin: Hirsch, *Second Ghetto*; Wilson, *Truly Disadvantaged*; Lugalia-Hollon and Cooper, *War on Neighborhoods*.

83. Amezcua, *Making Mexican Chicago*, 59.

84. Doussard, Peck, and Theodore, "After Deindustrialization," 184.

85. Peck and Theodore, "Contingent Chicago"; Theodore, "Day Labour"; Doussard, Peck, and Theodore, "After Deindustrialization."

86. Wacquant, *Urban Outcasts*, 234–36.

87. Peck and Theodore, "Contingent Chicago"; Theodore, "Day Labour."

88. Wilson, *When Work Disappears*; Wilson, *Truly Disadvantaged*.

89. Wilson, *When Work Disappears*, 35.

90. Oakley and Burchfield, "Out of the Projects, Still in the Hood."

91. J. Smith and Stovall, "'Coming Home.'"

92. Soss, Fording, and Schram, *Disciplining the Poor*.

93. Broder and Lessard, "Immigrant Eligibility."

94. Wacquant, *Urban Outcasts*, 85; Wilson, *When Work Disappears*, 49.

95. Lugalia-Hollon and Cooper, *War on Neighborhoods*.

96. Lugalia-Hollon and Cooper, *War on Neighborhoods*.

97. Lugalia-Hollon and Cooper, *War on Neighborhoods*, 35.

98. Theodore and Martin, "Migrant Civil Society."

99. Carrillo and Ipsen, "Worksites as Sacrifice Zones."

100. It is common to refer to these areas as "neighborhoods," but in fact, they are demarcations that were created in the 1920s by the University of Chicago Social Science Research Committee to facilitate the collection of crime statistics (Lugalia-Hollon and Cooper, *War on Neighborhoods*, 18). They have remained largely unchanged since the 1920s and are used in multiple data collection projects in the city. Often these areas encompass multiple smaller neighborhood groupings.

101. In table 0.1, total population estimates are based on 2020 census estimates. Unless otherwise specified, all other statistics for community areas are averaged estimates from 2017–2021 while Chicago-wide statistics are estimates for 2021. Vaccination rates are published by Chicago Department of Public Health at the zip code level, which does not align perfectly with these community areas. This table uses zip code 60625 to approximate Albany Park, zip code 60644 to approximate Austin, and zip code 60623 to approximate Little Village. These data were current as of July 18, 2023. Cal Garrett assembled the data for the table.

102. *Local Community Fact Book 1970 and 1980*.

103. Theodore and Martin, "Migrant Civil Society."

104. *Local Community Fact Book 1990.*

105. Naber et al., *Beyond Erasure.*

106. Theodore and Martin, "Migrant Civil Society."

107. Talen, "Design for Diversity."

108. *Local Community Fact Book 1970 and 1980.*

109. *Redlining* occurred when the Federal Housing Authority told banks not to insure or provide mortgages to residents in Black neighborhoods (Wilson, *When Work Disappears*, 47). *Blockbusting* occurs when real estate agents propagate fear of a "racial transition" to get white homeowners to sell at cheaper rates (Lugalia-Hollon and Cooper, *War on Neighborhoods*).

110. Lugalia-Hollon and Cooper, *War on Neighborhoods*; Austin Coming Together, "History of Austin."

111. Lugalia-Hollon and Cooper, *War on Neighborhoods.*

112. *Local Community Fact Book 1990.*

113. *Local Community Fact Book 1970 and 1980.*

114. *Local Community Fact Book 1990.*

115. *Local Community Fact Book 1970 and 1980.*

116. Reed, "South Lawndale."

117. Nixon, *Slow Violence*, 19. The epigraph that opens the section is from this same source; emphasis added.

118. Interview with Bernice, a Black woman from Austin, January 20, 2021.

119. Interview with Derek, a Black man from Austin, November 6, 2020.

120. Figure 0.2 was created by Iván Areñas based on data from Illinois Department of Public Health, Death Certificate Data Files. It also appears in Decoteau et al., *Deadly Disparities*, 59.

121. Cook County Government, "Homicides Drop."

122. Eldeib and Sanchez, "Opioid Overdoses."

123. Klinenberg, *Heat Wave.*

124. Interview with Mexican American alderperson, Latinx neighborhood, December 28, 2021.

125. Amezcua also discusses processes of ongoing gentrification and their impact on Pilsen and Little Village: Amezcua, *Making Mexican Chicago.*

126. Theodore, "Day Labour."

127. Yousef, "Rents May Be Going Up."

128. Decoteau, Golio, and Garrett, "Risks of Renting on the Margins."

129. Interview with housing attorney, October 25, 2021.

130. Figure 0.3 reports on data from the Household Pulse Survey (HPS), which is an experimental survey "designed to quickly and efficiently deploy data collected on how people's lives have been impacted by the coronavirus pandemic" (United States Census Bureau, "Household Pulse Survey Data Tables"). Survey responses were analyzed over time by race, tenure, and household income in the Chicago-Naperville-Elgin, IL-IN-WI Metropolitan Statistical Area (Chicagoland MSA). Disaggregated estimates tended to have small sample sizes, owing to the quick turnover in data collection, which limits overall sample sizes, especially at lower geographic levels. Data were compiled by Chris Poulos. The data are divided into two periods: week 15 (September 16, 2020–September 28, 2020) through week 31 (May 26–June 7, 2021) and week 32 (June 9–June 21, 2021) through week 48 (July 27–August 8, 2022). Standard errors were calculated using HPS replicate weights.

131. Reiley and Romm, "School Lunch Program"; Qiu, "Families Struggle."
132. Soglin, "Emergency SNAP Benefits Ending."
133. In table 0.3, *low food access* is defined as living more than one-half mile from a grocery store. In table 0.4, these measures are only available for zip codes and not neighborhoods. Zip code 60625 is used for Albany Park, 60644 and 60624 for Austin, and 60623 for Little Village. These zip codes have different geography and total population than the community areas themselves but are a close proxy. Cal Garrett assembled the data for tables 0.3 and 0.4.
134. Interview with Miguel, a Mexican immigrant man from Albany Park, August 14, 2020. This interview was conducted in Spanish by Yesenia Vargas and later translated into English.
135. Interview with Harold, a Black man from Austin, January 20, 2021. Emphasis added.
136. Interview with Carlos, a Mexican American man from Albany Park, February 27, 2021. Emphasis added.
137. Interview with Sharon, a Black woman from Austin, October 17, 2020.
138. Interview with member of mayor's racial equity team, March 24, 2021.
139. Kinder, Stateler, and Du, "Hazard Continues."
140. Interview with community organizer, Latinx neighborhood, December 17, 2021.

CHAPTER ONE

1. Bechteler and Kane-Willis, *Epidemic of Inequities.*
2. Interview with Shirley, a Black woman from Austin, October 31, 2020.
3. Interview with Marlin, a Black man from Austin, December 13, 2021.
4. Interview with Walter, a Black man from Austin, October 14, 2020.
5. Interview with Anthony, a Black man from Austin, February 25, 2022.
6. Vinicky, "Chicago Brings in National Guard."
7. Interview with Sholanda, a Black woman from Austin, January 28, 2022.
8. Wagner-Pacifici, "Are We in One?"
9. On Trump's downplaying of the pandemic, see Kolata and Rabin, "'Don't Be Afraid of Covid,' Trump Says." On "epistemology of ignorance," see Charles Mills, *Racial Contract*, 18.
10. Interview with Becky, a white woman from Albany Park, February 23, 2021.
11. Interview with Sholanda, January 28, 2022.
12. Interview with Keisha, a Black woman from Austin, October 17, 2020.
13. Interview with Kelly, a Black woman from Albany Park, January 26, 2021.
14. Hatch, "Data Will Not Save Us," 8.
15. See Reuters, "Trump Urges Slowdown," for an example.
16. Harell and Lieberman, "Race-Based Health Disparities."
17. Interview with Rodrigo, a Mexican American man from Little Village, May 18, 2021.
18. Interview with Ben, a Black man from Austin, January 20, 2021.
19. Interview with Charles, a Black man from Austin, November 1, 2020.
20. Schwartz, Bourdieu, and Auyero all discuss how making the oppressed wait is a core feature of domination. See Schwartz, "Waiting"; Bourdieu, *Pascalian Meditations*; Auyero, *Patients of the State.*

21. Bayne and Schumer, "What Happened May 30?"

22. Mortice, "Chicago's 1855 Beer Riot."

23. Interview with Annie, a Korean American woman from Albany Park, February 25, 2021.

24. Vinicky, "Chicago Brings in National Guard."

25. Interview with Kelly, January 26, 2021.

26. Interview with Lyla, an Arab American woman from Albany Park, January 27, 2021.

27. The Gold Coast, on the northeast side of Chicago, is one of the most expensive neighborhoods in the country.

28. Interview with Ebony, a Black woman from Austin, December 17, 2021.

29. Interview with Jada, a Black woman from Little Village, December 16, 2020.

30. Pathieu and Schulte, "More than $280M to CPD"; Byrne, "Activists Hammer Mayor."

31. Clarno, "Policing COVID."

32. Interview with Annie, January 7, 2022.

33. Interview with Sholanda, January 28, 2022.

34. J. Ferguson and Witzburg, *Response to George Floyd Protests*.

35. Cherone, "Police Botched Response."

36. Wall and Schulte, "Pritzker Signs Reform Bill."

37. Zapata, "We Are Adam."

38. Malagón, "Post-George Floyd Police Reforms."

39. Bouie, "Unleashed"; Metzl, *Dying of Whiteness*; Morrison, "Race War Evident"; Blake, "Angry White Man"; Taylor, "Bitter Fruits."

40. Interview with Tomás, a Mexican American man from Little Village, October 29, 2021.

41. Interview with Elena, a Mexican American woman from Little Village, November 23, 2021.

42. Interview with Sholanda, January 28, 2022.

43. Interview with Ebony, December 17, 2021.

44. Stokely Carmichael and Charles Hamilton explain that institutional racism is concealed from the public and thereby protects white supremacist domination. People who benefit from white supremacy may only "see" racism in individually violent acts, not the ongoing, mundane, ways in which institutions and structures protect white wealth and power. See Carmichael and Hamilton, *Black Power*.

45. Interview with Phyllis, a Black woman from Austin, February 18, 2022.

46. Interview with Walter, October 14, 2020.

47. Interview with Monique, a Black woman from Austin, December 3, 2020.

48. Interview with Reginald, a Black man from Austin, February 25, 2022.

49. Foucault, *Society Must Be Defended*, 254.

50. In fact, in *Society Must Be Defended*, Foucault traces the genealogy of state racism back to the sixteenth century and suggests that an earlier bifurcated "war of races" emerged between internal European enemies, initially articulated by challenges from the racially marginalized. It was then "tactically reversed" and co-opted by the state to control races deemed to be risky or dangerous to the optimization of the national norm. This original race war undergirds normative regulation in biopolitical societies.

51. Foucault, *Society Must Be Defended*, 246.

52. Agamben, *Homo Sacer*.

53. Weheliye, *Habeas Viscus*, 87.

54. Anderson, "Emergency Futures."

55. Keeanga-Yamahtta Taylor argues that the Black Lives Matter movement spotlights police violence and exposes the lie of colorblind racism (Taylor, *#BlackLivesMatter*).

56. Foucault, *Security, Territory, Population*.

57. Bourdieu, *Pascalian Meditations*.

58. Grove et al., "Uneven Distribution of Futurity."

59. Many scholars analyze how state actors manipulate time to control populations or forge a sense of national collectivity, including Foucault, *Discipline and Punish*; Bourdieu, *Pascalian Meditations*; Schwartz, "Waiting"; Anderson, "Governing Emergencies"; Auyero, *Patients of the State*. In her analysis of the restlessness of events, Robin Wagner-Pacifici recognizes that multiple temporalities can coexist, leading to a heightened sense of disorientation in the midst of ruptural events (Wagner-Pacifici, *What Is an Event?*).

60. See the timeline in appendix A for more details of both national and local events during the pandemic.

61. Interview with Camila, a Mexican American woman from Little Village, April 23, 2021.

62. Figures 1.1, 1.2, and 1.3 were created using the City of Chicago's COVID-19 Dashboard on October 17, 2022. Cal Garrett assembled the data.

63. Interview with Mary, a Black woman from Austin, March 2, 2022.

64. Interview with Federally Qualified Health Center (FQHC) provider in Latinx community, May 20, 2020.

65. Interview with Kelly, October 29, 2021.

66. White House, "Remarks by President Biden."

67. Interview with Shantal, March 2, 2022.

68. Interview with Willie, a Black man from Austin, February 5, 2022.

69. Interview with Ana, a Mexican American woman from Little Village, January 27, 2022.

70. Interview with Dolores, a Black woman from Austin, February 1, 2022.

71. Appendix A provides a timeline of COVID-19 events and shifting "best practices" advised by federal and local public health officials.

72. Interview with Dolores, February 1, 2022.

73. Biden, "Pandemic Is Over."

74. Interview with Annie, January 7, 2022.

75. Interview with Samira, a Black woman from Little Village, December 13, 2021.

CHAPTER TWO

1. On bodily weathering, see Geronimus, "Weathering"; James, "John Henryism"; Villarosa, *Under the Skin*. On interpersonal discrimination within health care settings, see Paradies et al., "Racism as a Determinant of Health"; Krieger, "Discrimination and Health Inequities"; Lundy et al., "Racial Categories." On residential segregation, see Klinenberg, *Heat Wave*; K. White, Haas, and Williams, "Role of Place"; Williams and Collins, "Racial Residential Segregation." On barriers to high-quality health care access, see Feagin and Bennefield, "Systemic Racism"; K. White, Haas, and Williams, "Role of Place"; Institute of Medicine, *Unequal Treatment*.

2. Jones, "Levels of Racism"; Bailey et al., "Structural Racism"; Viruell-Fuentes, Miranda, and Abdulrahim, "More Than Culture." Villarosa highlights the fact that racism negatively impacts the health of all racially marginalized Americans regardless of their class (Villarosa, *Under the Skin*).

3. Scholars who criticize the biologization of racial difference include Lundy et al., "Racial Categories"; Smedley and Smedley, "Race as a Social Problem."

4. Hammonds and Reverby, "Racial Health Disparities."

5. Starr, "Built to Last?"

6. Star, "Ethnography of Infrastructure"; Carse, "Keyword: Infrastructure."

7. Larkin, "Politics and Poetics of Infrastructure"; Anand, Gupta, and Appel, *Promise of Infrastructure*.

8. On critical or vital infrastructure, see Lakoff, *Unprepared*. On social infrastructure, see Klinenberg, *Palaces for the People*.

9. Lakoff, for example, pays scant attention to the ways in which race and class inequalities have been structured into emergency preparations (Lakoff, *Unprepared*).

10. On infrastructure as imperceptible and taken for granted, see Star, "Ethnography of Infrastructure," 380. On certain infrastructures being rendered invisible, see Larkin, "Politics and Poetics of Infrastructure"; Street, *Unstable Place*.

11. Parlapiano and Tankersley, "Biden's Infrastructure Plan." This bill went through multiple stages of revision. Part of this original act, signed into law in March 2021, was diverted toward new legislation passed in November 2021 called the Infrastructure Investment and Jobs Act. In 2022, when the Build Back Better Act was being considered by Congress, a compromise piece of legislation was passed, called the Inflation Reduction Act. This new act removed all attention to care infrastructure.

12. Snyder, "Shrinking Infrastructure Plan."

13. On illicit health economies, see Raudenbush, *Health Care Off the Books*.

14. Quadagno, "No National Health Insurance"; Quadagno, *One Nation Uninsured*; Gaffney, "Neoliberal Turn."

15. Williams and Collins, "Racial Residential Segregation"; Williams and Jackson, "Social Sources"; Bailey et al., "Structural Racism"; Ansell, *Death Gap*.

16. Gaffney and McCormick, "Affordable Care Act."

17. Decoteau et al., *Deadly Disparities*, 30.

18. Decoteau et al., *Deadly Disparities*, 30.

19. Martinez-Hume et al., "'They Treat You a Different Way'"; Maskovsky, "'Managing' the Poor."

20. Tolbert and Ammula, "Unwinding."

21. Cubanski et al., "Declarations End."

22. LaFraniere and Weiland, "End Public Health Emergency."

23. Presa, "Illinois Expansion." As of December 1, 2020, undocumented residents of Illinois who are aged sixty-five or older and living at or below the poverty level are eligible for Medicaid-like benefits under a program called Health Benefits for Immigrant Seniors (Illinois Department of Human Services, "New Health Benefit"). In May 2022, the program expanded to include anyone aged fifty-four or older. On undocumented immigrants' ineligibility for benefits under the ACA, see Artiga and Diaz, "Health Coverage and Care."

24. Illinois Department of Healthcare and Family Services. "Health Benefits for Immigrant Adults"; Petrella, "Costs Soaring."

25. Institute of Medicine, *Health Care Safety Net.*
26. Vargas, *Uninsured in Chicago.*
27. According to Trombetta ("Managed Care Medicaid," 199), "Managed care organizations of all varieties contract with state Medicaid agencies to deliver and manage the health-care benefits under the Medicaid programs in exchange for predetermined capitation revenue." Medicaid Managed Care was introduced to lower costs to the state associated with ACA expansion, but it has resulted in poorer outcomes for the most vulnerable Americans, especially those with chronic illnesses.
28. CountyCare is the largest Medicaid managed care plan in Chicago. It was created for patients in the Stroger/Cook County system.
29. Interview with FQHC administrator, April 16, 2021.
30. Interview with Ebony, December 17, 2021.
31. Martinez-Hume et al., "'They Treat You a Different Way.'"
32. Interview with FQHC provider, May 17, 2020.
33. Interview with FQHC provider, April 22, 2021.
34. Ansell, *County: Chicago's Public Hospital.*
35. Interview with FQHC provider, April 22, 2021.
36. Interview with Barbara, a Black woman from Austin, April 5, 2021.
37. Interview with FQHC provider, May 10, 2021.
38. Interview with FQHC provider, April 22, 2021.
39. Interview with FQHC provider, March 18, 2021.
40. Interview with FQHC administrator, April 16, 2021.
41. Interview with Brenda, a Black woman from Austin, November 25, 2021.
42. Interview with Terrance, a Black man from Austin, October 20, 2020.
43. Interview with Marlin, April 21, 2021.
44. Tung et al., "Geographic Access."
45. Interview with Gabriela, a Mexican American woman from Little Village, March 8, 2021.
46. Interview with William, a Black man from Austin, October 31, 2020.
47. Interview with FQHC provider, May 17, 2021.
48. Interview with Bernice, January 20, 2021.
49. Interview with Marlin, December 13, 2021.
50. Interview with Ebony, December 17, 2021.
51. Interview with Jada, December 16, 2020.
52. Interview with Miguel, August 14, 2020. This interview was conducted in Spanish by Yesenia Vargas and was later translated.
53. Eldeib et al., "COVID-19 Took Black Lives First."
54. Interview with FQHC provider, May 20, 2021.
55. Interview with Walter, October 14, 2020.
56. Ansell, *County: Chicago's Public Hospital.*
57. Interview with physician and hospital administrator, March 23, 2021.
58. Schorsch, "Another Gap."
59. St. Clair, "Financial Brink."
60. Chase, "South Side Hospitals Call Off Merger."
61. Schencker, "Mercy Hospital Closing."
62. Interview with Marlin, April 21, 2021.
63. Interview with FQHC administrator, April 16, 2021.

64. Chicago Department of Public Health, *Mental Health Services Report.*

65. Collaborative for Community Wellness, *Mental Health Service Access.*

66. Collaborative for Community Wellness, *Uplifting Voices*; Rembis, "New Asylums." This correlation was also expressed in my interview with a behavioral health specialist in Austin, November 4, 2021.

67. Black, "Time to Reopen Mental Health Clinics."

68. Spielman, "Lightfoot Announces $8 Million in Grants."

69. Cherone, "Chicago to Boost Mental Health Spending."

70. Spielman, "Lightfoot Announces $8 Million in Grants"; Cherone, "Chicago to Boost Mental Health Spending." In the wake of increasing mental illness related to the pandemic, Lightfoot added $1.2 million in mental health treatment support (Cherone, "Chicago to Boost Mental Health Spending"). She also invested $3.5 million in a pilot project pairing mental health providers with police responders to 911 calls (Struett and Schuba, "Mental Health Clinicians").

71. Interview with psychiatric physician assistant (PA) at FQHC, May 27, 2021.

72. Interview with psychiatric PA, May 27, 2021.

73. Interview with public mental health care provider, Albany Park, June 17, 2021.

74. Interview with psychiatric PA, May 27, 2021.

75. Interview with public mental health care provider, Austin, November 4, 2021.

76. Interview with psychiatric PA, May 27, 2021.

77. Interview with Armando, an undocumented Mexican man from Little Village, October 17, 2020.

78. Interview with Shantal, September 17, 2020.

79. Interview with Marlin, April 21, 2021.

80. Interview with FQHC provider, May 17, 2021.

81. Interview with FQHC administrator, April 16, 2021.

82. Interview with Ana, January 27, 2022.

83. Interview with Kelly, October 29, 21.

84. Foucault, "Birth of Social Medicine."

85. Colgrove, *Epidemic City.*

86. Markel and Stern, "Foreignness of Germs."

87. Shah, *Contagious Divides*; A. White, *Epidemic Orientalism.*

88. Molina, *Fit to Be Citizens*, 2.

89. Shah, *Contagious Divides*; Molina, *Fit to Be Citizens*; Schlabach, "Influenza Epidemic."

90. Shah, *Contagious Divides*; Gamble, "Wasn't a Lot of Comfort"; Schlabach, "Influenza Epidemic."

91. Molina, *Fit to Be Citizens*, 3–4.

92. Schlabach, "Influenza Epidemic."

93. Schlabach, "Influenza Epidemic."

94. Gamble, "Wasn't a Lot of Comfort."

95. Reverby, "Ethical Failures."

96. Susser and Susser, "Choosing a Future for Epidemiology."

97. Starr, *Social Transformation.*

98. Colgrove, Markowitz, and Rosner, *Contested Boundaries.*

99. Colgrove, *Epidemic City.*

100. Colgrove, *Epidemic City.*

101. Shah, *Contagious Divides*.

102. Colgrove, *Epidemic City*.

103. Reubi, "Genealogy of Epidemiological Reason."

104. Ehrenreich, *Making of a Pandemic*, 88.

105. Weisz, *Chronic Disease*.

106. Wahlberg and Rose, "Governmentalization of Living."

107. Ehrenreich, *Making of a Pandemic*, 89.

108. Colgrove, Markowitz, and Rosner, *Contested Boundaries*, 9.

109. Watkins-Hayes, *Remaking a Life*.

110. Levi et al., *Investing In America's Health*; Faberman and Krawchenko, *Impact of Chronic Underfunding*.

111. Chicago for the People, *Building Bridges*.

112. Interview with CDPH official, November 2, 2021.

113. Interview with RERRT epidemiologist, April 27, 2021.

114. Interview with CDPH epidemiologist, March 2, 2021.

115. Interview with CDPH epidemiologist, March 9, 2021.

116. Interview with CDPH epidemiologist, March 2, 2021.

117. Interview with CDPH epidemiologist, March 2, 2021.

118. Interview with CDPH epidemiologist, March 9, 2021.

119. Clarno, "Policing COVID."

120. Garrett and Decoteau, "Data Citizenship."

121. Interview with CDPH epidemiologist, March 2, 2021.

122. Interview with CDPH official, February 10, 2021.

123. Krupar and Ehlers, "Biofutures."

124. Interview with CDPH epidemiologist, March 2, 2021.

125. Interview with hospital administrator and member of RERRT, May 11, 2021.

126. Interview with chief equity officer, Mayor's Office, April 27, 2021.

127. Interview with Isaiah, a Black man from Austin, October 20, 2020.

CHAPTER THREE

1. Zamudio, "70% of Deaths."

2. Spielman, "Lightfoot 'Red Alarm.'"

3. Interview with Chicago Department of Public Health (CDPH) expert, November 2, 2021.

4. Omi and Winant, *Racial Formation*, 211. See also Bonilla-Silva, *Racism without Racists*.

5. Carmichael and Hamilton, *Black Power*.

6. Interview with Sholanda, January 28, 2022.

7. Interview with community organizer, Austin, November 18, 2021.

8. Hansen, "Datafication of Governance"; Adams, *Metrics*; Garrett and Decoteau, "Data Citizenship."

9. On numbers as exclusionary, see Espeland and Stevens, "Sociology of Quantification"; Scheel, "Biopolitical Bordering."

10. Zuberi, *Thicker Than Blood*.

11. Zuberi, *Thicker Than Blood*.

12. Chowkwanyun and Reed, "Caution and Context."

13. Interview with CDPH epidemiologist, March 9, 2021; Benjamin, *Race after Technology*.

14. Benjamin, "Catching Our Breath."

15. Hatch, "Data Will Not Save Us," 2.

16. Bourdieu, "Rethinking the State."

17. Cherone, "67% of Chicagoans Vaccinated." A non-peer-reviewed study published in September 2021 on medRxiv made the local news when it claimed that 118 lives could have been saved in Chicago if vaccines had been rolled out more effectively from the outset (Zeng et al., "Vaccine Allocation Inequity").

18. Interview with FQHC provider, April 16, 2021; Esposito and Chase, "Equitable Distribution."

19. Povinelli, *Economies of Abandonment*.

20. Garrett and Decoteau, "Data Citizenship."

21. Drake and Cayton, *Black Metropolis*; Wacquant, *Urban Outcasts*; Wilson, *Truly Disadvantaged*; Krause, *Model Cases*.

22. Henricks et al., *Three Cities*.

23. Simpson, *Rogues, Rebels, and Rubber Stamps*, Fishman, "How It Works."

24. Interview with alderperson in Albany Park, May 4, 2021.

25. Interview with community organizer, December 17, 2021.

26. Doussard, Peck, and Theodore, "After Deindustrialization."

27. Wacquant, *Urban Outcasts*, 82–83.

28. Morrell, "Activists Slam Chicago Mayor."

29. Interview with Albany Park alderperson, May 4, 2021.

30. Interview with Albany Park alderperson, May 4, 2021.

31. Institute for Housing Studies, "Policy Interventions."

32. US Department of the Treasury, *Recovery Funds 2021 Interim Final Rule*, 16.

33. Civic Federation, "City Continues 'Scoop and Toss Borrowing.'"

34. Cherone, "Cancel 'Scoop and Toss' Borrowing."

35. Cherone, "Cancel 'Scoop and Toss' Borrowing." Lightfoot took this approach after she was criticized for planning to use ARPA funds to pay off debt directly (Ramos, "Feds Urged to Investigate").

36. City of Chicago public record request, May 26, 2023, Reference # X047469-052623.

37. Interview with Albany Park alderperson, May 4, 2021.

38. In Philadelphia, for example, $10 million was dispersed to four thousand households in 2020 (Reina and Lee, "Emergency Rental Assistance," 211–12). On Seattle, see King County, *Homelessness Response*. See also Haskins, Parilla, and Bauer, "Local Governments Finalize Priorities."

39. Interview with Mayor's Office RERRT official, April 27, 2021.

40. Interview with RERRT leader, May 11, 2021.

41. Interview with Mayor's Office RERRT official, April 27, 2021.

42. Interview with community organizer, December 17, 2021.

43. Interview with CDPH infectious disease expert, February 10, 2021.

44. Interview with Mayor's Office RERRT official, April 27, 2021.

45. Interview with Illinois equity official, May 20, 2021.

46. Interview with RERRT community organizer, Little Village, October 25, 2021.

47. Institute for Housing Studies, "Policy Interventions."

48. Illinois Housing Development Authority, *Illinois Emergency Assistance.*
49. Illinois Housing Development Authority, *Illinois Rental Repayment Program.*
50. Reina and Lee, "Emergency Rental Assistance," 211.
51. Reina and Lee, "Emergency Rental Assistance."
52. Interview with Mayor's Office equity official, March 24, 2021.
53. Interview with community organizer, December 17, 2021.
54. Interview with Rodrigo, April 19, 2022.
55. Office of Governor Gavin Newsom, "Governor Newsom Visits." King County, Washington, also instituted policies wherein the homeless were given hotel rooms, paid for by ARPA funds (King County, *Homelessness Response*).
56. Flores, "Austin City Council."
57. Interview with CDPH official, March 29, 2021.
58. Interview with CDPH official, March 29, 2021.
59. In fact, the battles between Mayor Lightfoot and the Chicago Teachers Union (CTU) were legion during the first year of the pandemic—in part because CTU refused to allow its teachers to work in unsafe work environments, effectively shutting down public schools for an entire year. This book does not address the constraints residents faced in securing education and childcare for vulnerable children, which undoubtedly contributed to pandemic precarity among Black and Latinx Chicagoans. Please see the following resources for further information on these important topics: Office for Civil Rights, *Education in a Pandemic*; Oberg et al., "Impact of COVID-19 on Children's Lives"; Parolin, *Poverty in the Pandemic.*
60. Interview with Austin community organizer, November 18, 2021.
61. Interview with Marlin, April 21, 2021.
62. Interview with Marlin, December 13, 2021.
63. Interview with Little Village testing provider, October 29, 2021.
64. Interview with Little Village community organizer, October 25, 2021.
65. Interview with Little Village testing provider, October 29, 2021.
66. Interview with Little Village community organizer, October 25, 2021.
67. Garrett and Decoteau, "Data Citizenship."
68. Interview with RERRT official, May 24, 2021.
69. Interview with RERRT epidemiologist, April 27, 2021.
70. Garrett and Decoteau, "Data Citizenship."
71. Interview with CDPH epidemiologist, March 9, 2021.
72. Interview with CDPH epidemiologist, March 9, 2021.
73. Interview with CDPH epidemiologist, March 2, 2021.
74. Interview with CDPH epidemiologist, March 2, 2022.
75. Mandavilli, "New Infectious Threats"; LaFraniere, "Lack of Data." When an outbreak of mpox emerged among predominantly Black populations in Africa in 2022, mpox was initially referred to as *monkeypox*, the name it was given in 1970 because the virus that causes the disease in humans had first been discovered in captive monkeys in 1958. The World Health Organization (WHO), which was already reconsidering the naming of "all orthopoxvirus species," hastened the renaming process after "racist and stigmatizing language online, in other settings and in some communities was observed and reported to WHO," and on November 28, 2022, it began to use *mpox* as its preferred term while phasing out the former name over a one-year period (WHO, "WHO Recommends New Name").

76. On "vital infrastructure," see Lakoff, *Unprepared*.

77. Interview with Illinois equity official, May 20, 2021.

78. Interview with Tomás, October 29, 2021.

79. Interview with Illinois equity official, May 20, 2021.

80. Interview with CDPH epidemiologist, March 9, 2021.

81. Klinenberg, *Heat Wave*.

82. City of Chicago, "COVID-19 Dashboard."

83. Interview with RERRT community organizer, October 15, 2021.

84. On "hotspotting," see Krupar and Ehlers, "Biofutures."

85. Interview with CBO activist, December 17, 2021.

86. Interview with RERRT community organizer, December 13, 2021.

87. Interview with RERRT community organizer, October 25, 2021.

88. Interview with CDPH epidemiologist, March 9, 2021.

89. Interview with South Shore community organizer, November 9, 2021.

90. Interview with Sophia, November 23, 2021.

91. Interview with Charles, November 1, 2020.

92. Interview with Joseph, a Black man from Austin, January 27, 2022.

93. Morgan and Campbell, *Delegated Welfare State*.

94. Soss, Fording, and Schram, *Disciplining the Poor*.

95. Morgan and Campbell, *Delegated Welfare State*, 223.

96. Interview with State of Illinois human services official, October 14, 2021.

97. Interview with community organizer, December 17, 2021.

98. Interview with Albany Park alderperson, May 4, 2021.

99. Interview with community organizer, predominantly Black neighborhood, October 5, 2021.

100. Interview with Shantal, September 17, 2020.

101. Interview with Shantal, February 3, 2022.

102. Mayor's Press Office, "$56m Grant."

103. Interview with CDPH official, February 10, 2021. Emphasis added.

104. Interview with CDPH official, March 19, 2021.

105. Interview with CBO activist, December 16, 2021.

106. Reina and Lee, "Emergency Rental Assistance," 211.

107. Joint Center for Housing Studies, *America's Rental Housing*.

108. Institute for Housing Studies, "State of Rental Housing."

109. Reina and Lee, "Emergency Rental Assistance," 210.

110. Wacquant, *Punishing the Poor*; Soss, Fording, and Schram, *Disciplining the Poor*.

111. United States Department of Labor Employment and Training Administration, *Pandemic Unemployment Assistance*.

112. Weisenstein and Andriesen, "Illinoisans Await Calls."

113. Interview with Sholanda, January 28, 2022.

114. Interview with Kelly, October 29, 2021.

115. Interview with Rodrigo, April 19, 2022.

116. Interview with Department of Housing official, May 4, 2021.

117. Figure 3.1 compares all renters with renters whose household income is below $50,000 per year. See endnote 130 on page 226 for details on how data was assembled from the Housing Pulse Survey (HPS). HPS data were used to create figures 3.1 and 3.2. The census began asking about rental assistance on week 34 (July 21-August 2, 2021).

We pooled these estimates into one period: week 34 through week 48. Chris Poulos calculated these figures, and AJ Golio created the charts.

118. These data are also analyzed in Decoteau, Golio, and Garrett, "Risks of Renting."

119. Interview with Luis, an undocumented Mexican man from Albany Park, April 13, 2021. This interview was conducted in Spanish by Cindy Brito and later translated.

120. Interview with Luis, April 13, 2021.

121. Interview with State of Illinois human services official, October 14, 2021.

122. Interview with Tomás, October 17, 2020.

123. Interview with community organizer, December 17, 2021.

124. Interview with RERRT organizer, October 25, 2021.

125. Qin, "Cook County Evictions."

126. This story was reported on by NBC news in Chicago in January 2021 (Sutter, "Activist Seeks Help").

127. Interview with Albany Park alderperson, May 4, 2021.

128. Garrett and Decoteau, "Data Citizenship."

129. Interview with Marlin, April 21, 2021.

CHAPTER FOUR

1. Interview with Juan, a Mexican American man from Austin, February 8, 2021.

2. Camarillo, "Opioid Deaths."

3. Interview with Marlin, December 13, 2021.

4. Marcelo, "Hospital COVID Payments."

5. Interview with Shantal, September 17, 2020.

6. Interview with Marlin, December 13, 2021.

7. Povinelli, *Economies of Abandonment*, 144.

8. Nixon, "Neoliberalism, Slow Violence."

9. Carmichael and Hamilton argue that institutionalized forms of racism fade into the background and are easily ignored by those who benefit from white supremacy (Carmichael and Hamilton, *Black Power*).

10. Villarosa, *Under the Skin*; James, "John Henryism"; Geronimus, "Weathering."

11. On slow death, see Berlant, "Slow Death"; Berlant, *Cruel Optimism*; Anderson, "Emergency Futures." On slow violence, see Nixon, "Neoliberalism, Slow Violence."

12. Berlant, "Slow Death," 759, 754.

13. Berlant, *Cruel Optimism*.

14. Interview with Reginald, February 25, 2022.

15. Interview with Reginald, February 25, 2022.

16. Interview with Reginald, February 25, 2022. Emphasis added.

17. Interview with Reginald, February 25, 2022.

18. Lugalia-Hollon and Cooper, *War on Neighborhoods*.

19. Gowan and Whetstone, "Criminal Addict"; Kaye, "Rehabilitating the 'Drugs Lifestyle'"; Stuart, "From 'Rabble Management' to 'Recovery Management.'"

20. Interview with Reginald, February 25, 2022.

21. Interview with Clayton, a Black man from Austin, February 10, 2022.

22. Interview with Clayton, February 10, 2022.

23. Interview with Andre, a Black man from Austin, February 4, 2022.

24. Interview with Andre, February 4, 2022.

25. Villarosa, *Under the Skin*, 3.

26. Gowan and Whetstone, "Criminal Addict"; Kaye, "Rehabilitating the 'Drugs Lifestyle.'"

27. On labor requirements for receiving social welfare, see Soss, Fording, and Schram, *Disciplining the Poor*.

28. Nixon, "Neoliberalism, Slow Violence," 454.

29. Chicago Housing Authority (CHA) provides traditional public housing, mixed-income developments, and Housing Choice Voucher (HCV) and Project-Based Voucher (PBV) programs. Both voucher programs, together, account for the Section 8 population. Section 8 vouchers are programs funded by the US Department of Housing and Urban Development that are administered by CHA and fund residents to access housing on the private market. See Chicago Housing Authority, "Housing Choice Voucher (HCV) Program"; Chicago Housing Authority, "Project Based Voucher."

30. Interview with Phyllis, February 18, 2022.

31. Interview with Phyllis, February 18, 2022.

32. Interview with Phyllis, February 18, 2022.

33. Board of Governors, *Report on Economic Well-Being*.

34. Interview with Dolores, February 1, 2022.

35. The City of Chicago generates tremendous profit from traffic and parking violation tickets and fees on failure to pay, but debt from traffic and parking violations is unequally distributed. Black residents of Chicago suffer disproportionately from this debt, often causing loss of transportation and bankruptcy (Sanchez and Kambhampati, "Chicago Ticket Debt").

36. Claire Mills et al., *Low-Income America*.

37. Interview with Dolores, February 1, 2022. Emphasis added.

38. Interview with Marlin, December 13, 2021.

39. Interview with Luis, November 17, 2021.

40. Interview with Luis, April 13, 2021.

41. Interview with Lorenzo, an undocumented Mexican man from Little Village, March 30, 2021. This interview was conducted in Spanish by Cindy Brito and later translated.

42. Interview with Lorenzo, March 30, 2021.

43. Interview with Lorenzo, November 16, 2021.

44. Casselman and DePillis, "Poverty Rate Soared."

45. Berlant, *Cruel Optimism*.

46. Interview with Samira, December 13, 2021.

47. Interview with Samira, December 13, 2021.

48. Interview with Samira, February 23, 2021.

49. Interview with Samira, December 13, 2021.

50. Interview with Samira, December 13, 2021.

51. Interview with Samira, December 13, 2021.

52. Interview with Kelly, October 29, 2021.

53. Interview with Kelly, October 29, 2021.

54. Interview with Miguel, March 8, 2022.

55. Interview with Miguel, March 8, 2022.

56. Interview with Miguel, March 8, 2022.

57. Interview with Miguel, March 8, 2022.

58. Interview with Miguel, March 8, 2022. Emphasis added.

59. Anderson, "Emergency Futures," 472.

60. Ferguson, *Aberrations in Black*.

61. Interview with Shanice, a Black woman from Austin, July 8, 2022.

62. The focus group discussion was held on July 8, 2022, in Austin and included fifteen participants. Quotations from the discussion that follow are from participants, who were promised anonymity.

63. Interview with Shanice, July 8, 2022.

64. Interview with Marlin, July 8, 2022.

65. Interview with Marlin, July 8, 2022.

66. Interview with Shanice, July 8, 2022.

CHAPTER FIVE

1. Robinson, *Black Marxism*.

2. Interview with Rodrigo, May 18, 2021.

3. Interview with Rodrigo, April 19, 2022.

4. Interview with Rodrigo, May 18, 2021.

5. I quoted Rodrigo in chapter 3 when he discussed how the city of Austin, Texas, and certain regions of California provided housing to the undocumented to stop the spread of infection among those most vulnerable. I explained that the city council in Austin, Texas, paid six local hotels for rooms to house frontline workers who needed to quarantine in the early months of the pandemic (Flores, "Austin City Council"). The State of California secured hotel and motel rooms to house the homeless in the early months of the pandemic in order to protect them from widespread infections in communal spaces (Office of Governor Gavin Newsom, "Governor Newsom Visits").

6. Interview with Rodrigo, April 19, 2022.

7. Wacquant, *Punishing the Poor*.

8. Marx, *Capital*, 257.

9. Robinson, *Black Marxism*, 2.

10. Lowe, *Intimacies*; Clarno, *Neoliberal Apartheid*; Pulido, "Geographies of Race"; Danewid, "Fire This Time."

11. Melamed, "Racial Capitalism," 77.

12. Gilmore, *Golden Gulag*; Danewid, "Fire This Time"; Keegan, "Essential Agriculture."

13. Golash-Boza, *Deported*.

14. Golash-Boza, *Deported*; Amezcua, *Making Mexican Chicago*.

15. On necropolises, see Pulido, "Flint."

16. Olayo-Méndez et al., "Essential, Disposable, and Excluded."

17. Keegan, "Essential Agriculture."

18. Keegan, "Essential Agriculture."

19. Carrillo and Ipsen, "Worksites as Sacrifice Zones."

20. Carrillo and Ipsen, "Worksites as Sacrifice Zones."

21. Marx, *Capital*, 693.

22. Marx, *Capital*, 785.

23. Decoteau, *Ancestors and Antiretrovirals*; Hong, *Death beyond Disavowal*.

24. Olayo-Méndez et al., "Essential, Disposable, and Excluded."

25. In figures 5.1 and 5.2, unemployment rates were calculated using the Basic Monthly Current Population Survey, a survey on labor force participation that is co-sponsored by the US Census Bureau and the US Bureau of Labor Statistics. Monthly samples were pooled into annual estimates. These data were calculated by Chris Poulos.

26. Interview with Lorenzo, March 30, 2021.

27. Figure 5.3 reports on Household Pulse Survey data. See endnote 130 on page 226 for a description of the HPS, and how its data were pooled and analyzed by Chris Poulos.

28. United States Census Bureau, "Household Pulse Survey Data Tables."

29. Figure 5.4 reports on Household Pulse Survey data. It was only in April 2021 when the Household Pulse Survey began asking childcare disruption questions. Likely, during 2020–21, when public schools in Chicago were closed, parents struggled in similar ways to meet childcare needs. The data for figure 5.4 were assembled by Chris Poulos.

30. United States Census Bureau, "Household Pulse Survey Data Tables."

31. Rho et al., "Workers in Frontline Industries."

32. Rho et al., "Workers in Frontline Industries."

33. Decoteau et al., *Deadly Disparities*, 102. Iván Arenas created figure 5.5, and the data were pooled by Chris Poulos. A minimal percentage of respondents indicated "Other" as their racial category, which is why the percentages for each column do not quite total 100. The Brookings Institution found in 2020 that *nationally* frontline workers tended to be less educated and earn lower wages compared with all US workers, regardless of their race or ethnicity. Latinx and Black Americans constituted 33.8 percent of all frontline workers, but 61.1 percent were white, and 5.1 percent were Asian. Black and Latinx workers were concentrated in truck operation, slaughterhouses and meatpacking, nursing care, and corrections. See Tomer and Kane, "Protect Frontline Workers." Asian workers were concentrated in health care and nursing care. See Guevarra, "Frontline Filipinx/a/os Health Care Workers"; Kinder and Ford, "Black Essential Workers' Lives Matter."

34. Henricks et al., *Three Cities*.

35. Ross, Bateman, and Friedhoff, "Low-Wage Workforce." As of 2022, in the Chicago Metropolitan Area (CMA), 16 percent of the population is Black and 23 percent is Latinx; therefore, a disproportionate number of Black and Latinx residents of the CMA are lower-income workers. For demographics on the CMA, see Census Reporter, "Chicago Metro Area."

36. University of Chicago Urban Labs Poverty Lab, *COVID-19: Most At-Risk Workers*.

37. Chicago Metropolitan Agency for Planning, "Chicago's Essential Workers."

38. Rosenfeld and Tienda, "Mexican Immigration."

39. Illiois.gov, "Pritzker Announces Stay at Home Order"; Pritzker, *Executive Order*.

40. Interview with FQHC provider in Latinx neighborhood, March 8, 2021.

41. Interview with Gabriela, March 8, 2021.

42. Illiois.gov, "Pritzker Announces Restore Illinois."

43. Byrne and Pearson, "Chicago Will Join."

44. Interview with Gabriela, March 8, 2021.

45. Interview with Ana, January 27, 2022.

46. Ramirez-Rosa et al., "Mayor Prioritizing the Wealthy."

47. Whoriskey, Stein, and Jones, "Thousands of OSHA Complaints."

48. Kinder and Ford, "Black Essential Workers' Lives Matter."

49. University of Chicago Urban Labs Poverty Lab, *COVID-19: Most At-Risk Workers*; Asfaw, "Disparities in Teleworking."

50. Interview with Kim, a Filipina American woman from Albany Park, March 5, 2021.

51. Interview with Kelly, January 26, 2021.

52. Interview with Sholanda, January 28, 2022.

53. St. Clair, Mahr, and Schencker, "'This Is the Norm.'"

54. Interview with Sara, a Pakistani American woman from Albany Park, February 24, 2021.

55. Interview with Sara, January 7, 2022.

56. Interview with Sara, January 7, 2022.

57. Interview with Cheryl, a Black woman from Austin, November 25, 2020.

58. Interview with Gabriela, March 8, 2021.

59. Interview with Miguel, March 8, 2022.

60. Interview with Luis, November 17, 2021.

61. Interview with Tomás, October 17, 2020.

62. Interview with Tomás, October 17, 2020.

63. Interview with Tomás, October 29, 2021.

64. Interview with Maria, an undocumented Mexican woman from Little Village, November 30, 2021. This interview was conducted in Spanish by Cindy Brito and later translated.

65. Interview with Rodrigo, April 19, 2022.

66. Interview with Luis, November 17, 2021.

67. Interview with Luis, November 17, 2021.

68. Interview with Luis, November 17, 2021.

69. Duncan and Horton, "Immigrant Health."

70. On the policy retraction by the Biden administration, see Garrity, "DHS Unwinds Trump-Era Rule." On immigrants' fear of being exposed to immigration enforcement while using Medicaid, see Duncan and Horton, "Immigrant Health." For further information on how local, state and federal policies penalize immigrants who use public assistance, leading to poor health outcomes, see Van Natta et al., "Stratified Citizenship."

71. United States Census Bureau, "Report on Health Insurance."

72. Interview with Luis, November 17, 2021.

73. López-Cevallo, "Why COVID-19 Disproportionately Impacts Latino Communities."

74. Carrillo and Ipsen, "Worksites as Sacrifice Zones," 734.

75. On the invisibility of "doubling up," see Latino Policy Forum, *Long-Term Socioeconomic Consequences of COVID*.

76. Interview with Camila, Little Village, November 23, 2021.

77. Interview with Camila, November 23, 2021.

78. Interview with Camila, November 23, 2021.

79. Interview with Camila, November 23, 2021.

80. Interview with Camila, November 23, 2021.

81. Loustaunau et al., "Dimensions of Precarity."

82. Interview with Shantal, March 2, 2022.

83. Interview with Candice, February 22, 2022.

84. Interview with Candice, February 22, 2022.

85. Interview with Sholanda, January 28, 2022.

86. Interview with Dolores, February 1, 2022.

87. Interview with Isa, a Filipina American woman from Albany Park, February 27, 2021. "CDC's guidelines" refers to the official guidelines issued by the US Centers for Disease Control and Prevention.

88. Office of the Mayor, "City Announces Vaccine Requirements."

89. Interview with Sara, January 7, 2022.

90. Pulido, "Flint," 1.

91. Interview with Linda, a Black woman from Austin, January 26, 2021.

92. Interview with Linda, January 26, 2021.

93. Interview with Linda, January 26, 2021.

CHAPTER SIX

1. On racially marginalized populations' broad sentiments of distrust, see S. Smith, "Race and Trust"; Wilkes, "Re-thinking the Decline in Trust." On their distrust of the state, see Koch, "Racial Minorities' Trust." On their distrust of the medical establishment, see Benjamin, "Race for Cures"; Vargas, *Uninsured in Chicago*.

2. Notable exceptions include Freimuth et al., "Determinants of Trust"; Decoteau and Sweet, "Vaccine Hesitancy." *Vaccine hesitancy* refers to the broad array of context-specific doubts and concerns people may have about vaccines, despite their availability (Yaqub et al., "Attitudes to Vaccination").

3. There are numerous examples of this trend, but a few examples include Frenkel, "Communities Grapple with Vaccine Misinformation"; Kelley and Stone, "Anti-Vaccine Film"; Loomba et al., "Impact of Vaccine Misinformation"; Pertwee, Simas, and Larson, "Epidemic of Uncertainty."

4. In an article exploring vaccine distrust among Somali refugees, another racially marginalized group in the US, I also found that concerns about vaccines do not always lead to vaccine refusal (Decoteau and Sweet, "Vaccine Hesitancy").

5. Ndugga et al., "Vaccinations by Race/Ethnicity."

6. Figure 6.1 was created using the city of Chicago's COVID-19 dashboard on October 17, 2022. The data are not weighted for population. This means that the low daily vaccinations for Asian residents of Chicago are attributable to their relatively small share of the city's population compared with Black, Latinx, or white residents. Cal Garrett assembled the data.

7. City of Chicago, "COVID-19 Dashboard." These data were gathered on March 23, 2023.

8. For the first booster, the daily average number of booster doses given to white residents peaked at over 4,400 in December 2021 but had averaged over 3,000 doses per day since the end of October. Meanwhile, the average daily booster doses received by Latinx residents peaked at just over 2,700 in December 2021, and the peak for Black residents was just over 2,000 average doses per day in that same month. For the second booster, which became available in September 2022, the racial disparities in vaccination rates were even more pronounced. For approximately two months, from September to

November, the average daily number of boosters going to white residents never dipped
below 2,000 doses. Meanwhile, the daily average doses for Black residents peaked at
just over 1,200 in October and at just under 1,200 for Latinx residents at that same time
(City of Chicago, "COVID-19 Dashboard," retrieved March 23, 2023).

9. Padamsee et al., "Changes in COVID-19 Vaccine Hesitancy."

10. Padamsee et al., "Changes in COVID-19 Vaccine Hesitancy."

11. LaFraniere and Weiland, "End Public Health Emergency."

12. Benjamin, "Organized Ambivalence." Literature on vaccine distrust among white
groups in the US focuses on the link between conservative ideologies, distrust of public
health advice, and vaccine or mask noncompliance. See Shepherd, MacKendrick, and
Mora, "Pandemic Politics"; Latkin et al., "Trust: Socio-Ecological Perspective."

13. Latkin et al., "Trust: Socio-Ecological Perspective"; Butler et al., "COVID-19 Vaccination Readiness"; Nah et al., "Social Media Use."

14. Urena, "Relational Risk"; Sweet, *Politics of Surviving*; Kaye, *Enforcing Freedom*.

15. Tuskegee refers to an experiment that ran from 1932 to 1972, conducted by the
US Public Health Service, wherein six hundred Black men were recruited to study the
long-term effects of untreated syphilis. When penicillin became readily available as a
treatment for syphilis, it was withheld from the men in the study, who believed they
were receiving treatment. My respondents often understand the Tuskegee experiment
as a case in which the government knowingly infected men with syphilis, rather than
that the government failed to treat their already existing syphilis.

16. Interview with Bernice, October 22, 2020.

17. Interview with Alicia, a Black woman from Austin, December 2, 2020.

18. Interview with Shantal, February 3, 2022.

19. Interview with Phyllis, February 18, 2022.

20. Interview with Dolores, February 1, 2022.

21. Interview with Dolores, February 1, 2022.

22. Vargas, *Uninsured in Chicago*.

23. Interview with Reginald, February 25, 2022.

24. J. Moore et al., "Correlates of COVID-19 Vaccine Hesitancy."

25. Hamel et al., "COVID-19 Vaccine Monitor."

26. Interview with community organizer from a predominantly Black neighborhood
in Chicago, October 15, 2021.

27. Interview with Monique, October 23, 2020.

28. Interview with Adela, a Mexican American woman from Little Village, January
13, 2022.

29. Interview with Phyllis, February 18, 2022.

30. Latkin et al., "Trust: Socio-Ecological Perspective"; Butler et al., "COVID-19
Vaccination Readiness."

31. Interview with Deion, a Black man from Austin, October 13, 2020.

32. Interview with Maria, November 30, 2021.

33. Interview with Maria, November 30, 2021.

34. Interview with health ambassador from Austin, July 8, 2022.

35. Urena, "Relational Risk."

36. Interview with Rodrigo, April 19, 2022.

37. Interview with community organizer from Auburn Gresham, October 25, 2021.

38. Collins et al., "Male Fertility."

39. Interview with community organizer from Little Village, October 25, 2021.

40. Regarding lack of evidence for testicular swelling, see Collins et al., "Male Fertility." Regarding disruptions to menstruation, see Wong et al., "Menstrual Irregularities."

41. Interview with Auburn Gresham community organizer, October 25, 2021.

42. Interview with community organizer from Austin, December 13, 2021.

43. Interview with Rodrigo, May18, 2021.

44. Armstrong, "Cause of Death."

45. Interview with Marlin, December 13, 2021.

46. Interview with Shanice, July 8, 2022.

47. Naloxone is a treatment for opioid overdose, given in an emergency.

48. Interview with Marlin, December 13, 2021.

49. Interview with Shanice, July 8, 2022.

50. Focus group discussion with Destiny, a Black woman from Austin, July 8, 2022.

51. Focus group discussion with Jamilah, a Black woman from Austin, July 8, 2022.

52. Focus group discussion with Tanisha, a Black woman from Austin, July 8, 2022.

53. Decoteau, *Western Disease*.

54. Interview with Marlin, December 13, 2021. PubMed is a vast online repository of biomedical literature maintained by the National Institutes of Health National Library of Medicine.

55. Focus group discussion with Jamilah, July 8, 2022.

56. Interview with Marlin, July 8, 2022.

57. Interview with Shanice, July 8, 2022.

58. Focus group discussion with Tanisha, July 8, 2022.

59. Interview with Marlin, April 21, 2021.

60. Marlin kept naloxone (the generic name for opioid overdose treatment), or Narcan (the first name-brand widely available), in his office for this purpose.

61. Interview with Marlin, December 13, 2021.

CODA

1. A. White, *Epidemic Orientalism*.

2. Villarosa, *Under the Skin*, 163.

3. Decoteau, "Specter of AIDS."

4. Decoteau and Garrett, "Disease Surveillance Infrastructure."

5. Cubanski et al., "Declarations End"; Stolberg and Weiland, "Covid Emergency Ends."

6. In Illinois, 47,625 Illinois residents lost Medicaid coverage in May 2023. Most were still eligible but had to go through the bureaucratic hassle of renewing their applications. Residents of other states were not so lucky. Conservative states that did not expand Medicaid coverage after the passage of the Affordable Care Act rolled back Medicaid coverage for the poor. As of August 2023, 3.8 million people across the nation had lost their Medicaid coverage when the COVID-19 health emergency was terminated. See Schencker, "Residents Lose Medicaid."

7. Fadulu, "New York to Drop Requirement."

8. *New York Times*, "Track Covid-19."

9. Stolberg and Weiland, "Covid Emergency Ends"; Centers for Disease Control and Prevention, "COVID Data Tracker."

10. Centers for Disease Control and Prevention, "One in Five Have 'Long COVID.'"

11. Martinchek et al., *Food Insecurity Increased*; Casselman and DePillis, "Poverty Rate Soared."

12. Thrasher, *Viral Underclass.*

13. Interview with Kelly, October 29, 2021.

14. Sewell, *Logics of History*, 250–51.

15. Roy, "Pandemic Is a Portal."

16. Desmond, "Disgraced Class."

17. Parolin, *Poverty in the Pandemic*, 16.

18. Desmond, "Disgraced Class."

19. Casselman and DePillis, "Poverty Rate Soared."

20. Interview with Kelly, October 29, 2021. Emphasis added.

21. Sontag, *Illness as Metaphor.*

22. Interview with Annie, January 7, 2022.

23. The US Congress failed to pass a bipartisan bill to establish a National Covid Commission to analyze the US policy response to the pandemic and make recommendations for preparing for future outbreaks (Bergen, "Unnecessary Price").

24. Elliott, "Lightfoot's Resounding Loss."

25. Bosman and Smith, "Lightfoot Loses Bid for Re-election"; Weinberg, "Chicago Voters."

26. Elliott, "Lightfoot's Resounding Loss."

27. Charles Mills, *Racial Contract*, 18.

28. On "officially sanctioned" reality, see Charles Mills, *Racial Contract.*

29. Agamben, *Homo Sacer*; Decoteau, *Ancestors and Antiretrovirals.*

30. Nash, *Birthing Black Mothers.*

APPENDIX B

1. We ended up not using video platforms for resident interviews because so few people had access to Zoom. All resident interviews were conducted by phone, and expert interviews were conducted on Zoom.

2. Pritzker, *Executive Order.*

REFERENCES

Aaron, Henry J. "The Social Safety Net: The Gaps the COVID-19 Spotlights." Brookings Institution. June 23, 2020. https://www.brookings.edu/articles/the-social-safety-net-the-gaps-that-covid-19-spotlights/.

Adams, Vincanne, ed. *Metrics: What Counts in Global Health*. Durham, NC: Duke University Press, 2016.

Agamben, Giorgio. *Homo Sacer: Sovereign Power and Bare Life*. Translated by Daniel Heller-Roazen. Stanford, CA: Stanford University Press, 1998.

Amezcua, Mike. *Making Mexican Chicago: From Postwar Settlement to the Age of Gentrification*. Chicago: University of Chicago Press, 2022.

Anand, Nikhil, Akhil Gupta, and Hannah Appel, eds. *The Promise of Infrastructure*. Durham, NC: Duke University Press, 2018.

Anderson, Ben. "Emergency Futures: Exception, Urgency, Interval and Hope." *Sociological Review* 65, no. 3 (2017): 463–77.

Anderson, Ben. "Governing Emergencies: The Politics of Delay and the Logic of Response." *Transactions of the Institute of British Geographers*, no. 41 (2016): 14–26.

Anderson, Ben, Kevin Grove, Lauren Rickards, and Matthew Kearnes. "Slow Emergencies: Temporality and the Racialized Biopolitics of Emergency Governance." *Progress in Human Geography* 44, no. 4 (2020): 621–39.

Ansell, David. *County: Life, Death and Politics at Chicago's Public Hospital*. Chicago: Academy Chicago Publishers, 2013.

Ansell, David. *The Death Gap: How Inequality Kills*. Chicago: University of Chicago Press, 2017.

Armstrong, David. "The COVID-19 Pandemic and Cause of Death." *Sociology of Health and Illness*, no. 43 (2021): 1614–26.

Artiga, Samantha, and Martha Diaz. "Health Coverage and Care of Undocumented Immigrants." KFF (Kaiser Family Foundation). July 15, 2019. https://www.kff.org/racial-equity-and-health-policy/issue-brief/health-coverage-and-care-of-undocumented-immigrants/.

Asfaw, Abay. "Racial and Ethnic Disparities in Teleworking Due to the COVID-19 Pandemic in the United States: A Mediation Analysis." *International Journal of Environmental Research and Public Health* 19, no. 8 (2022): 4680.

Attwood, James, and Isis Almeida. "US Sees First Food-Worker Deaths." *Bloomberg*, April 7, 2020. https://www.bloomberg.com/news/articles/2020-04-08/pence-tells-u-s-food-workers-to-do-your-job-as-some-fall-ill#xj4y7vzkg.

Austin Coming Together. "History of Austin." Accessed December 15, 2022. https://austincomingtogether.org/history/.

Auyero, Javier. *Patients of the State: The Politics of Waiting in Argentina*. Durham, NC: Duke University Press, 2012.

Bailey, Zinzi D., Nancy Krieger, Madina Agénor, Jasmine Graves, Natalia Linos, and Mary T. Bassett. "Structural Racism and Health Inequities in the USA: Evidence and Interventions." *Lancet*, no. 389 (2017): 1453–63.

Bayne, Martha, and Jason Schumer. "What Happened May 30?" *Southside Weekly*, June 11, 2020. https://protesttimeline.southsideweekly.com.

Bechteler, S., and K. Kane-Willis. *An Epidemic of Inequities: Structural Racism and COVID-19 in the Black Community*. With Kareem Butler and Iliana Espinoza-Ravi. Chicago: Chicago Urban League, May 12, 2020. https://chiul.org/wp-content/uploads/2020/05/ChicagoUrbanLeague_An-Epidemic-of-Inequities_5-12-20.pdf.

Benjamin, Ruha. "Catching Our Breath: Critical Race STS and the Carceral Imagination." *Engaging Science, Technology and Society*, no. 2 (2016): 145–56.

Benjamin, Ruha. "Organized Ambivalence: When Sickle Cell Disease and Stem Cell Research Converge." *Ethnicity & Health* 16, no. 4–5 (2011): 447–63.

Benjamin, Ruha. *Race after Technology: Abolitionist Tools for the New Jim Code*. New York: Polity Press, 2019.

Benjamin, Ruha. "Race for Cures: Rethinking the Racial Logics of 'Trust' in Biomedicine." *Sociology Compass* 8, no. 6 (2014): 755–69.

Bergen, Peter. "Opinion: The Unnecessary Price of COVID-19." CNN. April 24, 2023. https://www.cnn.com/2023/04/24/opinions/covid-unnecessary-price-bergen/index.html.

Berlant, Lauren. *Cruel Optimism*. Durham, NC: Duke University Press, 2011.

Berlant, Lauren. "Slow Death: Sovereignty, Obesity, Lateral Agency." *Critical Inquiry*, no. 33 (2007): 754–80.

Betancur, John, Teresa Cordova, and Maria de los Angeles Torres. "Economic Restructuring and the Process of Incorporation of Latinos into the Chicago Economy." In *Latinos in a Changing US Economy: Comparative Perspectives on Growing Inequality*, edited by Rebecca Morales and Frank Bonilla, 109–32. New York: Sage, 1993.

Biden, Joe. "The Pandemic Is Over." Interview on *60 Minutes*, September 19, 2022. https://www.cbsnews.com/video/president-biden-the-pandemic-is-over-60-minutes/.

Bitler, Marianne P., Hilary W. Hoynes, and Diane Whitmore Schanzenbach. "Suffering, the Safety Net, and Disparities During COVID-19." *RSF: The Russell Sage Foundation Journal of the Social Sciences* 9, no. 3 (2023): 32–59.

Black, Curtis. "It's Time to Reopen Chicago's Closed Mental Health Clinics." *Chicago Reporter*, May 9, 2019. https://www.chicagoreporter.com/its-time-to-reopen-chicagos-closed-mental-health-clinics/.

Blake, John. "There's Nothing More Frightening in America Today Than an Angry White Man." CNN. Updated November 21, 2021. https://www.cnn.com/2021/11/20/us/angry-white-men-trials-blake-cec/index.html.

Board of Governors of the Federal Reserve System. *Report on the Economic Well-Being of US Households in 2020*. Washington, DC: Federal Reserve Board, May 2021. Accessed https://www.federalreserve.gov/publications/files/2020-report-economic-well-being-us-households-202105.pdf.

Bonilla, Yarimar. "The Coloniality of Disaster: Race, Empire, and the Temporal Logics of Emergency in Puerto Rico, USA." *Political Geography*, no. 78 (2020): 1–12.

Bonilla-Silva, Eduardo. *Racism without Racists: Color-Blind Racism and the Persistence of Inequality in America.* 5th ed. Lanham, MD: Rowman and Littlefield, 2017.

Bosman, Julie, and Mitch Smith. "Mayor Lori Lightfoot of Chicago Loses Her Bid for Reelection." *New York Times*, February 28, 2023. https://www.nytimes.com/2023/02/28/us/chicago-mayoral-election-lightfoot-vallas.html.

Bouie, Jamelle. "What We Have Unleashed." *Slate*, June 1, 2017. https://slate.com/news-and-politics/2017/06/this-years-string-of-brutal-hate-crimes-is-intrinsically-connected-to-the-rise-of-trump.html.

Bourdieu, Pierre. *Pascalian Meditations.* Stanford, CA: Stanford University Press, 2000.

Bourdieu, Pierre. "Rethinking the State: Genesis and Structure of the Bureaucratic Field." Translated by Loïc Wacquant and Samar Farage. In *State/Culture: State-Formation after the Cultural Turn*, edited by George Steinmetz, 53–75. Ithaca, NY: Cornell University Press, 1999.

Braudel, Fernand. "Histoire et sciences sociales: La longue durée." *Annales: Économies, Sociétés, Civilisations* 13 (1958): 725–53.

Broder, Tanya, and Gabrielle Lessard. "Overview of Immigrant Eligibility for Federal Programs." National Immigration Law Center, October 2023. https://www.nilc.org/issues/economic-support/overview-immeligfedprograms/#_ftn1.

Butler, Jonathan, Mariam Carson, Francine Rios-Fetchko, Roberto Vargas, Abby Cabrera, Angela Gallegos-Castillo, Monique LeSarre, Michael Liao, Kent Woo, Randi Ellis, Kirsten Lui, Arun Burra, Mario Ramirez, Brittney Doyle, Lydia Leung, Alicia Fernandez, and Kevin Grumbach. "COVID-19 Vaccination Readiness among Multiple Racial and Ethnic Groups in the San Francisco Bay Area: A Qualitative Analysis." *PLOS ONE* 17, no 5 (2022): e0266397. https://doi.org/10.1371/journal.pone.0266397.

Byrne, John. "Activists Hammer Mayor Lori Lightfoot for Spending $281.5 Million in Federal COVID-19 Money on Chicago Police Payroll." *Chicago Tribune*, February 18, 2021. https://www.chicagotribune.com/politics/ct-chicago-lightfoot-covid-19-police-spending-reaction-20210218-lhieyxoz3zgcjdl6g37aknfzem-story.html.

Byrne, John, and Rick Pearson. "Chicago Will Join Rest of Illinois in Advancing to Next Phase in Coronavirus Reopening on Friday." *Chicago Tribune*, June 22, 2020. https://www.chicagotribune.com/coronavirus/ct-chicago-coronavirus-lori-lightfoot-phase-four-opening-rules-20200622-3jkjdonsc5etlisgtdzr3xw3zi-story.html.

Camarillo, Emmanual. "Opioid Deaths in Chicago on Pace to Reach Similar Levels as Record-Setting 2021." *Chicago Sun-Times*, November 15, 2022. https://chicago.suntimes.com/2022/11/15/23461285/opioid-deaths-chicago-drug-overdoses-record-pace.

Carmichael, Stokely, and Charles V. Hamilton. *Black Power: The Politics of Liberation in America.* New York: Vintage Books, 1967.

Carse, Ashley. "Keyword: Infrastructure; How a Humble French Engineering Term Shaped the Modern World." In *Infrastructure and Social Complexity: A Companion*, edited by Penny Harvey, Casper Bruun Jensen, and Atsuro Morita, 27–39. London: Routledge, 2016.

Carrillo, Ian R., and Annabel Ipsen. "Worksites as Sacrifice Zones: Structural Precarity and COVID-19 in US Meatpacking." *Sociological Perspectives* 64, no. 5 (2021): 726–46.

Casselman, Ben, and Lydia DePillis. "Poverty Rate Soared in 2022 as Aid Ended and Prices Rose." *New York Times*, September 12, 2023. https://www.nytimes.com/2023/09/12/business/economy/income-poverty-health-insurance.html.

Census Reporter. "Chicago-Naperville-Elgin, IL-IN-WI Metro Area." US Census Bureau. Accessed January 22, 2024. https://censusreporter.org/profiles/ 31000US16980-chicago-naperville-elgin-il-in-wi-metro-area/.

Centers for Disease Control and Prevention. "COVID Data Tracker." February 16, 2024. https://covid.cdc.gov/covid-data-tracker/#datatracker-home.

Centers for Disease Control and Prevention. "Nearly One in Five American Adults Who Have Had COVID-19 Still Have 'Long COVID.'" June 22, 2022. https://www.cdc.gov/ nchs/pressroom/nchs_press_releases/2022/20220622.htm.

Chase, Brett. "With No State Help Forthcoming, 4 South Side Hospitals Call Off Merger, Predict Service Cuts." *Chicago Sun-Times*, May 26, 2020. https:// chicago.suntimes.com/2020/5/26/21271216/hospitals-merger-advocate -trinity-mercy-south-shore-st-bernard-health.

Cherone, Heather. "Chicago Police Botched Response to Protests, Unrest after George Floyd's Death: Watchdog." WTTW. February 18, 2021. https://news.wttw.com/ 2021/02/18/chicago-police-botched-response-protests-unrest-after-george-floyd -s-death-watchdog.

Cherone, Heather. "Chicago to Boost Mental Health Spending by $1.2 M to Help Those Struggling during the Pandemic." WTTW. May 21, 2020. https://news .wttw.com/2020/05/21/chicago-boost-mental-health-spending-12m-help-those -struggling-during-pandemic.

Cherone, Heather. "67% of Chicagoans Vaccinated Are White, Asian: City Data." WTTW. January 25, 2021. https://news.wttw.com/2021/01/25/67 -chicagoans-vaccinated-are-white-asian-city-data.

Cherone, Heather. "Use Half of Federal Relief Package to Cancel 'Scoop-and-Toss' Borrowing, Chief Financial Officer Urges." WTTW. April 14, 2021. https://news .wttw.com/2021/04/14/use-half-federal-relief-package-cancel-scoop-and-toss -borrowing-chief-financial-officer.

Chicago Department of Public Health (CDPH). *Mental Health Services Report.* Chicago: CDPH, June 2014. https://www.chicago.gov/content/dam/city/depts/cdph/clinical _care_and_more/CDPH_MHRepJun112014.pdf.

Chicago for the People. *Building Bridges and Growing the Soul of Chicago: A Blueprint for Creating a More Just and Vibrant City for All.* Transition Team Report to Mayor Brandon Johnson. July 2023. https://www.chicago.gov/content/dam/city/depts/ mayor/TransitionReport/TransitionReport.07.2023.pdf.

Chicago Health Atlas. "Chicago Health Atlas: Access Health Data for Chicago and Your Community." Accessed July 28 and 31, 2023. https://chicagohealthatlas.org/.

Chicago Housing Authority. "Housing Choice Voucher (HCV) Program." Accessed November 14, 2023. https://www.thecha.org/residents/housing -choice-voucher-hcv-program.

Chicago Housing Authority. "Project Based Voucher." Accessed November 14, 2023. https://www.thecha.org/landlords/project-based-voucher.

Chicago Metropolitan Agency for Planning (CMAP). "Metropolitan Chicago's Essential Workers Disproportionately Low-Income, People of Color." April 24, 2020. https:// www.cmap.illinois.gov/updates/all/-/asset_publisher/UIMfSLnFfMB6/content/ metropolitan-chicago-s-essential-workers-disproportionately-low-income-people -of-color.

Chowkwanyun, Merlin, and Adolph Reed. "Racial Health Disparities and COVID-19— Caution and Context." *New England Journal of Medicine* 383, no. 3 (2020): 201–3.

City of Chicago. "COVID-19 Dashboard." Accessed October 17, 2022. https://www
.chicago.gov/city/en/sites/covid-19/home/covid-dashboard.html.

City of Chicago. "COVID-19 Vaccine Coverage by Geography." Accessed July 18, 2023.
https://www.chicago.gov/city/en/sites/covid-19/home/covid-dashboard/covid19
-vaccine-coverage-geography.html.

Civic Federation. "City Continues 'Scoop and Toss Borrowing' to Balance the Budget."
Civic Federation Blog, November 5, 2014. https://www.civicfed.org/civic-federation/
blog/city-continues-scoop-toss-borrowing-balance-budget.

Clarno, Andy. *Neoliberal Apartheid: Palestine/Israel and South Africa after 1994*. Chicago:
University of Chicago Press, 2017.

Clarno, Andy. "Policing COVID in Chicago, Expert Commentary." In Decoteau et al.,
Deadly Disparities in the Days of COVID-19, 61–63.

Colgrove, James. *Epidemic City: The Politics of Public Health in New York*. New York:
Russell Sage Foundation, 2011.

Colgrove, James, Gerald Markowitz, and David Rosner, eds. *The Contested Boundaries of American Public Health*. New Brunswick, NJ: Rutgers University Press, 2008.

Collaborative for Community Wellness. *Mental Health Service Access in Chicago:
Findings from a City-Wide Survey*. Chicago: Center for Community Wellness,
2021. https://www.collaborativeforcommunitywellness.org/_files/ugd/c29cfd
_62f4f9e5c33943d298b00687d980bbb3.pdf.

Collaborative for Community Wellness. *Uplifting Voices to Create New
Alternatives: Documenting the Mental Health Crisis for Adults on Chicago's Southwest Side*. Chicago: Saint Anthony Hospital–Center for Community Wellness,
2018. https://www.collaborativeforcommunitywellness.org/_files/ugd/c29cfd
_542f04d11bf744c3a338ef3be8dbf6f6.pdf.

Collins, Alexander, Lei Zhao, Ziwen Zhu, Nathan Givens, Qian Bai, Mark Wakefield, and
Yujiang Fang. "Impact of COVID-19 on Male Fertility." *Urology* 164 (2022): 33–39.

Cook County Government. "Homicides Drop While Opioid Overdose Deaths Continue
to Break Records in Cook County: Medical Examiner's Office Releases Preliminary
2022 Data." January 3, 2023. https://www.cookcountyil.gov/news/homicides-drop
-while-opioid-overdose-deaths-continue-break-records-cook-county.

Corallo, Bradley, and Sophia Moreno. "Analysis of National Trends in Medicaid and
CHIP Enrollment during the 2019 COVID Pandemic." KFF (Kaiser Family Foundation). April 4, 2023. https://www.kff.org/coronavirus-covid-19/issue-brief/
analysis-of-recent-national-trends-in-medicaid-and-chip-enrollment/.

Cubanski, Juliette, Jennifer Kates, Jennifer Tolbert, Madeline Guth, Karen Pollitz, and
Meredith Freed. "What Happens When COVID-19 Emergency Declarations End?
Implications for Coverage, Costs and Access." KFF (Kaiser Family Foundation).
Updated January 31, 2023. https://www.kff.org/coronavirus-covid-19/issue-brief/
what-happens-when-covid-19-emergency-declarations-end-implications-for
-coverage-costs-and-access/.

Danewid, Ida. "The Fire This Time: Grenfell, Racial Capitalism and the Urbanisation of
Empire." *European Journal of International Relations* 26, no. 1 (2020): 289–313.

Davis, Angelique M., and Rose Ernst. "Racial Spectacles: Promoting a Colorblind
Agenda through Direct Democracy." *Law, Politics and Society*, no. 55 (2011):
133–71.

Decoteau, Claire L. *Ancestors and Antiretrovirals: The Biopolitics of HIV/AIDS in
Post-Apartheid South Africa*. Chicago: University of Chicago Press, 2013.

Decoteau, Claire L. "Exclusionary Inclusion and the Normalization of Biomedical Culture." *American Journal of Cultural Sociology* 1, no. 3 (2013): 403–30.

Decoteau, Claire L. "The Specter of AIDS: Testimonial Activism in the Aftermath of the Epidemic." *Sociological Theory* 26, no. 3 (September 2008): 230–57.

Decoteau, Claire L. *The Western Disease: Contesting Autism in the Somali Diaspora.* Chicago: University of Chicago Press, 2021.

Decoteau, Claire L., and Cal L. Garrett. "Disease Surveillance Infrastructure and the Economisation of Public Health." *Sociology of Health and Illness* 44, no. 8 (2022): 1251–69.

Decoteau, Claire L., Cal L. Garrett, Cynthia Brito, Fructoso M. Basaldua Jr., and Iván Arenas. *Deadly Disparities in the Days of COVID-19: How Public Policy Fails Black and Latinx Chicagoans.* Chicago: Institute for Research on Race and Public Policy, 2021.

Decoteau, Claire L., AJ Golio, and Cal L. Garrett. "The Risks of Renting on the Margins: Housing Informality and State Legibility in the COVID-19 Pandemic." Unpublished manuscript, last modified April 29, 2024. Microsoft Word file.

Decoteau, Claire L., and Paige L. Sweet. "Vaccine Hesitancy and the Accumulation of Distrust." *Social Problems.* Published ahead of print, March 3, 2023. https://doi.org/10.1093/socpro/spad006.

Desmond, Matthew. "America is in a Disgraced Class of Its Own." *New York Times*, March 16, 2023. https://www.nytimes.com/2023/03/16/opinion/poverty-abolition-united-states.html.

Doussard, Marc, Jamie Peck, and Nik Theodore. "After Deindustrialization: Uneven Growth and Economic Inequality in 'Postindustrial' Chicago." *Economic Geography* 85, no. 2 (2009): 183–207.

Drake, St. Clair, and Horace Cayton. *Black Metropolis: A Study of Negro Life in a Northern City.* Chicago: University of Chicago Press, 1993.

DuBois, W. E. B. *Black Reconstruction in America, 1860–1880.* New York: Free Press, 1998.

Duncan, Whitney L., and Sarah B. Horton. "Serious Challenges and Potential Solutions for Immigrant Health During COVID-19." *Health Affairs*, April 18, 2020. https://www.healthaffairs.org/do/10.1377/hblog20200416.887086/full/.

Ehrenreich, John. *The Making of a Pandemic.* Berlin: Springer Nature, 2022.

Eldeib, Duaa, Adriana Gallardo, Akilah Johnson, Annie Waldman, Nina Martin, Talia Buford, and Tony Briscoe. "COVID-19 Took Black Lives First. It Didn't Have To." ProPublica Illinois, May 9, 2020. https://features.propublica.org/chicago-first-deaths/covid-coronavirus-took-black-lives-first/.

Eldeib, Duaa, and Melissa Sanchez. "Opioid Overdoses Keep Surging in Chicago, Killing Black People on the West Side." ProPublica. July 14, 2020. https://www.propublica.org/article/opioid-overdoses-keep-surging-in-chicago-killing-black-people-on-the-west-side.

Elliott, Philip. "Lori Lightfoot's Resounding Loss in Chicago Holds Lessons for Democrats Everywhere." *Time*, March 1, 2023. https://time.com/6259485/lori-lightfoot-loss-chicago-lessons-democrats/.

Espeland, Wendy N., and Mitchell L. Stevens. "A Sociology of Quantification." *European Journal of Sociology* 49, no. 3 (2008): 401–36.

Esposito, Stefano, and Brett Chase. "Mayor Touts 'Major Improvements' in Equitable Distribution of COVID-19 Vaccine as Positivity Rate Drops

to Lowest Level Ever." *Chicago Sun-Times*, February 19, 2021. https://chicago
.suntimes.com/coronavirus/2021/2/19/22291148/chicago-covid-19-vaccine
-racial-equity-improving-mayor-lightfoot-coronavirus.

Eubanks, Virginia. *Automating Inequality: How High-Tech Tools Profile, Police, and Punish the Poor*. New York: St. Martin's Press, 2017.

Ewing, Mike. "Memes of Mayor Lightfoot Enforcing Stay-at-Home Orders Bring Light to Dark Times." WGN, March 30, 2020. https://wgntv.com/news/memes-of-mayor-lightfoot-enforcing-stay-at-home-order-bring-light-to-dark-times/.

Faberman, Rhea, and Katiana Krawchenko. *The Impact of Chronic Underfunding on America's Public Health System: Trends, Risks, and Recommendations, 2022*. Washington, DC: Trust for America's Health, July 2022. https://www.tfah.org/wp-content/uploads/2022/07/2022PublicHealthFundingFINAL.pdf.

Fadulu, Lola. "New York State to Drop Requirement That Masks Be Worn in Hospitals." *New York Times*, February 10, 2023. https://www.nytimes.com/2023/02/10/nyregion/mask-mandate-hospitals-new-york.html.

Feagin, Joe, and Zinobia Bennefield. "Systemic Racism and U.S. Health Care." *Social Science & Medicine*, no. 103 (2014): 7–14.

Ferguson, Joseph, and Deborah Witzburg. *Report on Chicago's Response to George Floyd Protests and Unrest*. City of Chicago Office of Inspector General, February 18, 2021. https://igchicago.org/2021/02/18/report-on-chicagos-response-to-george-floyd-protests-and-unrest/.

Ferguson, Roderick A. *Aberrations in Black: Toward a Queer of Color Critique*. Minneapolis: University of Minnesota Press, 2004.

Fernández, Lilia. *Brown in the Windy City: Mexicans and Puerto Ricans in Postwar Chicago*. Chicago: University of Chicago Press, 2012.

Fishman, Elly. "How It Works: Chicago's City Council and the Mayor's Office." WBEZ Chicago. June 7, 2021. https://www.wbez.org/stories/how-it-works-chicagos-city-council-and-the-mayors-office/c9bb4591-ec03-422c-bb84-0a62f46c551c.

Flores, Christian. "Austin City Council Possibly Considering Converting Another Hotel into COVID-19 Shelter." CBS Austin (Texas). November 11, 2020. https://cbsaustin.com/news/local/austin-city-council-possibly-considering-converting-another-hotel-into-covid-19-shelter.

Flynn, Meagan. "'Those Numbers Take Your Breath Away.'" *Washington Post*, April 7, 2020. https://www.washingtonpost.com/nation/2020/04/07/chicago-racial-disparity-coronavirus/.

Foucault, Michel. "The Birth of Social Medicine." In *The Essential Foucault: Selections from the Essential Works of Foucault, 1954–1984*, rev. ed., edited and with an introduction by Paul Rabinow and Nikolas Rose, 319–37. New York: New Press, 2003.

Foucault, Michel. *Discipline and Punish: The Birth of the Prison*. Translated by Alan Sheridan. New York: Vintage Books, 1995.

Foucault, Michel. *History of Sexuality*. Vol. 1. Translated by Robert Hurley. New York: Vintage, 1990.

Foucault, Michel. *Power/Knowledge: Selected Interviews and other Writings, 1972–1977*. New York: Pantheon Books, 1980.

Foucault, Michel. *Security, Territory, Population: Lectures at the Collège de France, 1977–1978*. Translated by Graham Burchell. New York: Picador, 2007.

Foucault, Michel. *"Society Must be Defended": Lectures at the Collège de France, 1975–1976*. Translated by David Macey. New York: Picador, 2003.

Freimuth, Vicki S., Amelia Jamison, Ji An, Gregory Hancock, and Sandra C. Quinn. "Determinants of Trust in the Flu Vaccine for African Americans and Whites." *Social Science & Medicine* 193 (2017): 70–79.

Frenkel, Sheera. "Black and Hispanic Communities Grapple with Vaccine Misinformation." *New York Times*, updated September 29, 2021. https://www.nytimes .com/2021/03/10/technology/vaccine-misinformation.html.

Gaffney, Adam. "The Neoliberal Turn in American Health Care." *International Journal of Health Services* 45, no. 1 (2015): 33–52.

Gaffney, Adam, and Danny McCormick. "The Affordable Care Act: Implications for Health-Care Equity." *Lancet* 389, no. 10077 (2017): 1442–52.

Gamble, Vanessa N. "'There Wasn't a Lot of Comfort in Those Days': African Americans, Public Health and the 1918 Influenza Epidemic." *Public Health Reports* 125 (2010): 114–22.

Garrett, Cal L., and Claire L. Decoteau. "Data Citizenship: Quantifying Structural Racism in COVID-19 and Beyond." *Big Data & Society* 10, no. 2 (2023). https://doi .org/10.1177/20539517231213821.

Garrity, Kelly. "DHS Unwinds Trump-Era 'Public Charge' Rule for Immigrants." *Politico*. September 8, 2022. https://www.politico.com/news/2022/09/08/trump -public-charge-rule-immigrants-biden-00055505.

Geronimus, Arline T. "The Weathering Hypothesis and the Health of African-American Women and Infants: Evidence and Speculations." *Ethnicity and Disease* 2, no. 3 (1992): 207–21.

Gilmore, Ruth Wilson. *Golden Gulag: Prisons, Surplus, Crisis, and Opposition in Globalizing California*. Berkeley: University of California Press, 2007.

Giordano, Cristiana. *Migrants in Translation: Caring and the Logics of Difference in Contemporary Italy*. Berkeley: University of California Press, 2014.

Golash-Boza, Tanya Maria. *Deported: Immigrant Policing, Disposable Labor, and Global Capitalism*. New York: New York University Press, 2015.

Goldberg, David Theo. *The Racial State*. Hoboken, NJ: Blackwell, 2002.

Gowan, Teresa, and Sarah Whetstone. "Making the Criminal Addict: Subjectivity and Social Control in a Strong-Arm Rehab." *Punishment and Society* 14, no. 1 (2012): 69–93.

Grove, Kevin, Lauren Rickards, Ben Anderson, and Matthew Kearnes. "The Uneven Distribution of Futurity: Slow Emergencies and the Event of COVID-19." *Geographical Research* 60 (2022): 6–17.

Guevarra, Anna. "Frontline Filipinx/a/os Health Care Workers." In Decoteau et al., *Deadly Disparities in the Days of COVID-19*, 49–52.

Hamel, Liz, Lunna Lopes, Grace Sparks, Ashley Kirzinger, Audrey Kearnet, Mellisha Stokes, and Mollyann Brodie. "KFF COVID-19 Vaccine Monitor: September 2021." KFF (Kaiser Family Foundation). September 28, 2021. https://www.kff.org/ coronavirus-covid-19/poll-finding/kff-covid-19-vaccine-monitor-september-2021/.

Hammonds, Evelynn, and Susan Reverby. "Toward a Historically Informed Analysis of Racial Health Disparities." *American Journal of Public Health* 109, no. 10 (2019): 1348–49.

Hansen, Hans Krause. "Numerical Operations, Transparency Illusions and the Data-fication of Governance." *European Journal of Social Theory* 18, no. 2 (2015): 203–20.

Harell, Allison, and Evan Lieberman. "How Information about Race-Based Health Disparities Affects Policy Preferences: Evidence from a Survey Experiment about the COVID-19 Pandemic in the United States." *Social Science & Medicine* 277 (2021): 113884.

Haskins, Glencora, Joseph Parilla, and Julia Bauer. "As Local Governments Finalize their American Rescue Plan Priorities, Some Dollars Have Become Easier to Spend." Brookings Institution, April 17, 2023. https://www.brookings.edu/articles/as-local-governments-finalize-their-american-rescue-plan-priorities-some-dollars-have-become-easier-to-spend/.

Hatch, Anthony R. *Blood Sugar: Racial Pharmacology and Food Justice in Black America*. Minneapolis: University of Minnesota Press, 2016.

Hatch, Anthony R. "The Data Will Not Save Us: Afropessimism and Racial Antimatter in the COVID-19 Pandemic." *Big Data & Society* 9, no. 1 (2022): 20539517211067948.

Henricks, Kasey, Amanda E. Lewis, Iván Arenas, and Deana Lewis. *A Tale of Three Cities: State of Racial Justice in Chicago Report*. Chicago: Institute for Research on Race and Public Policy, 2017.

Hirsch, Arnold. *Making the Second Ghetto: Race and Housing in Chicago, 1940–1960*. Cambridge: Cambridge University Press, 1983.

Hong, Grace Kyungwon. *Death beyond Disavowal: The Impossible Politics of Difference*. Minneapolis: University of Minnesota Press, 2015.

Illinois Department of Healthcare and Family Services. "Health Benefits for Immigrant Adults." Accessed December 1, 2020. https://hfs.illinois.gov/medicalclients/coverageforimmigrantseniors/healthbenefitsforimmigrants.html.

Illinois Department of Human Services. "New Health Benefit Coverage for Immigrant Seniors." May 30, 2020. https://www.dhs.state.il.us/page.aspx?item=128154.

Illiois.gov. "Governor Pritzker Announces Restore Illinois: A Public Health Approach to Safely Reopen Our State." Press release, May 5, 2020. https://www.illinois.gov/news/press-release.21509.html.

Illiois.gov. "Gov. Pritzker Announces Statewide Stay at Home Order to Maximize COVID-19 Containment, Ensure Health Care System Remains Fully Operational." Press release, March 20, 2020. https://www.illinois.gov/news/press-release.21288.html.

Illinois Housing Development Authority. *Illinois Emergency Rental and Mortgage Assistance Fact Book*. Chicago: State of Illinois, 2021.

Illinois Housing Development Authority. *Illinois Rental Repayment Program: Round 1 Fact and Information Booklet*. Chicago: State of Illinois, 2021.

Institute for Housing Studies. "Policy Interventions to Respond to the Housing Impacts of COVID-19." *Institute for Housing Studies at DePaul University* (blog), June 5, 2020. https://www.housingstudies.org/blog/covid-policy-interventions/.

Institute for Housing Studies. "2021 State of Rental Housing in Cook County." DePaul University. September 30, 2021. https://www.housingstudies.org/releases/state-rental-2021/.

Institute of Medicine. *Unequal Treatment: Confronting Racial and Ethnic Disparities in Health Care*. Washington, DC: National Academies Press, 2003.

Institute of Medicine (US) Committee on the Changing Market, Managed Care, and the Future Viability of Safety Net Providers. *America's Health Care Safety Net: Intact but Endangered.* Washington, DC: National Academies Press, 2000.

James, Sherman. "John Henryism and the Health of African Americans." *Culture, Medicine and Psychiatry* 18 (1994): 163–82.

Johnson, Cedric. "The Triumph of Black Lives Matter and Neoliberal Redemption." *Nonsite,* June 9, 2020. https://nonsite.org/the-triumph-of-black-lives-matter-and-neoliberal-redemption/.

Joint Center for Housing Studies. *America's Rental Housing 2020.* Cambridge, MA: Harvard University, 2020. https://www.jchs.harvard.edu/sites/default/files/reports/files/Harvard_JCHS_Americas_Rental_Housing_2020.pdf.

Jones, Camara Phyllis. "Levels of Racism: A Theoretical Framework and a Gardener's Tale." *American Journal of Public Health* 90 (2000): 1212–15.

Kaye, Kerwin. *Enforcing Freedom: Drug Courts, Therapeutic Communities, and the Intimacies of the State.* New York: Columbia University Press, 2019.

Kaye, Kerwin. "Rehabilitating the 'Drugs Lifestyle': Criminal Justice, Social Control, and the Cultivation of Agency." *Ethnography* 14, no. 2 (2012): 207–32.

Keegan, Caroline. "Essential Agriculture, Sacrificial Labor, and the COVID-19 Pandemic in the US South." *Journal of Agrarian Change,* no. 23 (2022): 611–21.

Kelley, Mary L., and Will Stone. "An Anti-Vaccine Film Targeted to Black Americans Spreads Vaccine Misinformation." NPR. June 8, 2021. https://www.npr.org/transcripts/1004214189.

Kinder, Molly, and Tiffany Ford. "Black Essential Workers' Lives Matter. They Deserve Real Change, not Just Lip Service." Brookings Institution, June 24, 2020. https://www.brookings.edu/articles/black-essential-workers-lives-matter-they-deserve-real-change-not-just-lip-service/.

Kinder, Molly, Laura Stateler, and Julia Du. "The COVID-19 Hazard Continues, but the Hazard Pay Does Not." Brookings Institution, October 29, 2020. https://www.brookings.edu/articles/the-covid-19-hazard-continues-but-the-hazard-pay-does-not-why-americas-frontline-workers-need-a-raise/.

King County. *Homelessness Response: King County Revive & Thrive Recovery Plan 2022.* Seattle: King County, 2022. https://kingcounty.gov/~/media/depts/executive/performance-strategy-budget/budget/COVID-19/Homelessness-Response-2022-Recovery-Plan.ashx?la=en.

Klinenberg, Eric. *Heat Wave: A Social Autopsy of Disaster in Chicago.* 2nd ed. Chicago: University of Chicago Press, 2015.

Klinenberg, Eric. *Palaces for the People: How Social Infrastructure Can Help Fight Inequality, Polarization and the Decline of Civic Life.* New York: Broadway Books, 2018.

Koch, Jeffrey W. "Racial Minorities' Trust in Government and Government Decision-makers." *Social Science Quarterly* 100, no. 1 (2019): 19–37.

Kolata, Gina, and Roni Caryn Rabin. "'Don't Be Afraid of Covid,' Trump Says, Undermining Public Health Messages." *New York Times,* October 5, 2020. https://www.nytimes.com/2020/10/05/health/trump-covid-public-health.html.

Kotsko, Adam. "What Happened to Giorgio Agamben?" *Slate,* February 20, 2022. https://slate.com/human-interest/2022/02/giorgio-agamben-covid-holocaust-comparison-right-wing-protest.html.

Krause, Monika. *Model Cases: On Canonical Research Objects and Sites*. Chicago: University of Chicago Press, 2021.

Krieger, Nancy. "Discrimination and Health Inequities." *International Journal of Health Service*, no. 44 (2014): 643–710.

Krupar, Shiloh, and Nadine Ehlers. "Biofutures: Race and the Governance of Health." *Environment and Planning D: Society and Space* 35, no. 2 (2017): 222–40.

LaFraniere, Sharon. "'Very Harmful' Lack of Data Blunts US Response to Outbreaks." *New York Times*, September 20, 2022. https://www.nytimes.com/2022/09/20/us/politics/covid-data-outbreaks.html.

LaFraniere, Sharon, and Noah Weiland. "U.S. Plans to End Public Health Emergency for Covid in May." *New York Times*, January 30, 2023. https://www.nytimes.com/2023/01/30/us/politics/biden-covid-public-health-emergency.html.

Lakoff, Andrew. *Unprepared: Global Health in a Time of Emergency*. Berkeley: University of California Press, 2017.

Larkin, Brian. "The Politics and Poetics of Infrastructure." *Annual Review of Anthropology*, no. 42 (2013): 327–43.

Latino Policy Forum. *Long-Term Socioeconomic Consequences of COVID in the Latino Community: Creating a Path Forward*. Chicago: Latino Policy Forum, 2022. Published in collaboration with Illinois Unidos. With foreword by Brookings Institution. https://www.latinopolicyforum.org/publications/briefs/document/Long-Term-Socioeconomic-Consequences-of-COVID-in-the-Latino-Community-1.pdf.

Latkin, Carl A., Lauren Dayton, Grace Yi, Arianna Konstantopoulos, and Basmattee Boodram. "Trust in COVID-19 Vaccine in the US: A Socio-Ecological Perspective." *Social Science & Medicine* 270 (2021): 113684.

Levi, Jeffrey, Laura Segal, Rebecca Laurent, and Albert Lang. *Investing in America's Health: A State-by-State Look at Public Health Funding and Key Health Facts*. Princeton, NJ: Robert Wood Johnson, Trust for America's Health, 2013.

Local Community Fact Book: Chicago Metropolitan Area: Based on the 1970 and 1980 Censuses. Chicago: Chicago Review Press, 1984.

Local Community Fact Book: Chicago Metropolitan Area, 1990. Chicago: University of Illinois at Chicago, 1995.

Loomba, Sahil, Alexandre de Figueiredo, Simon J. Piatek, Kristen de Graaf, and Heidi J. Larson. "Measuring the Impact of COVID-19 Vaccine Misinformation on Vaccination Intent in the UK and USA." *Nature Human Behavior* 5 (2021): 337–48.

López-Cevallo, Daniel. "Why COVID-19 Disproportionately Impacts Latino Communities." Interview by Noel King. NPR. July 1, 2020. https://www.npr.org/2020/07/01/885878571/why-covid-19-disproportionately-impacts-latino-communities.

Loustaunau, Lola, Lina Stepick, Ellen Scott, Larissa Petruccim, and Miriam Henifin. "No Choice but to Be Essential: Expanding Dimensions of Precarity During COVID-19." *Sociological Perspectives* 64, no. 5 (2021): 857–75.

Lowe, Lisa. *The Intimacies of Four Continents*. Durham, NC: Duke University Press, 2015.

Lugalia-Hollon, Ryan, and Daniel Cooper. *The War on Neighborhoods: Policing, Prison and Punishment in a Divided City*. Boston: Beacon Press, 2018.

Lundy, Braun, Anne Fausto-Sterling, Duana Fullwiley, Evelynn M. Hammonds, Alondra Nelson, William Quivers, Susan M. Reverby, and Alexandra E. Shields.

"Racial Categories in Medical Practice: How Useful Are They?" *PLOS Medicine* 4, no. 9 (2007): 1423–28.

Malagón, Elvia. "Post-George Floyd Police Reforms in Chicago 'Disappointing,'" Community Leaders Say." *Chicago Sun-Times*, May 22, 2021. https://chicago .suntimes.com/politics/2021/5/22/22442122/protests-chicago-george-floyd -anniversary-police-reforms.

Mandavilli, Apoorva. "New Infectious Threats Are Coming: The U.S. Probably Won't Contain Them." *New York Times*, September 29, 2022. https://www.nytimes .com/2022/09/29/health/pandemic-preparedness-covid-monkeypox.html.

Marcelo, Philip. "Hospital COVID Payments Tied to Patient Treatment, Not Deaths." Associated Press (AP). March 9, 2023. https://apnews.com/article/ fact-check-covid-pandemic-hospitals-medicare-157398144949.

Markel, Howard, and Alexandra M. Stern. "The Foreignness of Germs: The Persistent Association of Immigrants with Disease in American Society." *Millbank Quarterly* 80, no. 4 (2002): 757–88.

Martinchek, Kassandra, Poonam Gupta, Michael Karpman, and Dulce Gonzalez. *As Inflation Squeezed Family Budgets, Food Insecurity Increased between 2021 and 2022: Findings from the Well-Being and Basic Needs Survey*. Washington, DC: Urban Institute, March 2023. https://www.urban.org/sites/default/files/2023-03/ As%20Inflation%20Squeezed%20Family%20Budgets%20Food%20Insecurity %20Increased%20between%202021%20and%202022.pdf.

Martinez-Hume, Anna C., Allison M. Baker, Hannah S. Bell, Isabel Montemayor, Kristan Elwell, and Linda M. Hunt. "'They Treat You a Different Way': Public Insurance, Stigma, and the Challenge to Quality Health Care." *Culture, Medicine, and Psychiatry*, no. 41 (2017): 161–80.

Marx, Karl. *Capital: A Critique of Political Economy*. Edited by Friedrich Engels. New York: Modern Library, 1906.

Maskovsky, Jeff. "'Managing' the Poor: Neoliberalism, Medicaid HMOs and the Triumph of Consumerism among the Poor." *Medical Anthropology* 19, no. 2 (2000): 121–46.

Mayor's Office of Violence Reduction. "Violence and Victimization Trends." Accessed February 16, 2023. https://www.chicago.gov/city/en/sites/vrd/home/violence -victimization.html.

Mayor's Press Office. "Mayor Lightfoot and CDPH Announce $56m Grant to Chicago Cook Workforce Partnership and Partners to Bolster Contact Tracing Efforts for COVID-19 Cases in Chicago." Press release, June 30, 2020. https://www.chicago .gov/city/en/depts/mayor/press_room/press_releases/2020/june/GrantChicago CookWorkforcePartnership.html.

Melamed, Jodi. "Racial Capitalism." *Critical Ethnic Studies* 1, no. 1 (2015): 76–85.

Metzl, Jonathan. *Dying of Whiteness: How the Politics of Racial Representation Is Killing America's Heartland*. New York: Basic Books, 2019.

Miller, Claire C., and Alicia Parlapiano. "The U.S. Built a European-Style Welfare State: It's Largely Over." *New York Times*, Updated May 11, 2023. https://www.nytimes .com/interactive/2023/04/06/upshot/pandemic-safety-net-medicaid.html.

Milloy, Courtland. "The Cure for Racial Disparities in Health Care Is Known: It's the Willingness to Fix It That's Lagging." *Washington Post*, April 21, 2020. https:// www.washingtonpost.com/local/the-cure-for-racial-disparities-in-health-care-is -known-its-the-willingness-to-fix-it-thats-lagging/2020/04/21/1ed28610-83c7 -11ea-878a-86477a724bdb_story.html.

Mills, Charles W. *The Racial Contract*. Ithaca, NY: Cornell University Press, 1997.

Mills, Claire K., Rebecca Landau, Belicia Rodriguez, and Joelle Scally. *The State of Low-Income America: Credit Access and Debt Payment*. Federal Reserve Bank of New York, March 2022. https://www.newyorkfed.org/medialibrary/media/press/ the-state-of-low-income-america-credit-access-debt-payment-march-2022.

Moffitt, Robert A., and James P. Ziliak. "COVID-19 and the US Safety Net." *Fiscal Studies* 41, no. 3 (2020): 515–48.

Molina, Natalia. *Fit to Be Citizens: Public Health and Race in Los Angeles, 1879–1939*. Berkeley: University of California Press, 2006.

Moore, Justin Xavier, Keon L. Gilbert, Katie L. Lively, Christian Laurent, Rishab Chawla, Cynthia Li, Ryan Johnson, Robert Petcu, Mehul Mehra, Antron Spooner, Ravindra Kolhe, and Christy J. W. Ledford. "Correlates of COVID-19 Vaccine Hesitancy among a Community Sample of African Americans Living in the Southern United States." *Vaccines* 9, no. 8 (2021): 879–94.

Moore, Natalie Y. *The South Side: A Portrait of Chicago and American Segregation*. New York: Picador, 2016.

Morgan, Kimberly J., and Andrea Louise Campbell. *The Delegated Welfare State: Medicare, Markets, and the Governance of Social Policy*. Oxford: Oxford University Press, 2011.

Morrell, Claudia. "Activists Slam Chicago Mayor Lori Lightfoot for Directing Millions in COVID-19 Relief Money to Police." WBEZ Chicago. February 18, 2021. https://www.wbez.org/stories/activists-slam-chicago-mayor-lori-lightfoot-for -directing-millions-in-covid-19-relief-money-to-police/1570442b-927f-46bc-9717 -a2763649910e.

Morrison, Aaron. "Analysis: A Race War Evident Long before the Capitol Siege." Associated Press (AP). February 5, 2021. https://apnews.com/article/donald-trump-us -news-race-and-ethnicity-conspiracy-theories-philanthropy-f8f793b94b0dd7e8e c62957dcbeb53d8.

Mortice, Zach. "Chicago's 1855 Beer Riot Is a Bridge to the Unrest of 2020." Bloomberg CityLab. August 14, 2020. https://www.bloomberg.com/news/articles/2020-08-14/ in-chicago-unrest-echoes-of-a-1855-beer-riot.

Murphy, Michelle. *The Economization of Life*. Durham, NC: Duke University Press, 2017.

Naber, Nadine, Nicole Nguyen, Chris D. Poulos, Iván Arenas, Louise Cainkar, Nazek Sankari, Amanda E. Lewis, Nina Shoman-Dajani, and Zeina Zaatari. *Beyond Erasure and Profiling: Cultivating Strong and Vibrant Arab American Communities in Chicagoland*. Chicago: Institute for Research on Race and Public Policy, 2023.

Nah, Soya, Lillie Williamson, Lee Ann Kahlor, Lucy Atkinson, Sean Upshaw, and Jean-Louis Ntang-Beb. "The Roles of Social Media Use and Medical Mistrust in Black Americans' COVID-19 Vaccine Hesitancy: The RISP Perspective." *Health Communication*. Published online, August 8, 2023. https://doi.org/10.1080/10410236.2023 .2244169.

Nash, Jennifer. *Birthing Black Mothers*. Durham, NC: Duke University Press, 2021.

Ndugga, Nambi, Latoya Hill, Samantha Artiga, and Sweta Haldar. "Latest Data on COVID-19 Vaccinations by Race/Ethnicity." KFF (Kaiser Family Foundation). July 14, 2022. https://www.kff.org/coronavirus-covid-19/issue-brief/ latest-data-on-covid-19-vaccinations-by-race-ethnicity/.

New York Times. "Track Covid-19 in the U.S." Accessed May 11, 2023. https://www .nytimes.com/interactive/2023/us/covid-cases.html.

Nguyen, Vinh-Kim. "Government-By-Exception: Enrollment and Experimentality in Mass HIV Treatment Programmes in Africa." *Social Theory and Health* 7, no. 3 (2009): 196–217.

Nixon, Rob. "Neoliberalism, Slow Violence, and the Environmental Picaresque." *MFS Modern Fiction Studies* 55, no. 3 (2009): 443–67.

Nixon, Rob. *Slow Violence and the Environmentalism of the Poor.* Cambridge, MA: Harvard University Press, 2011.

Noble, Safiya U. "Teaching Trayvon: Race, Media and the Politics of Spectacle." *Black Scholar* 44, no. 1 (2014): 12–29.

Nowicki, Jerry. "Amid Apparent Virus Plateau, Pritzker Stays the Course." Capitol News Illinois. May 6, 2020. https://www.capitolnewsillinois.com/NEWS/amid-apparent-virus-plateau-pritzker-says-stay-the-course.

Oakley, Dierdre, and Keri Burchfield. "Out of the Projects, Still in the Hood: The Spatial Constraints on Public-Housing Residents' Relocation in Chicago." *Journal of Urban Affairs* 31, no. 5 (2009): 589–614.

Oberg, Charles, H. R. Hodges, Sarah Gander, Rita Nathawad, and Diana Cutts. "The Impact of COVID-19 on Children's Lives in the United States: Amplified Inequities and a Just Path to Recovery." *Current Problems in Pediatric Adolescent Health Care* 52, no. 7 (2022): 101181.

Office for Civil Rights (OCR). *Education in a Pandemic: The Disparate Impacts of COVID-19 on America's Students.* Washington, DC: US Department of Education, 2021. https://www2.ed.gov/about/offices/list/ocr/docs/20210608-impacts-of -covid19.pdf.

Office of Governor Gavin Newsom. "Governor Newsom Visits Project Roomkey Site in Santa Clara County to Highlight Progress on the State's Initiative to Protect Homeless Individuals from COVID-19." April 18, 2020. https://www.gov.ca.gov/2020/04/18/ governor-newsom-visits-project-roomkey-site-in-santa-clara-county-to-highlight -progress-on-the-states-initiative-to-protect-homeless-individuals-from-covid-19/.

Office of the Mayor. "City of Chicago Announces Vaccine Requirements for Restaurants, Bars, Gyms, and Other Indoor Public Places." Press release, December 21, 2021. https://www.chicago.gov/city/en/depts/mayor/press_room/press_releases/2021/ december/VaccineRequirementsIndoorPublicPlaces.html.

Office of the Mayor. "Mayor Lightfoot and Chicago Department of Public Health Jointly Declare Racism a Public Health Crisis in Chicago." Press release, June 17, 2021. https://www.chicago.gov/city/en/depts/mayor/press_room/press_releases/2021/ june/RacismPublicHealthCrisis.html.

Olayo-Méndez, Alejandro, María Vidal De Haymes, Maricela García, and Llewellyn Joseph Cornelius. "Essential, Disposable, and Excluded: The Experience of Latino Immigrant Workers in the US during COVID-19." *Journal of Poverty* 25, no. 7 (2021): 612–28.

Omi, Michael, and Howard Winant. *Racial Formation in the United States.* 3rd ed. New York: Routledge, 2014.

Padamsee, Tasleem J., Robert M. Bond, Graham N. Dixon, Shelly R. Hovick, Kilhoe Na, Erik C. Nisbet, Duane T. Wegener, and R. Kelly Garrett. "Changes in COVID-19 Vaccine Hesitancy Among Black and White Individuals in the US." *JAMA Network Open* 5, no. 1 (2022): e2144470. https://doi.org/10.1001/jamanetworkopen.2021.44470.

Paradies, Yin, Jehonathan Ben, Nida Denson, Amanuel Elias, Naomi Priest, Alex Pieterse, Arpana Gupta, Margaret Kelaher, and Gilbert Gee. "Racism as a

Determinant of Health: A Systemic Review and Meta-Analysis." *PLOS ONE* 10, no. 9 (2015): e0138511. https://doi.org/10.1371/journal.pone.0138511.

Parlapiano, Alicia, and Jim Tankersley. "What's in Biden's Infrastructure Plan?" *New York Times*, March 31, 2021. https://www.nytimes.com/interactive/2021/03/31/upshot/whats-in-bidens-infrastructure-plan.html.

Parolin, Zachary. *Poverty in the Pandemic: Policy Lessons from COVID-19*. New York: Russell Sage Foundation, 2023.

Pathieu, Diane, and Sarah Schulte. "More than $280M from COVID Relief Funding Went to CPD, New Report Finds." *ABC7 Eyewitness News*, February 18, 2021. ABC WLS-TV Chicago (website). https://abc7chicago.com/covid-relief-cpd-budget-lightfoot-chicago-police/10350078/.

Peck, Jamie, and Nik Theodore. "Contingent Chicago: Restructuring the Spaces of Temporary Labor." *International Journal of Urban and Regional Research* 25, no. 3 (2001): 471–96.

Pertwee, Ed, Clarissa Simas, and Heidi J. Larson. "An Epidemic of Uncertainty: Rumors, Conspiracy Theories and Vaccine Hesitancy." *Nature Medicine*, no. 28 (2022): 456–59.

Petrella, Dan. "With Costs Soaring, Gov. J.B. Pritzker to Close Enrollment for Many in Insurance Program for Immigrants." *Chicago Tribune*, June 16, 2023. https://www.chicagotribune.com/politics/ct-immigrant-health-care-program-rules-20230616-744x5byoi5ccvfw72d7lyvwnj4-story.html.

Piven, Frances F., and Richard A. Cloward. *Regulating the Poor: The Functions of Public Welfare*. Updated ed. New York: Vintage, 1993.

Povinelli, Elizabeth A. *Economies of Abandonment: Social Belonging and Endurance in Late Liberalism*. Durham, NC: Duke University Press, 2011.

Presa, Laura Rodríguez. "Illinois Expansion of Health Coverage for Older Adults Living Illegally in US Is Expected to Benefit Thousands of Essential Workers at Risk." *Chicago Tribune*, August 24, 2021. https://www.chicagotribune.com/news/ct-healthcare-coverage-expansion-noncititzen-adults-illinois-20210824-x6yns6nw4zea3gihlfsohvy2eq-story.html.

Pritzker, JB. *Executive Order in Response to COVID-19 (COVID-19 Executive Order No. 8)*. Illinois.gov. https://www2.illinois.gov/IISNews/21288-Gov._Pritzker_Stay_at_Home_Order.pdf.

Pulido, Laura. "Flint, Environmental Racism and Racial Capitalism." *Capitalism Nature Socialism* 27, no. 3 (2016): 1–16.

Pulido, Laura. "Geographies of Race and Ethnicity II: Environmental Racism, Racial Capitalism and State-Sanctioned Violence." *Progress in Human Geography* 41, no. 4 (2017): 524–33.

Qin, Amy. "Cook County Evictions Reach their Highest Monthly Total in More than Four Years." WBEZ Chicago, June 26, 2023. https://www.wbez.org/stories/cook-county-evictions-back-to-pre-pandemic-levels/3e34bc0c-10b9-4e77-93be-4811ff6e541d.

Qiu, Linda. "Families Struggle as Pandemic Program Offering Free School Meals Ends." *New York Times*, January 22, 2023. https://www.nytimes.com/2023/01/22/us/politics/universal-school-meals-free-lunches.html.

Quadagno, Jill. *One Nation Uninsured: Why the US Has No National Health Insurance*. Oxford: Oxford University Press, 2005.

Quadagno, Jill. "Why the United States Has No National Health Insurance: Stakeholder Mobilization against the Welfare State, 1945–1996." *Journal of Health and Social Behavior* 45 (2004): 25–44.

Ramirez-Rosa, Carlos, Byron Sigcho-Lopez, Rossana Rodriguez-Sanchez, and Jeanette Taylor. "Chicago Mayor Lori Lightfoot Is Prioritizing a Coronavirus Recovery for the Wealthy, Not Average Chicagoans." *Jacobin*, May 19, 2020. https://jacobin .com/2020/05/chicago-mayor-lori-lightfoot-coronavirus-city-council.

Ramos, Manny. "Feds Urged to Investigate City's Use of COVID-19 Relief Funds." *Chicago Sun-Times*, January 10, 2022. https://chicago.suntimes.com/coronavirus/ 2022/1/10/22876635/chicago-coronavirus-relief-debt-lightfoot-budget-schools -cps-covid-teachers-union-remote-learning.

Raudenbush, Danielle T. *Health Care Off the Books: Poverty, Illness and Strategies for Survival in Urban America*. Berkeley: University of California Press, 2020.

Reed, Christopher R. "South Lawndale." In *The Electronic Encyclopedia of Chicago*. Chicago: Chicago Historical Society, 2005. http://www.encyclopedia.chicagohistory .org/pages/1174.html.

Reiley, Laura, and Tony Romm. "Pandemic Expansion of School Lunch Program Appears Slated to End Suddenly." *Washington Post*, March 7, 2022. https://www .washingtonpost.com/business/2022/03/07/school-nutrition-program-covid-waivers/.

Reina, Vincent J., and Yeonhwa Lee. "COVID-19 and Emergency Rental Assistance: Impact on Rent Arrears, Debt and the Well-Being of Renters in Philadelphia." *RSF: The Russell Sage Foundation Journal of the Social Sciences* 9, no. 3 (2023): 208–29.

Rembis, Michael. "The New Asylums: Madness and Mass Incarceration in the Neoliberal Era." In *Disability Incarcerated*, edited by Liat Ben-Moshe, Chris Chapman, and Allison C. Carey, 139–59. New York: Palgrave Macmillan, 2014.

Reubi, David. "A Genealogy of Epidemiological Reason: Saving Lives, Social Surveys and Global Population." *BioSocieties* 13 (2018): 81–102.

Reuters. "Trump Urges Slowdown in COVID-19 Testing, Calling it a 'Double-Edge Sword.'" June 21, 2020. https://www.reuters.com/article/us-health-coronavirus -trump-testing/trump-urges-slowdown-in-covid-19-testing-calling-it-a-double -edge-sword-idUSKBN23S0B4.

Reverby, Susan. "Ethical Failures and History Lessons: The US Public Health Service Research Studies in Tuskegee and Guatemala." *Public Health Reviews* 34, no. 1 (2012): 1–18.

Rho, Hye Jin, Hayley Brown, Shawn Fremstad, and Peter Creticos. "Workers in Frontline Industries in Chicago and Illinois." Center for Economic and Policy Research (CEPR). May 6, 2020. https://cepr.net/frontline-workers-chicago-and-illinois/.

Robinson, Cedric J. *Black Marxism: The Making of the Black Radical Tradition*. 3rd edition. Chapel Hill: University of North Carolina Press, 2020.

Rosenfeld, Michael J., and Marta Tienda. "Mexican Immigration, Occupational Niches, and Labor-Market Competition: Evidence from Los Angeles, Chicago and Atlanta, 1970 to 1990." In *Immigration and Opportunity: Race, Ethnicity and Employment in the United States*, edited by Frank D. Bean and Stephanie Bell-Rose, 64–107. Princeton, NJ: Russell Sage Foundation, 1999.

Ross, Martha, Nicole Bateman, and Alec Friedhoff. "Low-Wage Workforce." Brookings Institution. March 2020. https://www.brookings.edu/interactives/ low-wage-workforce/.

Roy, Arundhati. "The Pandemic Is a Portal." In "Teaching and Learning in the Pandemic." Special issue, *Rethinking Schools* 34, no. 4 (Summer 2020). https:// rethinkingschools.org/articles/the-pandemic-is-a-portal/.

Ruiz-Grossman, Sarah. "Undocumented Immigrants Won't Get Stimulus Checks—For Third Time Around." *Huffington Post*, March 9, 2021. https://www .huffpost.com/entry/undocumented-immigrants-no-stimulus-checks-coronavirus -again_n_6048025fc5b636ed3376acac.

Sanchez, Melissa, and Sandhya Kambhampati. "How Chicago Ticket Debt Sends Black Motorists into Bankruptcy." ProPublica Illinois. February 27, 2018. https://features .propublica.org/driven-into-debt/chicago-ticket-debt-bankruptcy/.

Scheel, Stephan. "Biopolitical Bordering: Enacting Populations as Intelligible Objects of Government." *European Journal of Social Theory* 23, no. 4 (2020): 571–90.

Schencker, Lisa. "More than 47,000 Illinois Residents Lose Medicaid as State Begins Asking Recipients to Prove Eligibility." *Chicago Tribune*, updated August 7, 2023. https://www.chicagotribune.com/business/ct-biz-illinois-medicaid-lost-coverage -redeterminations-20230802-kh74zazx5zcenpiyfzaqrnikba-story.html.

Schencker, Lisa. "Theodore Roosevelt was Treated at Mercy Hospital, Mayor Richard M. Daley Was Born There: Now After More Than 150 Years on the South Side, It Is Closing." *Chicago Tribune*, July 29, 2020. https://www.chicagotribune.com/2020/07/29/ theodore-roosevelt-was-treated-at-mercy-hospital-mayor-richard-m-daley-was -born-there-now-after-more-than-150-years-on-the-south-side-its-closing/.

Schlabach, Elizabeth. "The Influenza Epidemic and Jim Crow Public Health Policies and Practices in Chicago, 1917–1921." *Journal of African American History* 104, no. 1 (2019): 31–58.

Schorsch, Kristen. "The Pandemic Revealed Another Gap in Chicago Health Care: Hospitals Are on Their Own to Transfer Patients." WBEZ Chicago. June 29, 2020. https://www.wbez.org/stories/one-chicago-hospital-called-for-8-hours-to-transfer -covid-19-patients-thats-problematic-for-future-outbreaks/1ecd60f3-f185-4deb -ae65-3e3ca25f0063.

Schwartz, Barry. "Waiting, Exchange and Power: The Distribution of Time in Social Systems." *American Journal of Sociology* 79, no. 4 (1974): 841–70.

Sewell, William. *Logics of History: Social Theory and Social Transformation*. Chicago: University of Chicago Press, 2005.

Shah, Nayan. *Contagious Divides: Epidemics and Race in San Francisco's Chinatown*. Berkeley: University of California Press, 2001.

Shepherd, Hana, Norah MacKendrick, and G. Christina Mora. "Pandemic Politics: Political Worldviews and COVID-19 Beliefs and Practices in an Unsettled Time." *Socius* 6 (2020): 1–18.

Simpson, Richard. *Rogues, Rebels, and Rubber Stamps: The Politics of the Chicago City Council, 1863 to the Present*. New York: Routledge Press, 2001.

Smedley, Audrey, and Brian D. Smedley. "Race as Biology Is Fiction, Racism as a Social Problem Is Real: Anthropological and Historical Perspectives on the Social Construction of Race." *American Psychologist* 60, no. 1 (2005): 16–26.

Smith, Janet J., and David Stovall. "'Coming Home' to New Homes and New Schools: Critical Race Theory and the New Politics of Containment." *Journal of Education Policy* 23, no. 2 (2008): 135–52.

Smith, Sandra S. "Race and Trust." *Annual Review of Sociology* 36 (2010): 453–75.

Snyder, Tanya. "Biden's Incredible Shrinking Infrastructure Plan." *Politico*. June 17, 2022. https://www.politico.com/news/2022/06/17/democrats-shrinking -infrastructure-plan-00039588.

Soglin, Talia. "Emergency SNAP Benefits Are Ending: Here's What That Means for Chicago Families." *Chicago Tribune*, February 15, 2023. https://www.chicagotribune.com/business/ct-biz-emergency-snap-benefits-ending-20230215-kvqha77fqvbszfyivcucagp45q-story.html.

Sontag, Susan. *Illness as Metaphor and AIDS and Its Metaphors*. New York: Picador, 2001.

Soss, Joe, Richard C. Fording, and Sanford F. Schram. *Disciplining the Poor: Neoliberal Paternalism and the Persistent Power of the State*. Chicago: University of Chicago Press, 2011.

Spielman, Fran. "Lightfoot Announces $8 Million in Grants to Strengthen Mental Health System." *Chicago Sun-Times*, October 6, 2020. https://chicago.suntimes.com/city-hall/2020/10/6/21504439/mental-health-clinics-chicago-mayor-lightfoot-8-million-grants.

Spielman, Fran. "Lightfoot Declares 'Public Health Red Alarm' about Racial Disparity in COVID-19 Deaths." *Chicago Sun-Times*, April 6, 2020. https://chicago.suntimes.com/coronavirus/2020/4/6/21209848/coronavirus-covid-19-deaths-racial-disparity-life-expectancy-arwady-lightfoot.

Star, Susan Leigh. "The Ethnography of Infrastructure." *American Behavioral Scientist* 43, no. 3 (1999): 377–91.

Starr, Paul. "Built to Last? Policy Entrenchment and Regret in Medicare, Medicaid and the Affordable Care Act." In *Medicare and Medicaid at 50*, edited by Alan Cohen, David Colby, Keith Wailoo, and Julian Zelizer, 319–40. Oxford: Oxford University Press, 2015.

Starr, Paul. *The Social Transformation of American Medicine*. New York: Basic Books, 1982.

St. Clair, Stacy. "Chicago Hospital on the Financial Brink: St. Anthony's Fights for Survival, Sues State for Money Owed." *Chicago Tribune*, May 18, 2020. https://www.chicagotribune.com/coronavirus/ct-coronavirus-hospital-medicaid-funding-st-anthony-chicago-20200518-nvjnpwwcoza27bjotoxsibc5au-story.html.

St. Clair, Stacy, Joe Mahr, and Lisa Schencker. "'This Is the Norm': How Early Vaccine Shots Went to Residents of Affluent Suburbs and Chicagoans in Low-Risk Areas, Despite City Push for Equity." *Chicago Tribune*, May 21, 2021. https://www.chicagotribune.com/coronavirus/vaccine/ct-coronavirus-chicago-vaccine-dose-inequity-suburbs-20210521-he7w4kyd7fdsnhtwtwe3vzxs4e-story.html.

Stolberg, Sheryl G., and Noah Weiland. "As Covid Emergency Ends, U.S. Response Shifts to Peacetime Mode." *New York Times*, May 10, 2023. https://www.nytimes.com/2023/05/10/us/politics/covid-public-health-emergency.html.

Stoler, Ann L. *Race and the Education of Desire: Foucault's "History of Sexuality" and the Colonial Order of Things*. Durham, NC: Duke University Press, 1996.

Street, Alice. *Biomedicine in an Unstable Place: Infrastructure and Personhood in a Papua New Guinea Hospital*. Durham, NC: Duke University Press, 2014.

Struett, David, and Tom Schuba. "Mental Health Clinicians Will Start Answering Some 911 Calls in Chicago—Instead of Cops." *Chicago Sun-Times*, July 13, 2021. https://chicago.suntimes.com/news/2021/7/13/22573899/mental-health-first-responder-police-alternative-response-lightfoot-crisis-response-care-911-cpd.

Stuart, Forrest. "From 'Rabble Management' to 'Recovery Management': Policing Homelessness in Marginal Urban Space." *Urban Studies* 51, no. 9 (2014): 1909–25.

Susser, Mervyn, and Ezra Susser. "Choosing a Future for Epidemiology: Eras and Paradigms." *American Journal of Public Health* 86, no. 5 (1996): 668–73.

Sutter, Lexi. "Chicago Activist Seeks Help for Mother Accused of Endangering her 7 Children." NBC Chicago. January 2, 2021. https://www.nbcchicago.com/news/local/chicago-activist-seeks-help-for-mother-accused-of-endangering-her-7-children/2406556/.

Sweet, Paige L. *The Politics of Surviving: How Women Navigate Domestic Violence and Its Aftermath*. Berkeley: University of California Press, 2021.

Talen, Emily. "Design for Diversity: Evaluating the Context of Socially Mixed Neighbourhoods." *Journal of Urban Design* 11, no. 1 (2006): 1–32.

Taylor, Keeanga-Yamahtta. "The Bitter Fruits of Trump's White-Power Presidency." *New Yorker*, January 21, 2021. https://www.newyorker.com/news/our-columnists/the-bitter-fruits-of-trumps-white-power-presidency.

Taylor, Keeanga-Yamahtta. "The Black Plague." *New Yorker*, April 16, 2020. https://www.newyorker.com/news/our-columnists/the-black-plague.

Taylor, Keeanga-Yamahtta. *From #BlackLivesMatter to Black Liberation*. Chicago: Haymarket Books, 2016.

Thebault, Reis, Andrew Ba Tran, and Vanessa Williams. "The Coronavirus Is Infecting and Killing Black Americans at an Alarming Rate." *Washington Post*, April 7, 2020. https://www.washingtonpost.com/nation/2020/04/07/coronavirus-is-infecting-killing-black-americans-an-alarmingly-high-rate-post-analysis-shows/.

Theodore, Nik. "Political Economies of Day Labour: Regulation and Restructuring of Chicago's Contingent Labour Markets." *Urban Studies* 40, no. 9 (2003): 1811–28.

Theodore, Nik, and Nina Martin. "Migrant Civil Society: New Voices in the Struggle over Community Development." *Journal of Urban Affairs* 29, no. 3 (2007): 269–87.

Thrasher, Steven W. *The Viral Underclass: The Human Toll When Inequality and Disease Collide*. New York: Celadon Books, 2022.

Tolbert, Jennifer, and Meghana Ammula. "10 Things to Know about the Unwinding of the Medicaid Continuous Enrollment Requirement." KFF (Kaiser Family Foundation). June 9, 2023. https://www.kff.org/medicaid/issue-brief/10-things-to-know-about-the-unwinding-of-the-medicaid-continuous-enrollment-requirement/.

Tomer, Adie, and Joseph Kane. "To Protect Frontline Workers during and after COVID-19, We Must Define Who They Are." Brookings Institution. June 10, 2020. https://www.brookings.edu/articles/to-protect-frontline-workers-during-and-after-covid-19-we-must-define-who-they-are/.

Trombetta, William. "Managed Care Medicaid." *International Journal of Pharmaceutical and Healthcare Marketing* 11, no. 2 (2017): 198–210.

Tung, Elizabeth L., David A. Hampton, Marynia Kolak, Selwyn O. Rogers, Joyce P. Yang, and Monica E. Peek. "Race/Ethnicity and Geographic Access to Urban Trauma Care." *JAMA Network Open* 2, no. 3 (2019): e190138. https://doi.org/10.1001/jamanetworkopen.2019.0138.

United States Census Bureau. "Census Bureau Releases New Report on Health Insurance by Race and Hispanic Origin." Press release no. CB22-TPS.100, November 22, 2022. https://www.census.gov/newsroom/press-releases/2022/health-insurance-by-race.html.

United States Census Bureau. "Household Pulse Survey Data Tables." Revised October 31, 2023. https://www.census.gov/programs-surveys/household-pulse-survey/data.html.

United States Department of Labor Employment and Training Administration. *Pandemic Unemployment Assistance*. Accessed January 18, 2024. https://oui.doleta.gov/unemploy/pdf/PUA_FactSheet.pdf.

University of Chicago Urban Labs Poverty Lab. *COVID-19: Understanding Where Chicago's Most At-Risk Workers Live*. Chicago: University of Chicago, 2020. https://urbanlabs.uchicago.edu/attachments/533072c72ce4e33dbdf761dd448f5932cca3bf2b/store/75009a89b8f4b85f84ac4abf365b3a8459113637aa415ca8f1cb58d16f26/06222020_COVID-19+Risk+Among+Workers+in+Chicago_vFINAL.pdf.

Urena, Anthony. "Relational Risk: How Relationships Shape Personal Assessments of Risk and Mitigation." *American Sociological Review* 87, no. 5 (2022): 723–49.

US Department of the Treasury. *Coronavirus State and Local Fiscal Recovery Funds 2021 Interim Final Rule: Frequently Asked Questions*. Updated August 2023. https://home.treasury.gov/system/files/136/SLFRPFAQ.pdf.

Van Natta, Meredith, Nancy J. Burke, Irene H. Yen, Mark D. Fleming, Christoph L. Hanssmann, Maryani Palupi Rasidjan, and Janet K. Shim. "Stratified Citizenship, Stratified Health: Examining Latinx Legal Status in the US Healthcare Safety Net." *Social Science & Medicine* 220 (2019): 49–55.

Vargas, Robert. *Uninsured in Chicago: How the Social Safety Net Leaves Latinos Behind*. New York: New York University Press, 2022.

Venkatesh, Sudhir. *The American Project: The Rise and Fall of an American Ghetto*. Cambridge, MA: Harvard University Press, 2002.

Villarosa, Linda. *Under the Skin: The Hidden Toll of Racism on Health in America*. New York: Anchor Books, 2022.

Vinicky, Amanda. "Chicago Brings in National Guard after Saturday Night Violence." WTTW. May 31, 2020. https://news.wttw.com/2020/05/31/chicago-brings-national-guard-after-saturday-night-violence.

Viruell-Fuentes, Edna, Patricia Miranda, and Sawsan Abdulrahim. "More Than Culture: Structural Racism, Intersectionality Theory, and Immigrant Health." *Social Science & Medicine* 75, no. 12 (2012): 2099–2106.

Wacquant, Loïc. *Punishing the Poor: The Neoliberal Government of Social Insecurity*. Durham, NC: Duke University Press, 2009.

Wacquant, Loïc J. *Urban Outcasts: A Comparative Sociology of Advanced Marginality*. Cambridge: Polity Press, 2008.

Wagner-Pacifici, Robin. "Theorizing the Restlessness of Events." *American Journal of Sociology* 115, no. 5 (2010): 1351–86.

Wagner-Pacifici, Robin. *What Is An Event?* Chicago: University of Chicago Press, 2017.

Wagner-Pacifici, Robin. "What Is an Event and Are We in One?" In "Against Disaster." Special issue, *Sociologica* 15, no. 1 (2021): 11–20.

Wahlberg, Ayo, and Nikolas Rose. "The Governmentalization of Living: Calculating Global Health." *Economy & Society* 44, no. 1 (2015): 60–90.

Wailoo, Keith. "Spectacles of Difference: The Racial Scripting of Epidemic." *Bulletin of the History of Medicine* 94, no. 4 (2020): 602–25.

Wall, Craig, and Sarah Schulte. "Pritzker Signs Sweeping Police Reform, Criminal Justice Bill, Despite Opposition From Law Enforcement." *ABC7 Eyewitness News*, February 22, 2021. ABC WLS-TV Chicago (website). https://abc7chicago.com/police-and-criminal-justice-reform-bill-pritzker-house-3653-accountability/10361126/.

Watkins-Hayes, Celeste. *Remaking a Life: How Women Living with HIV/AIDS Confront Inequality.* Berkeley: University of California Press, 2019.

Weheliye, Alexander. *Habeas Viscus: Racializing Assemblages, Biopolitics, and Black Feminist Theories of the Human.* Durham, NC: Duke University Press, 2014.

Weinbaum, Alys E. *The Afterlife of Reproductive Slavery: Biocapitalism and Black Feminism's Philosophy of History.* Durham, NC: Duke University Press, 2019.

Weinberg, Tessa. "Chicago Voters Resoundingly Rejected Mayor Lori Lightfoot's Reelection Bid." *Morning Edition*, March 1, 2023. NPR. https://www.npr.org/2023/03/01/1160297860/chicago-voters-resoundingly-rejected-mayor-lori-lightfoots-reelection-bid.

Weisenstein, Brad, and Patrick Andriesen. "Thousands of Illinoisans Await Calls from State Unemployment Agency." Illinois Policy. May 7, 2021. https://www.illinoispolicy.org/thousands-of-illinoisans-await-calls-from-state-unemployment-agency/.

Weisz, George. *Chronic Disease in the Twentieth Century: A History.* Baltimore: Johns Hopkins University Press, 2014.

White, Alexandre. *Epidemic Orientalism: Race, Capital and the Governance of Infectious Disease.* Stanford, CA: Stanford University Press, 2023.

White House. "Remarks by President Biden on the Status of the Country's Fight against COVID-19." March 30, 2022. https://www.whitehouse.gov/briefing-room/speeches-remarks/2022/03/30/remarks-by-president-biden-on-the-status-of-the-countrys-fight-against-covid-19/.

White, Kellee, Jennifer S. Haas, and David R. Williams. "Elucidating the Role of Place in Health Care Disparities: The Example of Racial/Ethnic Residential Segregation." *Health Services Research* 47, no. 3 (2012): 1278–99.

Whoriskey, Peter, Jeff Stein, and Nate Jones. "Thousands of OSHA Complaints Filed against Companies for Virus Workplace Safety Concerns, Records Show." *Washington Post*, April 16, 2020. https://www.washingtonpost.com/business/2020/04/16/osha-coronavirus-complaints/#.

Wilkes, Rima. "Re-thinking the Decline in Trust: A Comparison of Black and White Americans." *Social Science Research* 40 (2011): 1596–1610.

Williams, David R., and Chiquita Collins. "Racial Residential Segregation: A Fundamental Cause of Racial Disparities in Health." *Public Health Reports* 116 (2001): 404–16.

Williams, David R., and Pamela Braboy Jackson. "Social Sources of Racial Disparities in Health." *Health Affairs* 24, no. 2 (2005): 325–44.

Willse, Craig. *The Value of Homelessness: Managing Surplus Life in the United States.* Minneapolis: University of Minnesota Press, 2015.

Wilson, William Julius. *The Truly Disadvantaged: The Inner City, the Underclass and Public Policy.* Chicago: University of Chicago Press, 2012.

Wilson, William Julius. *When Work Disappears: The World of the New Urban Poor.* New York: Knopf, 1996.

Wong, Karen, Charles Heilig, Anne Hause, Tanya Myers, Christine Olson, Julianne Gee, Paige Marquez, Penelope Strid, and David Shay. "Menstrual Irregularities and Vaginal Bleeding after COVID-19 Vaccination Reported to V-Safe Active Surveillance, USA in December, 2020–January, 2022: An Observational Cohort Study." *Lancet Digital Health* 4 (2022): e667–e675. https://doi.org/10.1016/S2589-7500(22)00125-X.

World Health Organization (WHO). "WHO Recommends New Name for Monkey-pox Disease." News release, November 28, 2022. https://www.who.int/news/item/28-11-2022-who-recommends-new-name-for-monkeypox-disease.

Yaqub, Ohid, Sophie Castle-Clarke, Nick Sevdalis, and Joanna Chataway. "Attitudes to Vaccination: A Critical Review." *Social Science & Medicine* 112 (2014): 1–11.

Yousef, Odette. "Rents May Be Going Up, but Residents Say They're Not Going Anywhere." WBEZ Chicago. December 19, 2014. https://www.wbez.org/stories/rents-may-be-going-up-but-residents-say-theyre-not-going-anywhere/efi10c30-50c5-4d09-9103-d72412958e4c.

Zamudio, María Inés. "In Chicago, 70% of COVID-19 Deaths Are Black." WBEZ Chicago. April 5, 2020. https://www.wbez.org/stories/in-chicago-70-of-covid-19-deaths-are-black/dd3f295f-445e-4e38-b37f-a1503782b507.

Zamudio, María Inés. "Thousands of Undocumented Workers Face the Pandemic Without A Safety Net." NPR. March 27, 2020. https://www.npr.org/local/309/2020/03/27/822475329/thousands-of-undocumented-workers-face-the-pandemic-without-a-safety-net (content no longer available).

Zapata, Mateo. "Op-Ed: We Are Adam; For Many Youth across Chicago's South and West Sides, Adam Toledo's Life Trajectory Is Too Familiar." *Chicago Tribune*, April 15, 2021. https://www.chicagotribune.com/opinion/commentary/ct-opinion-adam-toledo-little-village-20210415-yfuxq4fz7jgtnl54bwn5w4ztw4-story.html.

Zeng, Sharon, Kenley M. Pelzer, Robert D. Gibbons, Monica E. Peek, and William F. Parker. "Consequences of COVID-19 Vaccine Allocation Inequity in Chicago." medRxiv, preprint, submitted September 23, 2021. https://www.medrxiv.org/content/10.1101/2021.09.22.21263984v1.full.

Zuberi, Tukufu. *Thicker Than Blood: How Racial Statistics Lie*. Minneapolis: University of Minnesota Press, 2001.

INDEX

Omi, Michael, 88–89
Omicron variant, 53, 56–57, 172
ontological insecurity, 7, 15–16, 35, 41–42, 48–51, 53–61, 63–65, 76–79, 90–91, 107. *See also* race and racism; segregation, racial
Operation Bootstrap, 17
opioid crisis, 27–28, 121–22
outsourcing, 92–94, 103–9, 119–20, 144–45, 187–88, 190–93. *See also* neoliberalism
overdetermination, 4, 54, 90–91

paid sick leave, 106–9, 129–30, 150, 171–74; Chicago's failure to provide, 2, 106–9
Parolin, Zachary, 196, 221n5
paternalism, 19–20, 92–93, 118, 123–24, 127–29, 149–52, 196. *See also* means testing; policing; surveillance; welfare safety net
Pence, Mike, 11
Perez, Bianca, 214
Personal Responsibility and Work Opportunity Reconciliation Act (PRWORA), 19–20
police reform, 47–48
policing, 6–9, 16–21, 24–25, 35, 40–53, 56, 83, 123–29, 151–52, 179–84
Poulos, Chris, 240n33
poverty rates, 19, 106, 126–27, 135–36; safety-net expansions and, 1
Povinelli, Elizabeth, 91–92
precarity convergence, 150, 193
Pritzker, JB, 11, 41–42, 45, 47–48, 156, 158
Protect Chicago Plus program, 56, 97–99
PRWORA. *See* Personal Responsibility and Work Opportunity Reconciliation Act (PRWORA)
Public Charge Rule, 167, 177–78
public health: history of, 77–81; HIV/AIDS and, 7–8, 194; Inflation Reduction Act and, 65; infrastructure of, 63–77, 81–86; neoliberal narrowing of, 10–11, 13–15, 35–36; racial ontologization and, 76–81, 85–86; racism as crisis of, 1,

39–42, 62–63; scarcity assumptions and, 92–93, 103–9; social determinants of, 11–16, 103–9, 113, 141–45

quantification, 88–93. *See also* data-driven decisions; invisibilizing dynamics; means testing; neoliberalism

race and racism: abandonment and, 62–63, 65–75, 81–86, 88–93, 119–20, 193, 195–97; accumulated vulnerability and, 2–5, 9–21, 26–35, 39–42, 65, 69–70, 77–87, 92–93, 99–103, 123–29, 133–36, 149–52, 190–91; backlash dynamics and, 48–51; biocapitalism and, 5–9, 41–42, 51–53, 60–61, 77–81, 123–24, 141–52, 198–99, 223n22; Chicago's history of, 1, 16–26, 65; colorblindness and, 66, 88–93; debt and, 130–34, 152–56, 164–65, 238n35; definitions of, 222n16; disproportionate impact on health outcomes, 1–2, 11, 16–21, 32–35, 42–43, 88–93, 144–45; distrust of state agents and, 49–50, 118, 124–26, 129, 175–89; epistemology of ignorance and, 42, 88–93, 198; essential workers and, 146–48, 170–74; gentrification and, 16–21; George Floyd protests and, 40, 48–51, 53, 56; health care services and, 65–68, 70–74, 77–81, 85–86, 129–36; infrastructure and, 123–29, 228n44; letting vs. making die and, 6; mental health care and, 74–77, 122, 134–35; neoliberal targeting and, 1, 11–16, 29, 50–51, 64–65, 97–99, 101–9, 124; as normative, 48–51; ontological insecurity and, 7, 15–16, 35, 41–42, 48–51, 53–61, 65, 76–77, 90–91, 107; policing and, 124–26, 179–84; as public health crisis, 1, 11–16; rental assistance and, 115–18; sacrificial logics and, 2, 8–9, 35–37, 39–45, 56–58, 91–93, 149–52, 154–56, 159–74; scientific objectivity and, 78–81; self-help logics and, 11–12; slow emergencies and, 123–24; social reproduction and, 8–9; symbolic capital available through, 11–16, 35–37,

Printed and bound by CPI Group (UK) Ltd, Croydon, CR0 4YY

09/06/2025

14685757-0001